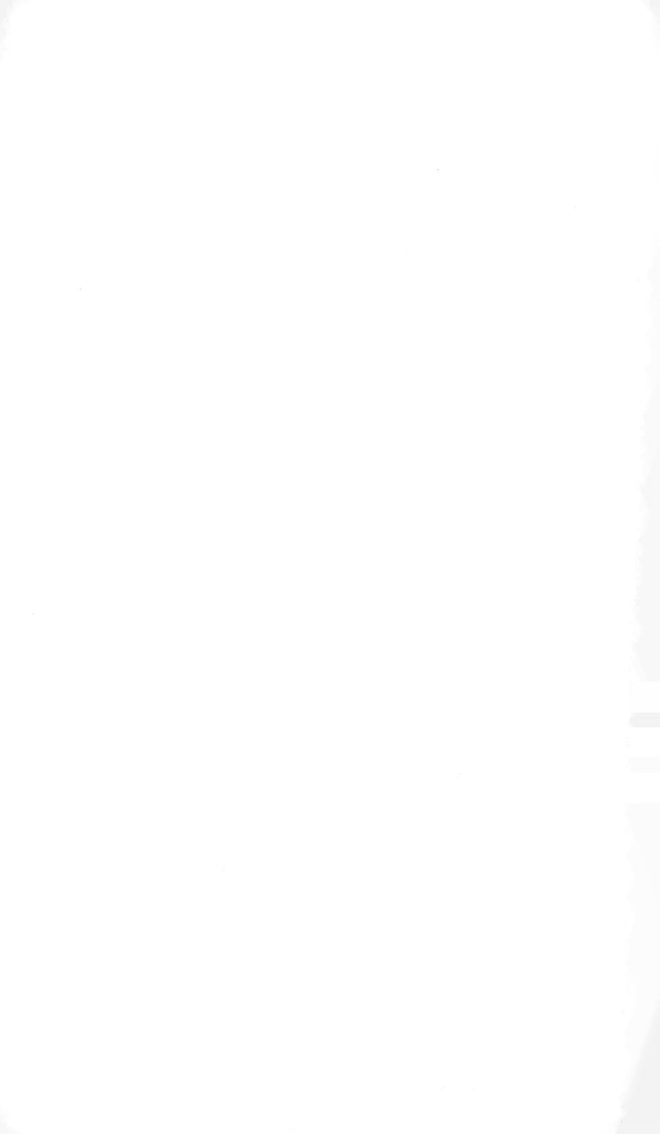

Springer Pocket Dictionary
Cardiology

Peter Reuter

Springer
Pocket Dictionary
Cardiology

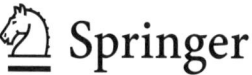
Springer

Peter Reuter, M.D.
Fort Myers, Florida, USA
reutermedical@comcast.net

ISBN 978 90 781 2294 4

© 2009 Springer Uitgeverij, Houten, The Netherlands
Translation: MediLingua, Leiden, The Netherlands
Cover design: Nout Design, Buren, The Netherlands
Projectmanager: Jean-Michel Butter, Houten, The Netherlands
Typesetting: wiskom e.K., Friedrichshafen, Germany

Translation from the German database:
Reuter Datenbank Medizin/Zahnmedizin
Copyright © Peter Reuter, Fort Myers, FL, USA
All Rights Reserved

No part of this publication may be reproduced, stored in a retrieval system or transmitted in any form or by any means electronic, mechanical, photocopying, recording or otherwise without the prior written permission of the copyright holder.
Although every effort has been made to ensure that drug doses and other information are presented accurately in this publication, the ultimate responsibility rests with the prescribing physician. Neither the publisher nor the authors can be held responsible for errors or for any consequences arising from the use of the information contained herein. Any product mentioned in this publication should be used in accordance with the prescribing information prepared by the manufacturers. No claims or endorsements are made for any drug or compound at present under clinical investigation.

Springer Uitgeverij bv, Het Spoor 2, 3994 AK Houten, The Netherlands
www.springeruitgeverij.nl

Preface

As editor-in-chief of the Spinger medical dictionaries it was my pleasure to select terminology for the *Springer Pocket Dictionary Cardiology*. The entries have been selected from an extensive medical and biomedical database, and have been edited for the target audience. Despite our efforts to provide most relevant terms this edition does not claim to be comprehensive and still contains inevitable errors. Therefore, we are looking forward to receiving comments as well as critical and positive feedback from our readers.

Fort Myers, Florida
July 2009

Peter Reuter

Using this Dictionary

Main entries are alphabetized using a letter-for-letter system.

As a rule multiple-word terms are given as subentries under the appropriate main entry. They are alphabetized letter by letter just like the main entries.

Different styles of type are used for different categories of information:

boldface for the main entry

lightface for subentries and entities within the definition

plainface for the definition

italic for restrictive labels and references

Various meanings of an entry are distinguished by use of Arabic numerals.

Cross-references within the A–Z vocabulary are indicated by an arrow [→].

Abbreviations used

approx.	approximately
e.g.	for example
esp.	especially
etc.	et cetera, and so forth, and so on
i.e.	id est, that is
i.m.	intramuscular; intramuscularly
i.v.	intravenous; intravenously
lab.	laboratory
s.a.	see also
s.u.	see under

A

abacterial *Syn: nonbacterial*; free from bacteria, sterile; (*illness*) not caused by bacteria

abciximab Fab fragment of one of the chimeric monoclonal antibodies 7E3 against the glycoprotein-IIb/IIIa receptor; acts as an inhibitor of thrombocyte aggregation, particularly in the coronary arteries; **usage**: unstable angina pectoris, infarction without ST-segment elevation; **side effects**: bleeding complications, thrombocytopenia, hypotension, bradycardia

ABC of resuscitation sequence of life-saving measures according to Safar and Gordon: Airway [opening of airways], Breathing [ventilation], Circulation [restoration of circulatory functions]

abdominal relating to the abdomen

abdominocardiac relating to abdomen and heart

abdominothoracic → *thoracoabdominal*

aberrant 1. in an atypical location, of atypical form **2.** abnormal, deviating from the norm

ablation removal, extirpation; separation, detachment

  catheter-induced ablation methods for targeted tissue injury using radio frequency current; used most commonly in heart rhythm disturbances due to accessory conduction bundles

ABPM → *ambulatory blood pressure monitoring*

absence lack, deficiency

  congenital absence of heart → *acardia*

acapnia diminished carbon dioxide content in the blood

acardia congenital absence of the heart

acardiac without heart

acardiacus → *acardius*

acardius *Syn: acardiacus*; duplication malformation with only one heart

accelerator a substance that accelerates

  serum prothrombin conversion accelerator → *factor VII*

accelerin *Syn: factor VI*; factor in the clotting cascade, which is formed

there from accelerator globulin

accessory additional, collateral, complementary

accident an incident resulting in injury

cerebrovascular accident *Syn: apoplectic fit, apoplectic stroke, apoplexia, apoplexy, cerebral crisis, cerebral apoplexy, encephalorrhagia, stroke syndrome*; symptomatic loss of central neural functions caused by acute ischemia [ischemic insult]; they are subdivided, depending upon the severity and duration of the symptoms, into: **1. transient ischemic attack** [TIA] with regression of the symptoms within 24 hours **2. prolonged reversible ischemic neurologic deficit** [PRIND] or **reversible ischemic neurologic deficit** [RIND] with completely reversible symptoms which persist for longer than 24 hours **3. partially reversible ischemic neurologic symptoms** [PRINS], which slowly evolves and is irreversible or only partially so **4. persistent cerebral infarct** with permanent neurologic injuries; the degree and extent of the ischemic infarct depend upon the localization of the vessel occlusion, the size of the vessel, and the presence of anastomoses; **therapy**: stroke is a medical emergency; the goal of the initial treatment is to stabilize and normalize the bodily functions [cardiovascular, breathing, fluid balance], and to admit the patient to a ward where targeted diagnostic and therapeutic measures can be instituted; timely intervention can prevent further progression, particularly in cases of mild, incomplete stroke or progressive insults that are still worsening; as soon as it is recognized that this acute phase is over [mostly within 24 h], patient rehabilitation must be begun; the best results are obtained with a combination of physiotherapy, logopathie, and medical treatments [treatment of the underlying disease(s); secondary prevention to reduce the risk of further ischemic episodes]

electrical accident accident in which electric current flows through the body; the severity of the accident or the extent of injury depends upon various factors [current strength, voltage, DC or AC current, duration of electrocution, current path, etc.]; **low voltage accidents** [voltage under 1000 V] can lead to prolonged muscle contractions and thereby muscle, joint, and bone injuries; usually, however, the cardiac and circulatory symptoms [ventricular fibrillation] are the most important; there are thermal burns at the entry and exit points of the current, as well as formation of the so-called **current marks**; **high voltage accidents** [voltage greater than 1000 V] usually lead to severe tissue destruction [2.-4. degree burns]; if the initial electrocution is survived, the prognosis depends upon the severity of the tissue injuries and the complications [renal insufficiency]

accidental coincidental (accessory or incidental), inadvertent

accretion pathologic adhesion, agglutination

   pericardial accretion adhesion of the parietal layer of the pericardial sac [pericardium] to the pleura; usually the result of inflammation of the pericardial sac that has run its course

acebutolol cardioselective beta-blocker

acenocoumarin → *acenocoumarol*

acenocoumarol *Syn: acenocoumarin*; coumarin derivative, vitamin K antagonist; anticoagulant

acetazolamide carbonic anhydrase inhibitor; **usage**: diuretic, management of glaucoma, acute pancreatitis; **side effects**: hyperuricemia, worsening of diabetes mellitus; **contraindications**: hypokalemia, renal insufficiency

acetosal → *acetylsalicylic acid*

α-acetyldigoxin cardiac glycoside; **usage**: cardiac insufficiency

β-acetyldigoxin cardiac glycoside; **usage**: cardiac insufficiency, supraventricular tachycardia, atrial fibrillation, and flutter in absolute arrhythmia

acetylsalicylic acid *Syn: aspirin, acetosal*; salicylate with antipyretic, analgesic, anti-inflammatory, and platelet aggregation inhibiting activity; it acts by inhibiting cyclooxygenase, which is responsible for the biosynthesis of prostaglandins and thromboxanes; **indications**: analgesic, antirheumatic, antipyretic, platelet aggregation inhibitor

acidosis disturbance in the acid-base balance with a decline in the blood pH below 7.36; **compensated acidosis** occurs as long as the body is capable of returning the pH to the normal range or having it approach the normal range; **decompensated acidosis** occurs when the compensatory mechanisms are exhausted

acromacria → *Marfan's disease*

acrotic without pulse, pulseless

acrotism absence of, or inability to feel a peripheral pulse

actinic relating to rays or radiation

actino- combining form denoting relation to a ray or radiation

Actinobacillus class of Gram-negative bacteria, which only rarely cause disease

   Actinobacillus actinomycetemcomitans a cause of endocarditis and wound infections following animal bites; *s.a. HACEK group*

action something done, act
   disordered action of the heart → *neurocirculatory asthenia*
activator a substance that activates; catalyzer
   recombined tissue plasminogen activator → *alteplase*
activity the state or quality of being active
   plasma renin activity *Syn: plasma renin assay*; the rate at which renin cleaves angiotensinogen to form angiotensin I per unit time; expressed in nanograms per milliliter per hour (ng/ml/hr); the normal adult value is 0.2 to 4 ng/ml/hr, depending on salt intake and the time the patient has been in an upright position before the test [an upright position raises production of renin, and a high salt intake lowers it]; PRA may be used to screen for renal hypertension or in the diagnosis of primary aldosteronism; it is also an independent predictor of cardiovascular morbidity and mortality
actomyosin a complex of actin and myosin
   platelet actomyosin glycoprotein complex of the thrombocyte membrane, which is important for contraction of the platelet plug; it is absent or the levels are reduced in thromboasthenia
acyanotic (proceeding) without cyanosis
acylaminopenicillins *Syn: ureidopenicillins*; group of parenteral penicillins with a broad action spectrum against gram-positive and gram-negative pathogens; it includes apalcillin, azlocillin, mezlocillin, and piperacillin
adaptative → *adaptive*
adaptive *Syn: adaptative*; based on adaptation
additive additional, accessory
adenosine nucleoside made from adenine and ribose; building block of the nucleic acids; possesses a vasodilating action on precapillary vessels, which can, for example, improve the coronary perfusion; used for this reason as an antiarrhythmic in AV-nodal re-entry tachycardias
adherent adherent, adhesive; stuck, tangled
adhesion the act, state or quality of adhering
   platelet adhesion *Syn: thrombocyte adhesion*; *s.u. thrombocyte aggregation*
   thrombocyte adhesion *Syn: platelet adhesion*; *s.u. thrombocyte aggregation*
adhesive adherent, sticky
adipo- combining form denoting relation to fat or lipids
adipolysis → *lipolysis*

adjuvant 1. a substance which helps another **2.** helping, supporting
adonitoxin cardioactive glycoside with positive inotropic action
adrenal 1. → *adrenal gland* **2.** situated near the kidney **3.** *Syn: adrenic*; relating to the adrenal gland
adrenaline → *epinephrine*
adrenalinemia *Syn: epinephrinemia*; elevated adrenaline content of the blood, e.g., in stress or pheochromocytoma
adrenergic produced by adrenaline, discharging adrenaline, responding to adrenaline
adrenic *Syn: adrenal*; relating to the adrenal gland
adreno- combining form denoting relation to the adrenal gland
adrenoceptive responding to adrenergic transmitters
adrenocorticotrophic → *adrenocorticotropic*
adrenocorticotropic *Syn: adrenocorticotrophic*; acting on the adrenal cortex
adrenogenic *Syn: adrenogenous*; caused by the adrenal gland(s), released by them, or arising from them
adrenogenous → *adrenogenic*
adrenolytic 1. an agent with adrenolytic properties **2.** enhancing the effects of adrenaline
adrenomimetic *Syn: sympatheticomimetic, sympathicomimetic, sympathomimetic*; **1.** an agent with adrenomimetic properties **2.** exciting the sympathetic system, having a stimulatory action on the sympathetic system
advancing → *progressive*
adventitia *Syn: adventitial coat*; outer connective tissue covering of vessels and organs
adventitial relating to the adventitia
adynamia → *asthenia*
aeremia → *aeroembolism*
aero- combining form denoting air/gas/mist
aerobic *Syn: aerophilic, aerophilous*; (*biology*) using oxygen to live, dependent upon oxygen; (*chemistry*) proceeding in the presence of oxygen, dependent upon oxygen
aeroembolism *Syn: aeremia, ebullism*; the release of bubbles of gas in the blood and body tissues when the pressure drops
aerogenic *Syn: aerogenous*; gas-producing
aerogenous → *aerogenic*
aerophagia → *aerophagy*

aerophagy *Syn: aerophagia, pneumophagia*; abnormal swallowing of air, which can provoke bloating, palpitations, and chest pain by overfilling of the stomach and small intestine with air

aerophilic *Syn: aerophilous*; living in oxygen; dependent upon oxygen

aerophilous → *aerophilic*

aerotolerant growing in the presence of oxygen; oxygen tolerant

afebrile *Syn: apyretic, apyrexial, athermic*; progressing without fever, not feverish

affected afflicted; touched by

afibrinogenemia *Syn: deficiency of fibrinogen, factor I deficiency*; congenital [autosomal recessive] or acquired absolute deficiency of fibrinogen, which leads to disturbances of clotting; **lab.**: TPZ, PTT, and PTZ are prolonged, determination of the fibrinogen level demonstrates none or very little

   acquired afibrinogenemia the most important causes are increased fibrinolysis [e.g., post-operative], consumptive coagulopathy, and impaired liver function

   congenital afibrinogenemia rare defect, which may present soon after birth with prolonged bleeding from the umbilical cord

afterload energy utilization of the heart muscle to overcome the resistance in the outflow tracts of the left ventricle and peripheral circulation; the action of vasodilators [Ca-antagonists, nitrates, dihydralazine, etc.] is based in large part upon a reduction in the afterload, which leads to unloading of the left ventricular muscle

agent a substance capable of producing an effect

   antimicrobial agent → *antibiotic*

   blocking agent → *blocker*

   calcium-blocking agent → *calcium antagonist*

   cardiovascular agents description of substances that influence the circulation, such as antihypertensives or antihypotensives

agglomerate *Syn: agglomerated*; accumulated, aggregated

agglomerated → *agglomerate*

agglutinable capable of agglutination

agglutinate *Syn: clumpy*; stuck together, adherent

agglutination *Syn: clumping*; the act or process of agglutinating

   platelet agglutination → *thromboagglutination*

aggravating exacerbated, intensifying

aggregate accumulated, cumulated, coalesced

aggregation accumulation, cumulation

platelet aggregation → *thrombocyte aggregation*

thrombocyte aggregation *Syn: platelet aggregation*; clumping of thrombocytes in the setting of hemostasis; thrombocytes stick to the connective tissue filaments at the wound margins; under the influence of von Willebrand factor, the thrombocytes adhere to the vessel wall [**thrombocyte adhesion**] and this leads to **reversible thrombocyte aggregation**, which is promoted by ADP and adrenalin; the emptying of the thrombocyte granules releases various factors, of which the **thrombospondin** from the α-granules is the main promoter of progression to **irreversible thrombocyte aggregation**

agitated excited, restless

agnogenic → *idiopathic*

air-borne (*pathogen*) transmitted via the air

air hunger → *Kussmaul-Kien respiration*

ajmaline alkaloid derived from **Rauwolfia serpentina**; antiarrhythmic with chinidine-type action; **usage**: paroxysmal tachycardias, ventricular tachycardia, pre-excitation syndromes; **contraindications**: AV-block, bradycardia, bundle branch block, cardiogenic shock

albumen → *albumin*

albumin *Syn: albumen*; water-soluble, globular protein, made predominantly in the liver; 120–200 mg/kg of albumin is produced daily in adults; the most important protein in the blood plasma [approx. 50–60% of the plasma proteins]; in reality, only approx. 40% of the total albumin is found in the blood plasma, the rest being mainly distributed in the extracellular compartment; albumins are probably present in all bodily fluids; their main role in the blood is the transport of non-esterified fatty acids, pharmaceuticals, vitamins, magnesium, calcium, trace elements, as well as maintenance of the colloid osmotic pressure at a constant level

    human albumin infusion solution used as a plasma substitute; **usage**: hypovolemic shock, hypoalbuminemia [predominantly burns]; **side effects**: allergic reactions, fever, hypotonia, shock

    plasma albumin *s.u. plasma protein*

albuminuria → *proteinuria*

aldosterone an adrenal cortical hormone of the mineralocorticoid group; together with angiotensin, it regulates sodium and water reabsorption in the kidney, ileum, and colon and thereby has considerable influence on water and electrolyte balance

aldosteronopenia → *hypoaldosteronism*

algesic → *algetic*

algesiogenic → *algogenic*

algetic *Syn: algesic*; painful, producing pain

algogenic *Syn: algesiogenic*; causing pain(s)

alimentary dependent upon nutrition, absorbed with food, dietary

aliskiren first oral direct renin inhibitor; decreases plasma renin activity by inhibiting conversion of angiotensinogen to angiotensin I within the renin-angiotensin-aldosterone system; **usage**: essential hypertension, alone or in combination with other antihypertensive agents

alkalemia elevation of the pH value of the blood; excessive alkali in the blood; often equated with decompensated alkalosis

alkalosis disturbance in the acid-base balance caused by an increase in the blood pH above 7.44; **compensated alkalosis** occurs as long as the body is capable of returning the pH to the normal range or having it approach the normal range; **decompensated** alkalosis occurs when the compensatory mechanisms are exhausted

allergy *Syn: acquired sensitivity, induced sensitivity*; a clinical picture caused by a hypersensitivity (reaction) to an allergen; the term is not clearly defined; this is due to some extent to the fact that a clinical differentiation between allergic [e.g., allergic contact dermatitis] and pseudoallergic diseases [e.g., toxic contact dermatitis] is often possible only with difficulty; allergic hypersensitivity reactions were divided by **Gell and Coombs** (1969) into four basic types, only two of which cause classic allergies: **1. anaphylactic reaction** or **immediate hypersensitivity**: the clinical disease is called an **immediate allergy** and the patients have a predisposition to develop the allergy [atopy]; this type includes, for instance, hay fever, bronchial asthma, urticaria, food allergies, allergy to insect stings, etc. **2. delayed-type** (or **delayed**) **hypersensitivity** or **cell-mediated hypersensitivity**: upon second contact with an allergen cytotoxic T lymphocytes cause a delayed reaction, which peaks after 48–72 hours; allergic contact dermatitis and the tuberculin test are examples of this type of hypersensitivity

penicillin allergy immediate or delayed allergy to penicillin or its degradation products

allo- combining form denoting a condition differing from the normal, or reversal, or referring to another

allodromy irregularity of rhythm appreciated by the patient; usually it is an extrasystole

allogeneic → *allogenic*

allogenic *Syn: allogeneic, homogenous, homological, homologous*; deriving from the same species

allomorphic occurring in various forms, with various forms

alloplastic made from foreign material

allorhythmia disturbance of the heart rhythm with regular extrasystoles, e.g., bigeminy, trigeminy

allorhythmic relating to or affected with allorhythmia

alpha-aminobenzylpenicillin → *ampicillin*

alpha-blocker *Syn: alpha blocking agent, alpha-adrenergic blocking agent, alpha-adrenergic blocking agent, alpha-adrenergic receptor blocking agent, alphalytic*; agent that competitively inhibits the α-receptors in the target organs; blockers of the $α_1$- and $α_2$-receptors in the vessel wall are clinically important since they are activated in, for example, disturbances of perfusion or disorders of bladder emptying

alpha-hemolysis *Syn: α-hemolysis*; bacterial growth with complete hemolysis of the erythrocytes in blood agar

alpha-hemolytic → *α-hemolytic*

alphalytic → *alpha-blocker*

alphamimetic *Syn: alpha sympathomimetic, alpha-sympathomimetic*; **1.** an agent with alphamimetic properties; stimulation causes contraction of the smooth muscles of skin vessels, bronchi, and bowels, of the dilatator muscle of pupil, etc. **2.** stimulating α-receptors of the sympathetic system

alpha-sympathomimetic → *alphamimetic*

alprenolol beta-blocker with weak cardioselective action

alprostadil *Syn: prostaglandin E_1*; prostaglandin with vasodilating action; **usage**: vasodilator, perfusion-enhancing agent

alteplase *Syn: recombined tissue plasminogen activator*; recombinant tissue plasminogen activator; **usage**: lytic therapy in acute myocardial infarction, deep vein thrombosis pulmonary embolism; **side effects**: bleeding at puncture sites, in the gastrointestinal tract, hematuria, gum and nose bleeding; **contraindications**: hemorrhagic diathesis, oral anticoagulant therapy, duodenal or pyloric ulcers, colitis, esophageal varices, aortic aneurysm, arterial hypertension, apoplectic insult, postoperatively, metastatic malignancies, pregnancy, immediate postpartum period

alterant → *alterative*

alterative *Syn: alterant*; changing, changeable

alternate alternating, reciprocal

alternating → *alternate*

alymphocytosis absolute deficiency of lymphocytes in the blood

ambulatory blood pressure monitoring a procedure where an automated electronic device is worn by the patient usually for a period of 24 hours; it measures blood pressure at regular intervals throughout the day and the night

amezinium metilsulfate sympathomimetic; **usage**: anti-hypotensive agent

amicrobic not caused by microbes

amikacin aminoglycoside antibiotic; **indications**: reserve antibiotic for severe infections with gram-negative pathogens

amiloride potassium-sparing diuretic

amine any of a class of compounds derived from ammonia by replacing one or more hydrogen atoms with organic groups
 biogenic amine → *bioamine*

α-aminobenzylpenicillin → *ampicillin*

aminoform → *hexamethylentetramine*

aminoglycoside → *aminoglycoside antibiotic*

aminopenicillins umbrella term for a number of penicillins, which are also effective against gram-negative bacteria; these include, e.g., ampicillin and amoxicillin

amiodarone class III antiarrhythmic; coronary vasodilator; **usage**: therapy-resistant ventricular and supraventricular arrhythmias; **contraindications**: sinus bradycardia, sick sinus syndrome, 2. and 3. degree AV-block, supraventricular disturbances of heart rhythm after myocardial infarction

amlodipine calcium antagonist, anti-hypertensive agent; **usage**: arterial hypertension, coronary heart disease, angina pectoris; **side effects**: flushing, allergy, headache, dizziness, muscle cramps

A-mode *s.u.* sonography

amoxicillin semisynthetic penicillin with a broad action spectrum; **indications**: gram-positive and gram-negative pathogens [primarily enterococci, Clostridium, Listeria, streptococci, Treponema, and Haemophilus influenzae]; it is less effective against Escherichia coli, Salmonella, Shigella, and Proteus

amphoric (*sound*) hollow sounding

amphorophony *Syn*: *amphoric respiration, amphoric resonance, cavernous resonance, bottle sound*; hollow-sounding breath sound audible over large lung cavities

ampicillin *Syn*: *α-aminobenzylpenicillin, alpha-aminobenzylpenicillin*;

acid-stable, semisynthetic penicillin with broad action spectrum; **indications**: gram-positive and gram-negative pathogens [primarily enterococci, Clostridium, Listeria, streptococci, Treponema, and Haemophilus influenzae]; it is less effective against Escherichia coli, Salmonella, Shigella, and Proteus **side effects**: gastrointestinal symptoms, diarrhea, allergy, urticaria, exanthem, leukopenia, thrombopenia, elevated AST

amrinone a rarely-used heart tonic

amyl nitrite *Syn: isoamyl nitrite*; ester of nitrous acid; volatile fluid that is explosive in air mixtures; produces vessel dilatation and a brief drop in blood pressure; **usage**: as inhalation therapy for angina pectoris

amyloidosis *Syn: Abercrombie's degeneration, Abercrombie's syndrome, amyloid degeneration, amyloid thesaurismosis, bacony degeneration, amylosis, cellulose degeneration, chitinous degeneration, hyaloid degeneration, lardaceous degeneration, Virchow's degeneration, waxy degeneration, Virchow's disease*; generic term for diseases caused by the deposition of amyloid; the deposition can affect particular organs [e.g., renal amyloidosis] or may occur in primary or secondary generalized forms; the amyloidoses can also be the nucleus for, e.g., secondary cardiomyopathy, hepatomegaly, malabsorption, worsening of renal function, macroglossia

amyloidosis of aging → *senile amyloidosis*

cardiopathic amyloidosis senile cardiac amyloidosis affecting mainly the cardiovascular system

idiopathic amyloidosis → *primary amyloidosis*

myocardial amyloidosis idiopathic or hereditary amyloidosis which leads to cardiomyopathy and chronic cardiac insufficiency

primary amyloidosis *Syn: idiopathic amyloidosis, paramyloidosis*; amyloidosis caused by the deposition of amyloid L, which affects multiple organs [heart, kidney, liver, spleen, muscle, vessels]; the causes include, among others, multiple myeloma, plasmacytoma, Waldenström's macroglobulinemia; in addition, there are also idiopathic forms

senile amyloidosis *Syn: amyloidosis of aging*; an amyloidosis caused by amyloid S with damage predominantly to the heart muscle and brain

systemic amyloidosis primary or secondary amyloidosis with deposition of amyloid in multiple organs or organ systems

amylosis → *amyloidosis*

anaemia → *anemia*

anaerobian → *anaerobic*

anaerobic *Syn: anaerobian, anaerobiotic*; living without oxygen, not dependent upon oxygen
anaerobiotic → *anaerobic*
analgesic → *analgetic*
analgetic *Syn: analgesic*; **1.** an agent with analgetic properties; pain reliever **2.** relieving pain **3.** not sensitive to pain, anesthetic
analysis determination of the component parts of a substance
  arrhythmia analysis generally computer-assisted [**arrhythmia computer**] analysis of disturbances of the heart rhythm, such as heart block, bradycardia, tachycardia
  analysis of blood → *hemanalysis*
  blood gas analysis quantitative measurement of the gases present in the arterial or venous blood; usually combined with a measurement of the acid-base balance
  dilution analysis analysis technique, which relies upon dilution of the concentration of a substance by mixing it with other substances; if, for example, a dye is injected into the bloodstream and then the concentration of dye in the blood is measured, this can be used to determine the total blood volume
  frequency analysis computer-assisted analysis of rhythmic biosignals; e.g., automated EEG or ECG analysis
analysor → *autoanalyzer*
analyzer → *autoanalyzer*
  blood gas analyzer apparatus for the determination of the gases present in arterial or venous blood
anaphylactic relating to anaphylaxis
anaphylactogenic *Syn: producing anaphylaxis*; causing anaphylaxis
anaphylactoid with the symptoms of anaphylaxis
anaphylatoxins substances belonging to the complement system, which, among other actions, provoke contraction of smooth muscle; generic term for the cleavage products C4a, C3a, and C5a that provoke an anaphylactic reaction
anaphylaxis *Syn: allergic shock, anaphylactic shock, generalized anaphylaxis, systemic anaphylaxis*; immediate allergy [hypersensitivity of anaphylactic type] to repeated antigen injection, mediated by IgE; leads to release of histamine, serotonin, heparin, and prostaglandins from mast cells; may lead to the development of **allergic** or **anaphylactic shock** with acute threat to life
  generalized anaphylaxis → *anaphylaxis*

systemic anaphylaxis →*anaphylaxis*

anastomosis 1. natural connection of two hollow organs, vessels, or nerves **2.** surgically created connection between hollow organs, vessels, or nerves

arterial anastomosis operative joining of arteries, e.g., to create a bypass or a shunt

arteriolovenular anastomosis →*arteriovenous anastomosis*

arteriovenous anastomosis *Syn: arteriolovenular anastomosis, AV anastomosis*; physiological connection of arteries and veins

AV anastomosis →*arteriovenous anastomosis*

bidirectional cavopulmonary anastomosis →*Glenn's operation*

Blalock-Taussig anastomosis *Syn: Blalock-Taussig operation*; operative anastomosis of the subclavian artery to the pulmonary artery in cases of congenital heart defects (e.g., Fallot's tetralogy)

cavopulmonary anastomosis →*Glenn's operation*

end-to-end anastomosis *Syn: terminoterminal anastomosis*; end-to-end suture of vessels, hollow organs, or nerves

end-to-side anastomosis *Syn: terminolateral anastomosis*; end-to-side anastomosis of vessels, hollow organs, or nerves, e.g., the efferent loop in a Roux-en-Y anastomosis

laterolateral anastomosis *Syn: side-to-side anastomosis*; side-to-side anastomosis of vessels, hollow organs, or nerves, e.g., the afferent and efferent intestinal loops in a Braun anastomosis

Nakayama anastomosis end-to-end anastomosis of small vessels by operative flange clinch sealing of the vessel stumps using tantalum rings; performed, e.g., when constructing a Cimino shunt for hemodialysis

precapillary anastomosis anastomosis of arterioles before the transition to capillaries

Riolan's anastomosis variable connection between the superior and inferior mesenteric artery

side-to-side anastomosis →*laterolateral anastomosis*

terminolateral anastomosis →*end-to-side anastomosis*

terminoterminal anastomosis →*end-to-end anastomosis*

ancrod fibrin splitting enzyme of the malayan pit viper **Agkistrodon rhodostoma**; usage: anticoagulant in deep vein thrombosis, disturbances of peripheral arterial perfusion or postoperative thromboprophylaxis

anemia *Syn: anaemia*; reduction of the hemoglobin concentration, erythrocyte count, and/or hematocrit to below the age- and gender-specific

anemia

normal values; the anemias can be categorized by morphologic features [hyperchromic anemia, megaloblastic anemia] or according to the causes [iron deficiency anemia, hemolytic anemia]; in Europe, the most common anemias are caused by absolute or relative iron deficiency

acquired anemia → *secondary anemia*

acquired sideroachrestic anemia *Syn: refractory sideroblastic anemia*; anemia caused by an acquired disturbance of iron utilization

acute posthemorrhagic anemia *Syn: hemorrhagic anemia*; acute anemia caused by massive blood loss

angiopathic hemolytic anemia hemolytic anemia caused by changes in blood vessels

anhemopoietic anemia anemia caused by an inborn [congenital dyserythropoietic anemia] or acquired disturbance of erythrocyte formation [erythropoiesis]

aplastic anemia *Syn: aregenerative anemia, Ehrlich's anemia, panmyelophthisis, refractory anemia*; anemia as a consequence of a congenital or acquired disturbance of blood formation; Fanconi anemia and Blackfan-Diamond anemia are forms of the rare **primary aplastic anemias**, among others; the more common **secondary aplastic anemias** are mainly caused by medications [analgesics, antirheumatics]

aregenerative anemia → *aplastic anemia*

autoimmune hemolytic anemia hemolytic anemia caused by autoimmune antibodies against erythrocytes

congenital aplastic anemia → *Fanconi's anemia*

congenital hypoplastic anemia → *Fanconi's anemia*

deficiency anemia *Syn: nutritional anemia*; anemia caused by inadequate intake of one or more essential nutrients

dilution anemia *Syn: hydremia, polyplasmia*; anemia caused by an increase in the plasma or blood fluid

Ehrlich's anemia → *aplastic anemia*

enzyme deficiency hemolytic anemia hemolytic anemia with inborn or acquired enzymopathy

Fanconi's anemia *Syn: congenital aplastic anemia, congenital hypoplastic anemia, congenital pancytopenia, constitutional infantile panmyelopathy, Fanconi's syndrome, Fanconi's pancytopenia, pancytopenia-dysmelia syndrome*; inherited disorder of hematopoiesis affecting all series in the bone marrow, i.e., it causes anemia, granulocytopenia, and thrombocytopenia; in addition, there are malformations [microcephaly, hypogonadism, hypo- or aplasia of the forearm or wrist]; bone marrow transplantation can cure the panmyelopathy, but most patients die from malformations of the internal organs or common malignancies [e.g., leukemia] before reaching adulthood

folic acid deficiency anemia megaloblastic anemia due to insufficient folic acid [alcoholism, malnourishment, dialysis], disturbances of reabsorption in the small intestine [sprue, celiac disease, oral contraceptives], increased requirements [pregnancy], or treatment with folate antagonists

hemolytic anemia *Syn: Abrami's disease*; anemia due to a pathologic increase in the disintegration of erythrocytes, i.e., increased hemolysis; as long as the bone marrow is capable of replacing the erythrocyte loss by producing more, this is described as **compensated increased hemolysis**; in **decompensated increased hemolysis**, the actual anemia develops; hemolytic anemias can be caused by a variety of factors; **corpuscular hemolytic anemia** groups together those hemolytic anemias whose cause lies in the erythrocytes; in central Europe, spherocytic anemia is the most common; **serogenic hemolytic anemia** is caused by antibodies against erythrocytes; **toxic anemias** relate to disorders of blood formation or direct injury to the erythrocytes

hemorrhagic anemia *Syn: posthemorrhagic anemia*; anemia caused by acute or chronic blood loss

hemotoxic anemia *Syn: toxanemia, toxic anemia*; anemia caused by toxic substances with disturbance of hematopoiesis or damage to erythrocytes

hyperchromatic anemia → *hyperchromic anemia*

hyperchromic anemia *Syn: hyperchromatic anemia*; anemia with elevated hemoglobin content in the erythrocytes

hypoferric anemia → *sideropenic anemia*

hypochromic anemia *Syn: hypochromemia*; anemia with diminished hemoglobin content in the erythrocytes

hypochromic microcytic anemia anemia with hypochromic microcytes

hypoplastic anemia anemia due to inadequate erythrocyte formation

idiopathic anemia → *primary anemia*

immune hemolytic anemia hemolytic anemia caused by antibodies against erythrocytes

infectious anemia normo- or hypochromic anemia in chronic infections [e.g., tuberculosis, rheumatoid arthritis]

infectious hemolytic anemia hemolytic anemia caused by a pathogen [e.g., plasmodia]

iron deficiency anemia → *sideropenic anemia*

isochromic anemia → *normochromic anemia*

macrocytic anemia *Syn: megalocytic anemia*; anemia with macrocytes in the blood smear

megaloblastic anemia hyperchromic anemia with megaloblasts in the bone marrow and in the peripheral blood; the most important causes are vitamin B_{12} deficiency, folic acid deficiency, metabolic disorders [hereditary orotic aciduria], goat's milk anemia, cytostatic therapy [inhibitors of purine or pyrimidine synthesis]

megalocytic anemia → *macrocytic anemia*

microangiopathic anemia → *thrombotic microangiopathy*

microangiopathic hemolytic anemia → *thrombotic microangiopathy*

microcytic anemia anemia with formation of microcytes

molecular anemia corpuscular hemolytic anemia due to pathologic hemoglobin [e.g., sickle cell anemia]

normochromic anemia *Syn: isochromic anemia*; anemia with normal hemoglobin content in the erythrocytes

normocytic anemia anemia with normally formed and pigmented erythrocytes

nutritional anemia → *deficiency anemia*

posthemorrhagic anemia anemia following acute or chronic blood loss

primary anemia *Syn: idiopathic anemia*; anemia of no apparent cause

protein deficiency anemia anemia due to severe protein deficiency and the resultant disturbance of hemoglobin formation; since there is usually a combined deficiency state, in which other substances are missing [vitamins, iron], there is no typical blood picture finding

refractory anemia → *aplastic anemia*

refractory sideroblastic anemia → *acquired sideroachrestic anemia*

secondary anemia acquired anemia

sideroachrestic anemia *Syn: sideroblastic anemia*; anemia due to congenital or acquired disturbances of iron utilization [iron deficiency without deficient iron]; characterized by frequent sideroblasts with coarse-grained iron deposition in ring shapes [**ring sideroblasts**]

sideroblastic anemia → *sideroachrestic anemia*

sideropenic anemia *Syn: hypoferric anemia, iron deficiency anemia*; most common form of anemia, due to congenital or acquired iron deficiency; the iron deficiency leads to disturbances of hemoglobin formation and thereby to the development of a hypochromic anemia; the accompanying disturbance of erythropoiesis leads to a reduction in the erythrocyte volume [microcytic anemia] and to the occurrence of anomalous erythrocyte forms [anulocytes] in the peripheral blood; the **clinical picture** is determined by the general symptoms of iron deficiency; the **blood picture** shows a reduction in the erythrocyte volume and hemoglobin content of the erythrocytes as well as aniso-, anulo- and poikilocytosis

toxic anemia → *hemotoxic anemia*

anemic relating to or characterized by anemia

anergic 1. inactive; without energy **2.** with reduced capacity for reaction

aneurysm circumscribed dilatation of the wall of an artery or the heart; congenital aneurysms may be solitary or multiple [**Bonnet-Dechaune-Blanc syndrome**] or occur together with other malformations [e.g., renal]; they are found most commonly as intracranial aneurysms; acquired aneurysms are caused by, among others, Marfan's syndrome, Ehlers-Danlos syndrome, arteriosclerosis, cystic medial necrosis, periarteritis nodosa, or trauma [including iatrogenic with catheters!]; depending upon their shape, aneurysms are classified as **fusiform** [spindle shaped], **saccular** [sac-like], **serpigiform** [snake-like], **cirsoid** [tendrillar], etc.; in **true aneurysms**, all layers of the wall are affected, whereas in **false aneurysms** the cause is a traumatic hematoma in the vessel; aneurysms in the upper and lower extremities are particularly commonly clinically silent for a long time; they act as sources of emboli and at the time of diagnosis the distal circulation may have been thromboembolically occluded, leading to loss of the limb; the more common aneurysms of the aorta can lead to dissection and then become surgical emergencies; **therapy** depends upon the location and size of the aneurysm as well as the histology; in general, both true and false aneurysms are treated expectantly and their course is observed

ampullary aneurysm *Syn: sacculated aneurysm, saccular aneurysm*; *s.u. aneurysm*

aortic aneurysm congenital or acquired saccular enlargement of the aorta, which can occur in all portions of the aorta; aneurysms of the ascending aorta and the thoracic descending aorta are frequently asymptomatic; aneurysms of the ascending aorta usually occur in the third to fifth decade of life and are normally the result of an idiopathic medial disease; aneurysms of the thoracic descending aorta, in con-

aneurysm

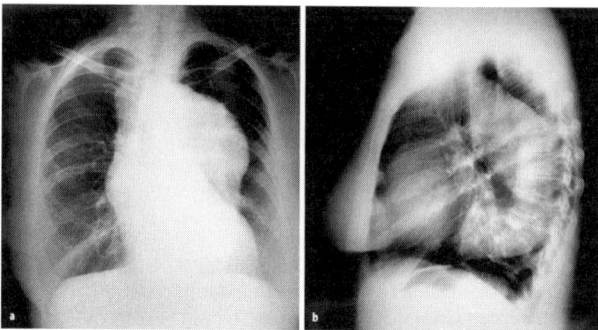

Aortic aneurysm. Aneurysm of the descending aorta

trast, often have an arteriosclerotic etiology especially and usually manifest themselves in the sixth to seventh decade of life; aneurysms of the aortic arch can cause symptoms by compressing the airways or the esophagus or by hoarseness due to pressure on the left recurrent nerve; **surgical treatment** is simplest for aneurysms of the descending aorta; the ascending aorta and primarily the aortic arch have a more complex anatomy and for this reason pose a number of challenges to the surgeon and have a higher mortality [up to 25%]; the selection of the surgical method [replacement with a tubular prosthesis, intraluminal stent] depends on the situation and the surgeon

arteriosclerotic aneurysm *Syn: atherosclerotic aneurysm*; an aneurysm caused by atherosclerosis, mainly affecting the abdominal aorta, femoral artery, or popliteal artery

arteriovenous aneurysm usually traumatic fistula between an artery and a vein

atherosclerotic aneurysm → *arteriosclerotic aneurysm*

cardiac aneurysm *Syn: false aneurysm of heart, myocardial aneurysm, ventricular aneurysm*; aneurysm of the heart wall, e.g., following infarction

cardiac valve aneurysm baggy bulging of the heart valve in inflammation or degeneration

cirsoid aneurysm *Syn: racemose aneurysm, diffuse arterial ectasia*; *s.u. aneurysm*

dissecting aneurysm *Syn: Shekelton's aneurysm*; aneurysm developing following the formation of fissures in the arterial wall

dissecting aortic aneurysm →*aortic dissection*

false aneurysm *Syn: spurious aneurysm, aneurysmal hematoma*; s.u. *aneurysm*

false aneurysm of heart →*cardiac aneurysm*

fusiform aneurysm *Syn: Richet's aneurysm*; s.u. *aneurysm*

intracranial aneurysm up to 90% of aneurysms of the brain arteries are congenital; the majority lie in the region of the skull base; [anterior communicating artery, 30%], the internal carotid artery or the middle cerebral artery; aneurysms with a diameter of more than 1 cm are described as **large aneurysms**, **giant aneurysms** have a diameter of more than 2.5 cm; aneurysms are a common cause of subarachnoid hemorrhage, but may also come to light by causing neurologic symptoms as a result of their position and size [e.g., oculomotor nerve palsy]; the operative disconnection of symptomatic or ruptured aneurysms is achieved by **clipping** [application of an aneurysm clip to the neck of the aneurysm; method of choice], **ligation of the neck of the aneurysm**, **trapping** [careful restriction of the blood flow to diminish the risk of rupture; rarely used today], **wrapping** [wrapping the aneurysm, e.g., with tendon or fascia] or **filling** [packing with inert material]

myocardial aneurysm →*cardiac aneurysm*

racemose aneurysm *Syn: diffuse arterial ectasia, cirsoid aneurysm*; s.u. *aneurysm*

Richet's aneurysm *Syn: fusiform aneurysm*; s.u. *aneurysm*

saccular aneurysm *Syn: ampullary aneurysm, sacculated aneurysm*; s.u. *aneurysm*

sacculated aneurysm *Syn: ampullary aneurysm, saccular aneurysm*; s.u. *aneurysm*

serpentine aneurysm s.u. *aneurysm*

Shekelton's aneurysm →*dissecting aneurysm*

spurious aneurysm *Syn: aneurysmal hematoma, false aneurysm*; s.u. *aneurysm*

true aneurysm s.u. *aneurysm*

ventricular aneurysm →*cardiac aneurysm*

aneurysmal →*aneurysmatic*

aneurysmatic *Syn: aneurysmal*; relating to an aneurysm

aneurysmectomy operative excision of an aneurysm; usually only performed for aneurysms of peripheral arteries or the aorta, the resected vessel segment generally being replaced with a tubular prosthesis

aneurysmorrhaphy suture of an aneurysm; generally combined with aneurysmoplasty to reconstitute the circulation

aneurysmotomy opening of an aneurysm

angi- combining form denoting relationship to a vessel, usually a blood vessel

angialgia *Syn: angiodynia*; pain in a blood vessel, e.g., phlebalgia

angiectasia → *angiectasis*

angiectasis *Syn: angiectasia*; inborn or acquired vessel dilatation

angiectatic *Syn: angioectatic*; relating to angiectasis

angiectomy operative excision of a blood vessel or blood vessel segment

angiitis *Syn: vasculitis, vascular inflammation*; inflammation of the (entire) vessel wall

   allergic granulomatous angiitis *Syn: Churg-Strauss syndrome, allergic granulomatosis*; systemic, necrotizing vasculitis of unknown etiology; the changes are similar to those in polyarteritis nodosa, but all vessels are affected with granuloma formation; eosinophilia and bronchial asthma also occur; **therapy**: prednisone, possibly in combination with cyclophosphamide; dose tapering only after 6–12 months of stable remission; prognosis: if untreated, the outcome is fatal in 50% within a year

   leukocytoclastic angiitis → *allergic vasculitis*

   necrotizing angiitis *Syn: necrotizing vasculitis*; necrotizing inflammation of a blood vessel

angina 1. severe constricting often spasmodic pain; usually referring to angina pectoris **2.** obsolete for sore throat

   abdominal angina *Syn: intestinal angina, Ortner's disease*; colicky abdominal pain with symptoms of the acute abdomen due to restriction of the perfusion of the small intestine due to arteriosclerosis of the mesenteric vessels; course, prognosis, and therapy depend upon the extent and duration of the ischemia

   crescendo angina secondary unstable angina pectoris with increasingly severe, longer lasting and more frequent attacks of pain

   angina cruris → *intermittent claudication*

   Heberden's angina → *angina pectoris*

   intestinal angina → *abdominal angina*

   angina pectoris *Syn: angina, angor, breast pang, cardiagra, Elsners asthma, coronarism, heart stroke, Heberden's angina, Heberden's asthma, Heberden's disease, Rougnon-Heberden disease, sternodynia, ster-*

nalgia, stenocardia; attack of pain in the vicinity of the heart caused by acute ischemia of the heart muscle with a characteristic feeling of constriction; generally brought on by physical or emotional stress; divided into: **1. stable** or **sporadic angina pectoris**: develops in relationship to stress with a relatively constant or variable stress threshold or at night [**angina decubitus**]; **2. unstable angina pectoris** [pre-infarction syndrome]: cardiologic emergency, which requires immediate observation and treatment as an inpatient; **3. vasospastic angina** or **Prinzmetal angina**: often occurs in the early morning with severe, spontaneous angina attacks with an otherwise good exercise capacity and mostly negative tests of ischemia; it carries a high risk of infarction, disturbances of heart rhythm, and sudden cardiac death

variant angina pectoris → *Prinzmetal's angina*

Prinzmetal's angina *Syn: variant angina pectoris*; severe, spontaneous angina attacks often occurring in the early morning in patients with otherwise good exercise tolerance and usually negative ischemia tests; there is a high risk of infarction, disturbances of heart rhythm, and sudden cardiac death; *s.a. angina pectoris*

anginose *Syn: anginous*; relating to or suffering from angina

anginous → *anginose*

angio- combining form denoting relationship to a vessel, usually a blood vessel

angioblast *Syn: vasofactive cell, vasoformative cell*; vessel forming cells

angioblastic relating to angioblasts

angioblastoma → *hemangioblastoma*

angiocardiogram X-ray contrast examination of the heart and great vessels

angiocardiographic relating to angiocardiography

angiocardiography X-ray contrast demonstration of the heart and great vessels

angiocardiopathic relating to angiocardiopathy

angiocardiopathy disease or malformation of the heart and great vessels

angiocarditic relating to or caused by angiocarditis

angiocarditis inflammation of the heart and the great vessels

angiodynia → *angialgia*

angiodysplasia defective formation of a blood vessel/vascular development

angiodystrophia → *angiodystrophy*

angiodystrophy *Syn: angiodystrophia*; inadequate nutrition of blood vessels

angioectatic → *angiectatic*

angioedema *Syn: angioneurotic edema*; subcutaneous swelling of the skin and mucous membranes caused by an allergic reaction; often combined with hives [urticaria]; rarer, but more dramatic, is the **hereditary angioedema** due to an autosomal dominant defect of the C1-esterase inhibitor and the angioedema of acquired defects in the enzyme; the cause of the swelling is not completely clear, but it relates to increased vascular permeability; **clinical**: the recurrent attacks impress by their sudden [within a few hours] drum-tight, cutaneous swelling, which mostly affects the facial areas and is accompanied by a risk of laryngeal edema and asphyxiation; the edema is painless, does not itch, and is not accompanied by urticaria; vomiting, abdominal colic, and diarrhea are signs of angioedema of the intestinal mucosa; **therapy**: C1-INH replacement; antihistamines and steroids are ineffective

    hereditary angioedema *Syn: hereditary angioneurotic edema, C1-inhibitor deficiency, C1-INH deficiency; s.u. angioedema*

angioedematous relating to angioedema

angioendothelioma → *hemangioendothelioma*

angiofibroma benign blood vessel tumor with connective tissue components

angiofollicular relating to lymphoid follicles and blood vessels

angiogenesis new formation of blood vessels

angiogenic relating to angiogenesis

angiogram *Syn: angiograph*; a contrast image of vessels acquired during angiography

    carotid angiogram X-ray contrast imaging of the internal carotid artery and its branches

angiogranuloma benign blood vessel tumor with granulation tissue

angiograph → *angiogram*

angiographic relating to angiography

angiography X-ray contrast demonstration of vessels; generic term for arteriography, phlebography, and lymphography; generally, renally excreted contrast agents are used, which can be given through catheters [catheter angiography] or injected directly into the vessel; in **retrograde angiography**, the contrast agent is injected against the flow, in **anterograde angiography** it flows in the same direction as the bloodstream

    angiography of the aortic arch *Syn: aortic arch angiography*; angio-

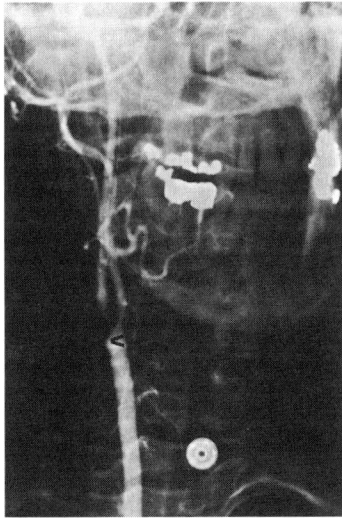

Carotid angiogram. Stenosis of the right internal carotid

graphic visualization of the aortic arch and the vessels arising from it

aortic arch angiography → *angiography of the aortic arch*

brachiocephalic angiography angiography of the brachiocephalic trunk and its branches in cases of suspected vascular malformation [aneurysm] or stenosis in the brachiocephalic region

carotid angiography X-ray contrast imaging of the internal carotid artery and its branches

catheter angiography angiography with contrast agent injection via a catheter

cerebral angiography X-ray contrast demonstration of the blood vessels to the brain, i.e., selective angiography of the internal and external carotid arteries as well as the vertebral artery with their branches; the injection of contrast agent is usually performed using a catheter introduced via the transfemoral [Seldinger-Judkins technique] or transbrachial [Seldinger-Sones technique] route, or [more rarely] by direct

puncture of the common carotid artery

coronary angiography X-ray demonstration of the coronary vessels of the heart; permits anatomic and functional assessment of the vessels

Doppler angiography *s.u. Doppler ultrasonography*

fluorescence angiography light examination [ophthalmoscopy] of the optic fundus following fluorescein injection

pulmonary angiography *Syn: pulmonary arteriography*; angiography of the pulmonary arteries; in **global pulmonary angiography** the contrast medium is injected into the pulmonary trunk; in **selective pulmonary angiography**, the contrast medium is injected only into the right or left pulmonary artery

radionuclide angiography angiography using radionuclides

renal angiography selective angiography of the renal arteries

selective angiography angiography of specific vessels by direct injection of contrast agent

angiohemophilia *Syn: constitutional thrombopathy, hereditary pseudohemophilia, Minot-von Willebrand syndrome, pseudohemophilia, von Willebrand's disease, vascular hemophilia, von Willebrand's syndrome, Willebrand's syndrome*; autosomal dominant deficiency of von Willebrand factor with a bleeding tendency, which leads to hemorrhages particularly in the spring and fall; **clinical**: recurrent skin and mucous membrane bleeding, hyper- and polymenorrhea; more rarely, joint hemorrhages; injury or operations can cause difficult to control bleeding; **lab.**: prolonged bleeding time, factor VIII under 25%; reduction in the ristocetin cofactor; **DD**: idiopathic thrombocytopenic purpura, thrombocytopenia; **therapy**: fresh frozen plasma, cryoprecipitate; **prognosis**: good; usually the bleeding tendency declines after the age of 20

angiohyalinosis hyalinosis with predominant involvement of the vessel wall

angiokinesis → *vasomotoricity*

angiokinetic → *vasomotor*

angiokymography kymographic demonstration of the flow rates in the arteries

angioleiomyolipoma *Syn: vascular leiomyolipoma*; benign mixed-tissue tumor with blood vessels, fatty tissue, and muscle tissue

angioleiomyoma → *angiomyoma*

angiolipoleiomyoma → *angiomyolipoma*

angiolipoma *Syn: nevoid lipoma, telangiectatic lipoma*; lipoma with numerous blood vessels

angiologia → *angiology*

angiologic relating to angiology

angiology *Syn: angiologia*; study of the blood vessels and their diseases

angiolopathies disease of the terminal arteries [arterioles]

angiolymphangioma angioma of the blood and lymphatic vessels

angioma *Syn: vascular tumor*; tumor-like new vessel formation or vessel malformation; known as **hemangioma** of blood vessels and as **lymphangioma** of lymphatic vessels

  hypertrophic angioma → *hemangioendothelioma*

  racemose angioma grape-shaped, subcutaneous hemangioma consisting of labyrinthine arteries and veins with multiple anastomoses; occur predominantly on the head and the extremities; **therapy**: sclerotization, excision of small lesions

angiomatosis development of multiple angiomas

angiomatous relating to or resembling an angioma

angiomegaly vessel enlargement, vascular dilatation

angiomyolipoma *Syn: angiolipoleiomyoma*; rare, benign kidney tumor with vascular, fat, and muscle tissue components; often occurs bilaterally and can lead to sudden internal hemorrhage; in larger, bilateral tumors, it is often difficult to preserve at least one kidney by means of angiographic embolization

angiomyoma *Syn: angioleiomyoma, vascular leiomyoma*; myoma with numerous blood vessels

angiomyoneuroma *Syn: glomangioma, glomus tumor*; slowly growing malignant tumor arising from a glomus

angiomyosarcoma malignant mixed-tissue tumor with angiomatous and sarcomatous components

angionecrosis necrosis of the wall of a blood or lymphatic vessel

angionecrotic relating to or marked by angionecrosis

angioneuralgia neuralgic vessel pain; mostly burning pain and swelling of the surrounding tissues

angioneurectomy combined excision of vessel and nerve

angioneuropathic relating to angioneuropathy

angioneuropathy disorder of perfusion caused by neural dysregulation

angioneurosis *Syn: vasoneurosis*; rarely used description of disorders of the vegetative regulation of vessels with disturbances of perfusion, e.g., Raynaud's syndrome

angioneurotic relating to angioneurosis

angioparalysis → *angioparesis*

angioparesis *Syn: angioparalysis, vasoparesis*; vasomotor paralysis due to disturbances of the nerve supply

angiopathic relating to or caused by angiopathy

angiopathy vascular disease; depending upon the size of the affected vessels, it can be subdivided into **microangiopathy** [e.g., capillaries, retinal vessels] and **macroangiopathy** [e.g., arteries, aorta]

  diabetic angiopathy most common long-term injury caused by poorly controlled diabetes mellitus; **diabetic macroangiopathy** mainly affects brain, heart, kidney, and peripheral vessels; **diabetic microangiopathy** is the cause of, among others, diabetic retinopathy, diabetic glomerulosclerosis, and diabetic neuropathy

  angiopathy of great vessels → *macroangiopathy*

angioplasty 1. plastic procedure on a blood vessel, as for example in bypass surgery **2.** stretching of a narrowed segment of a vessel, e.g., with a balloon catheter [**balloon angioplasty**] or catheters with increasing diameter [**Dotter technique**]; subdivided into **open** or **direct angioplasty**, which is usually performed intraoperatively, and **closed** or **indirect angioplasty** in which the catheter is introduced percutaneously

  balloon angioplasty stretching of a vessel using a balloon catheter

  coronary angioplasty widening of narrowed coronary arteries using a balloon catheter

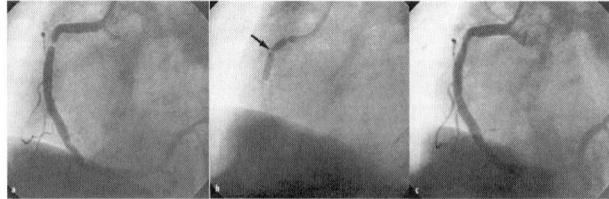

Coronary angioplasty. Stenosis of the right coronary artery before [a], during [b], and after [c] balloon inflation

  laser angioplasty angioplasty, in which the arteriosclerotic material is vaporized with a laser beam

  percutaneous transluminal coronary angioplasty widening of narrowed coronary arteries with a balloon catheter [**balloon angioplasty**];

angiotensins

standard method in heart surgery, which has a success rate of more than 90%; by additionally placing an intravascular stent, the restenosis rate of up to 50% is reduced to 20–30%; coronary dilatation is mainly indicated for angina pectoris and/or where there is confirmed ischemia and a related stenosis; however, where there is complex stenosis morphology, additional heart defects, renal insufficiency, or diabetes mellitus, most centers recommend a bypass procedure; in acute myocardial infarction, coronary angioplasty is nowadays preferred to thrombolytic treatment, since the reperfusion rate is directly comparable, but reperfusion is more complete and achieved more rapidly, and there are fewer bleeding complications [e.g., cerebral insult]

angiopoiesis *Syn: vasifaction, vasoformation*; vessel formation, new vessel formation

angiopoietic *Syn: vasifactive, vasoactive, vasoformative*; relating to or triggering angiopoiesis

angiorrhaphy suture of a vessel

angiosarcoma malignant tumor arising in [blood or lymphatic] vessels

angiosclerosis thickening and hardening of the wall of blood or lymphatic vessels

angiosclerotic relating to angiosclerosis

angioscope microscope for directly observing capillaries

angioscopic relating to angioscope or angioscopy

angioscopy 1. direct observation of surface capillaries with a capillary microscope **2.** endoscopy of vessels, e.g., for removal of thrombus

angiospasm *Syn: vasospasm*; vessel spasm caused by a reflex or by local irritation; is, e.g., the cause of angina pectoris

angiospastic *Syn: vasospastic*; relating to or triggering angiospasm

angiostenosis narrowing (of the lumen) of blood or lymphatic vessels

angiostenotic relating to or caused by angiostenosis

angiotensinase *Syn: angiotonase*; enzyme, which cleaves angiotensin II

angiotensinogen *Syn: angiotensin precursor*; inactive parent substance of the angiotensins; is converted from renin to angiotensin I by the renin-angiotensin-aldosterone system

angiotensins tissue hormone with a polypeptide structure; the inactive **angiotensin I** is converted by angiotensin converting enzyme into **angiotensin II**, which has powerful vasoconstrictor and blood pressure elevating actions; **angiotensin III** is an inactive breakdown product of angiotensin II, which plays an important role in the renin-angiotensin-aldosterone system

angiotomography combined angiography and tomography; e.g., for demonstration of hemangiomas, aneurysms, or tumors

angiotomy operative opening of a vessel

angiotonase → *angiotensinase*

angiotonia *Syn: vasotonia*; tone or tension of a vessel (wall)

angiotonic → *vasotonic*

angiotrophic *Syn: vasotrophic*; relating to vascular nutrition

angle area or point of intersection of borders or surfaces; corner; edge

   Pirogoff's angle → *venous angle*

   venous angle *Syn: Pirogoff's angle*; angle between the internal jugular vein and the subclavian vein; on the left side, it is the entry point of the thoracic duct

angor → *angina pectoris*

angulus angle; corner; edge

   angulus venosus → *venous angle*

anhydremia *Syn: anydremia*; water deficiency in the blood

aniso- combining form denoting relation to unequal or dissimilar

anisochromatic of variable color, non-uniformly pigmented

anistreplase inactive, fibrinolytic prodrug [APSAC, p-anisoylated lys-plasminogen-streptokinase-activator complex], which binds to fibrin in thrombus; spontaneous deacylation releases the enzymatically active lys-plasminogen-streptokinase complex, which converts plasminogen on and in the thrombus into plasmin and initiates fibrinolysis; **usage**: reperfusion therapy of occluded coronary arteries in acute myocardial infarction

annuloplasty → *anuloplasty*

annulus *Syn: anulus*; ring

   fibrous annulus *Syn: coronary tendon, fibrous ring of heart, Lower's ring*; fibrous ring around a heart orifice

anomaly marked deviation from the normal

   aortic arch anomalies malformations of the aortic arch, e.g., **double aortic arch** and **right aortic arch**

   Ebstein's anomaly *Syn: Ebstein's disease*; one of the rarer heart defects [less than 1% of all congenital heart defects] with displacement of the malformed tricuspid valve into the right ventricle; this leads to enlargement of the right atrium [**arterialization of the right ventricle**]; due to the insufficiency of the valve, there is retrograde flow of blood during systole [**pendular flow**]; in severe cases, impaired cardiac function, cyanosis, jugular pulse, and systolic murmurs are found

Uhl's anomaly congenital heart defect with underdevelopment of the muscles of the right ventricle

anoxemia high-grade oxygen deficiency in the blood

anoxemic relating to anoxemia

anoxia severe oxygen deficiency; the oxygen supply is significantly less than the tissue requirements and within a short time ischemia and tissue damage follow; the extent of damage and the general danger depend upon the degree and/or localization of the anoxia

anemic anoxia *Syn: anemic hypoxia*; anoxia in anemia

stagnant anoxia →*ischemic hypoxia*

anoxic relating to anoxia

antagonist a substance that tends to inhibit or nullify the action of another

aldosterone antagonists diuretic agents; block the aldosterone receptors in the tubular cells; this increases the excretion of water, sodium, and bicarbonate ions and reduces that of potassium ions; risk of hyperkalemia, gynecomastia, impaired potency, hirsutism, and amenorrhea

angiotensin II antagonist substances, which compete at the angiotensin II receptor and thereby act to reduce blood pressure

Ca antagonist →*calcium antagonist*

calcium antagonist *Syn: Ca antagonist, calcium channel blocker, calcium-blocking agent*; pharmaceuticals that inhibit the slow transmembranous influx of calcium into cells and thereby decouple the electric excitation and muscle contraction; this reduces the vascular resistance in the arterial system that reduces the afterload; calcium channel blockers improve the relationship between oxygen delivery and consumption, reduce the heart rate and inhibit AV conduction; **usage**: antiarrhythmic, antihypertensive, prophylaxis and therapy of angina pectoris, left heart insufficiency, disturbances of peripheral perfusion, migraine, tocolytic; **side effects**: headache, bradycardic disturbances of rhythm, hypotension, leg edema; **contraindications**: AV-block, severe hypertension, recent myocardial infarction

GP-IIb/IIIa antagonists new class of inhibitor of thrombocyte aggregation, which binds selectively to the glycoprotein-IIb/IIIa receptor on the thrombocytes; they reduce thrombocyte aggregation and the binding of fibrin to the thrombocyte surface; **usage**: unstable angina pectoris, management of acute myocardial infarction, possibly together with percutaneous transluminal coronary angioplasty [PTCA]

antecedent one that precedes another
plasma thromboplastin antecedent → *factor XI*
antegrade → *anterograde*
anterograde *Syn: antegrade*; (directed/running) to the front or forwards
anteroseptal situated in front of a septum
antesystole premature excitation of regions of the heart musculature
anthemorrhagic → *hemostatic*
anti- combining form denoting relation to counteracting, effective against, opposing, or opposite
antiadrenergic *Syn: antisympathetic, sympathicolytic, sympatholytic, sympathoparalytic*; **1.** an agent with antiadrenergic properties **2.** exciting the sympathetic system, having a stimulatory action on the sympathetic system increasing the action of adrenaline; inhibiting the sympathetic system
antiallergic directed against allergy
antianaphylactic directed against anaphylaxis
antiapoplectic preventing apoplexy, alleviating the symptoms of apoplexy
antiarrhythmic 1. *Syn: antiarrhythmic agent, antiarrhythmic drug, antidysrhythmic*; pharmaceuticals active against disturbances of heart rhythm classified into four classes after Vaughan Williams: **1. class I antiarrhythmics** [also called sodium antagonists or membrane stabilizers]: consists of the subgroups **class IA or chinidine type** [chinidine, procainamide, disopyramide, prajmalium, propafenone], **class IB or lidocaine type** [lidocaine, tocainide, mexiletine, phenytoin], and **class IC** [flecainide, propafenone]; their main action is to prolong the action potential and the **indication** for use is therefore the treatment of ventricular and supraventricular extrasystoles; **2. class II antiarrhythmics**: contains beta-blockers [metoprolol, atenolol, sotalol, oxyprenolol, acebutolol]; their **indications** for use are sinus tachycardia, supraventricular paroxysmal tachycardia, ventricular and supraventricular arrhythmias; **3. class III antiarrhythmics**: comprise calcium antagonists and beta-blockers with class III action [amiodarone, sotalol]; **indications**: ventricular and supraventricular disturbances of rhythm refractory to therapy; **4. class IV antiarrhythmics**: calcium antagonists with antiarrhythmic action [verapamil, diltiazem]; **indication**: tachycardic disturbances of rhythm **2.** *Syn: antidysrhythmic*; with actions against arrhythmias, preventing arrhythmias
antiarteriosclerotic agent for the prevention of atherosclerosis

antiatherogenic prevention of the formation of atheroma

antibacterial 1. an agent with antibacterial properties **2.** (acting) against bacteria

antibiogram testing of the antibiotic resistance of bacteria or fungi

antibiosis mutual inhibition of growth or killing of micro-organisms by excretion of antibiotics; rarely also a description of antibiotic therapy

antibiotic 1. any substance with the ability to destroy microorganisms [bacteria, viruses, fungi] [**bactericidal effect**] or inhibit their growth [**bacteriostasis**]; originally these were substances synthesized by living cells [bacteria, fungi, algae, plants] and were effective even in a minimal concentration; two-thirds of the approximately 7000 isolated natural antibiotics are synthesized by Actinomyces species; nowadays, however, synthetic or semisynthetic antibiotics are being used for the most part; in addition to the classic penicillin antibiotics, the following groups are differentiated: aminoglycoside antibiotics, cephalosporins, chloramphenicols, lincosamides, polyene antibiotics, gyrase inhibitors, macrolide antibiotics, nucleoside antibiotics, polypeptide antibiotics, tetracyclines, quinolones, and individual unclassified substances **2.** destructive to life

aminoglycoside antibiotic *Syn: aminoglycoside*; antibiotic group consisting of glycosidically linked amino sugars, with a usually broad action spectrum; these antibiotics are bactericidal inhibitors of protein synthesis and include, for example, amikacin, gentamicin, kanamycin, neomycin, netilmicin, streptomycin, and tobramycin

beta-lactam antibiotics *Syn: β-lactam antibiotics*; antibiotics with a β-lactam ring in the molecule, e.g., penicillins and cephalosporins

β-lactam antibiotics → *beta-lactam antibiotics*

broad-spectrum antibiotics antibiotic active against a number of pathogens, e.g., tetracycline

macrolide antibiotic antibiotic produced by Streptomyces species or synthetically, which contains a macrolide core [12- to 18-membered amino sugar]; macrolide antibiotics can be given orally but have only a narrow action spectrum [primarily gonococci, streptococci, pneumococci, rickettsia, and chlamydia]

prophylactic antibiotics → *antibiotic prophylaxis*

quinolone antibiotics → *gyrase inhibitors*

antibiotic-induced caused or induced by treatment with an antibiotic

antibiotic-resistant not able to be killed or to have their growth arrested by antibiotics

antibody *Syn: immunoglobulin*; any of numerous proteins produced by the body in response to the presence of specific foreign antigens; they consist of two pairs of polypeptide chains, heavy chains and light chains, that are arranged in a Y-shape; the two tips of the Y are the regions that bind to antigens and deactivate them

blood-group antibody specific antibodies directed against the blood group antigens, which cause blood group incompatibility; used to determine the blood group

anticholinergic *Syn: parasympatholytic, parasympathoparalytic*; **1.** an agent with anticholinergic properties **2.** impairing the action of acetylcholine; impairing the parasympathetic system

anticoagulant 1. substance which inhibits clotting; **1.** in laboratory tests or *in vitro* substances are applied that make the blood sample or conserved blood unclottable; most commonly, heparin or heparinoids [no change of the pH value] or substances that bind Ca ions [citrate, oxalate, EDTA, fluoride] are used **2.** to inhibit intravascular clotting, e.g., postoperatively, heparin or heparinoids, vitamin K antagonists [coumarin], and inhibitors of thrombocyte aggregation are used **2.** *Syn: anticoagulative*; impairing blood clotting

anticoagulated displaced by anticoagulants

anticoagulative *Syn: anticoagulant*; impairing blood clotting

antidiuresis reduction in the formation of urine in the kidney by reduction of water excretion or increased water reabsorption; physiologic mechanism in response to inadequate water intake

antidiuretic 1. an agent with antidiuretic properties **2.** impairing the excretion of water/diuresis in the kidney

antidromic conducting in the opposite direction

antidysrhythmic → *antiarrhythmic*

antifibrillatory 1. an agent with action against atrial or ventricular fibrillation **2.** active against cardiac fibrillation

antifibrinolytic 1. an agent with antifibrinolytic properties **2.** impairing fibrinolysis

antifungal → *antimycotic*

antigen any substance that can stimulate the production of antibodies and combine specifically with them

blood-group antigens genetically-determined macromolecules localized on erythrocytes and other cells, which are specific to the individual blood groups

erythrocyte antigens multiple substances lying on the surface of the erythrocyte cell membrane that act as antigens, of which the blood-group antigens are the most important

factor VIII-associated antigen *Syn: factor VIII:vWF, von Willebrand factor*; oligomeric glycoprotein, which occurs subendothelially and in thrombocytes; facilitates the adhesion of thrombocytes to the damaged vessel wall and protects blood clotting factor VIII from premature proteolysis; severe deficiency therefore leads to factor VIII deficiency and disturbances of secondary hemostasis

platelet antigens antigens located on the thrombocyte surface against which antibodies may be formed

antigenic *Syn: immunogenic*; possessing antigenic properties; acting as an antigen

antihemolytic *Syn: preventing hemolysis*; active against hemolysis, preventing hemolysis

antihemophilic active against hemophilia, preventing hemophilia

antihemorrhagic *Syn: hemostatic*; **1.** an agent with antihemorrhagic properties **2.** stopping hemorrhage

antiheparin *Syn: platelet factor 4*; substance contained in the blood platelets [thrombocytes], which inhibits the action of heparin

antihypertensive 1. an agent with antihypertensive properties **2.** acting against high blood pressure

antihypotensive medication that counteracts low blood pressure, blood pressure-increasing agent

anti-infectious → *anti-infective*

anti-infective 1. an agent with anti-infective properties **2.** *Syn: anti-infectious*; acting against infection or infectious agents

anti-inflammatory 1. an agent with anti-inflammatory properties **2.** acting against inflammation

antilipemic 1. an agent acting against elevated blood lipid levels **2.** reducing the lipid level

antimicrobial *Syn: antimicrobic*; **1.** an agent with antimicrobial properties **2.** acting against micro-organisms

antimicrobic → *antimicrobial*

antimycotic *Syn: antifungal*; acting against yeasts/fungi

antiphlogistic 1. an agent with antiphlogistic properties **2.** acting against inflammation and fever

antipyretic 1. *Syn: antifebrile, antithermic, febricide, febrifuge, defervescent*; an agent with antiphlogistic properties **2.** *Syn: antifebrile, antithermic, febricide, febrifugal, defervescent*; acting against fever,

antirheumatic 1. an agent with antirheumatic properties **2.** acting against rheumatic diseases

antiseptic 1. antiseptic agent; disinfectant for the prevention or treatment of wound infections [sepsis] **2.** relating to or producing antisepsis

antisympathetic → *antiadrenergic*

antithrombin physiologic plasma constituents, which inactivate or inhibit thrombin and thereby control blood clotting

   antithrombin I → *fibrin*

   antithrombin II immediate anti-thrombin made of heparin cofactor and α-heparin; promotes the action of antithrombin III

   antithrombin III enzyme inhibitor made in the liver and the vessel endothelium, which inhibit various blood clotting factors [factor Xa, IXa, XIa, plasmin]

   antithrombin IV immediate anti-thrombin derived from prothrombin

   antithrombin V anti-thrombin in the γ-globulin fraction occurring in chronic inflammation

   antithrombin VI immediate anti-thrombin deriving from fibrin and fibrinogen

antithrombotic 1. an agent with antithrombotic properties **2.** preventing or inhibiting thrombosis or thrombus formation; also used in the sense of inhibiting coagulation

antiviral *Syn: antivirotic*; **1.** an agent with antiviral properties **2.** targeted at viruses, killing viruses [**virucidal**], or inhibiting growth [**virustatic**]

antivirotic → *antiviral*

antivitamin the action of a substance which nullifies a vitamin; mostly a structural analog substance without vitamin action; used therapeutically, e.g., as anticoagulants [**vitamin K antagonist**] or cytostatics [**folic acid antagonists**]

anuloplasty *Syn: annuloplasty*; plastic heart valve operation with tightening of the annulus fibrosus cordis

anydremia → *anhydremia*

aort- combining form denoting relation to the aorta

aorta the major blood vessel arising from the left ventricle; it begins posterior to the aortic valve with the **ascending aorta**, which gives rise to the coronary arteries [right and left coronary arteries] within the pericardium; three large arteries [left subclavian artery, common carotid artery, brachiocephalic trunk] for the head and the upper extremities arise from the aortic arch running obliquely to the left; the **descending aorta** begins behind the aortic isthmus and consists of the **thoracic aorta** and **abdominal aorta**

abdominal aorta *Syn: abdominal part of aorta, aorta abdominalis*; portion of the aorta lying below the diaphragm; from it arise, among others, paired branches to the abdominal wall [lumbar arteries], the kidneys [renal arteries], and the adrenal glands [medial suprarenal artery], as well as unpaired branches to supply the abdominal organs [celiac trunk, superior and inferior mesenteric arteries]; at the level of the 4. lumbar vertebra, the aorta divides into the right and left common iliac arteries

aorta abdominalis → *abdominal aorta*

ascending aorta *Syn: aorta ascendens; s.u. aorta*

descending aorta *Syn: aorta descendens; s.u. aorta*

thoracic aorta *Syn: thoracic part of aorta, aorta thoracica*; portion of the aorta between the aortic isthmus and diaphragm; it gives rise to paired branches to supply the chest organs [bronchial, esophageal, mediastinal, and pericardiac branches] and the chest wall [intercostal arteries, posterior intercostal arteries]

aorta thoracica → *thoracic aorta*

aortal → *aortic*

aortalgia pain in the aorta

aortarctia → *aortic stenosis*

aortartia → *aortic stenosis*

aortectomy partial excision of the aorta, e.g., for aortic aneurysm; the resected segment is replaced by a tubular prosthesis

aortic *Syn: aortal*; relating to the aorta

aorticopulmonary *Syn: aortopulmonary*; relating to or associated with the aorta and pulmonary artery/pulmonary trunk

aorticorenal *Syn: aortorenal*; relating to aorta and kidneys

aortitic relating to aortitis

aortitis inflammation of the aorta or aortic wall; generally as a result of the spread of inflammation from the endocardium or the aortic valve

Döhle-Heller aortitis → *luetic mesaortitis*

luetic aortitis → *luetic mesaortitis*

syphilitic aortitis → *luetic mesaortitis*

aorto- combining form denoting relation to aorta

aortoangiography X-ray contrast demonstration of the aorta and the arteries arising from it

aortocoronary relating to aorta and coronary arteries
aortogram X-ray contrast film of the aorta and its branches
aortographic relating to aortography
aortography X-ray contrast demonstration of the aorta and its branches
aortoptosia → *aortoptosis*
aortoptosis *Syn: aortoptosia*; a sinking down of the abdominal aorta
aortopulmonary → *aorticopulmonary*
aortorenal → *aorticorenal*
aortorrhaphy suture of the aorta after operative or traumatic opening or rupture
aortosclerosis arteriosclerosis leading to calcification, affecting the aorta; arteriosclerosis leading to calcification; can lead to aortic insufficiency or aortic dissection
aortosclerotic relating to or caused by aortosclerosis
aortostenosis → *subvalvular aortic stenosis*
aortotomy opening of the aorta
apalcillin acylaminopenicillin with a broad action spectrum against gram-positive and gram-negative pathogens
apex tip

  apex of heart the rounded apex formed by the left ventricle
apexcardiogram *Syn: apex cardiogram*; mechano-cardiogram recorded over the cardiac apex
apexcardiographic relating to apexcardiography
apexcardiography form of the mechano-cardiogram when recorded over the cardiac apex
aplasia lack of development

  thymic-parathyroid aplasia → *DiGeorge syndrome*
apnea *Syn: cessation of breathing, respiratory arrest*; respiratory arrest resulting from central or peripheral respiratory paralysis or caused by an obstruction of the airways [e.g., by a foreign body]; it is also used to describe a prolonged respiratory pause in hypocapnia
apneic relating to or caused by apnea
apneumatic air-free; with air excluded
apo- combining form denoting relation to separate or derivation from
apoplectic relating to apoplexy
apoplectiform *Syn: apoplectoid*; having the form of an attack of apoplexy; apoplectic; similar to apoplexy
apoplectoid → *apoplectiform*
apoplexia → *cerebrovascular accident*

apoplexy a sudden, usually marked loss of bodily function due to rupture or occlusion of a blood vessel

cerebral apoplexy → *cerebrovascular accident*

thrombotic apoplexy apoplectic insult caused by thrombosis of a cerebral blood vessel in the brain

apparatus a group or combination organs having a particular function

Abbé-Zeiss apparatus → *Thoma-Zeiss counting cell*

respiratory apparatus → *respiratory tract*

apparent visible, manifest; evident, clear

approximal *Syn: approximate*; approaching, approximately

approximate → *approximal*

aprindine anti-arrhythmic; **usage**: long-term treatment of disturbances of ventricular rhythm

aprotinin inhibitor of protease and fibrinolysis, which inhibits various components of the clotting cascade

apyetous → *apyous*

apyogenous not caused by pus

apyous *Syn: apyetous*; non-purulent, without pus

apyretic → *afebrile*

apyrexial → *afebrile*

apyrogenic not provoking fever

arachnodactylia → *Marfan's disease*

arachnodactyly → *Marfan's disease*

congenital contractural arachnodactyly *Syn: Beals' syndrome*; autosomal dominant malformation syndrome with Marfanoid body habitus, arachnodactyly with contractures, kyphoscoliosis, mitral valve prolapse, and malformation of the helix of the ear ["crumpled ears"]

arch a curved structure

aortic arch *Syn: arcus aortae*; arch situated between the ascending and descending aorta, gives rise to the brachiocephalic trunk and the left common carotid and left subclavian arteries

double aortic arch congenital malformation in which the ascending aorta anterior to the trachea divides into a right and left aortic arch, which pass by the aorta on both sides; clinical symptoms [stridor, dyspnea, barking cough] develop even in early infancy due to compression of the trachea; **diagnosis**: esophagogram, angiocardiography; **therapy**: resection of the smaller arch [usually the left]

right aortic arch malformation in which the aortic arch passes by the trachea on the right and descends to the right of the spinal column;

it usually remains clinically asymptomatic; **diagnosis**: esophagogram, angiocardiography, echocardiography; **therapy**: requires treatment only in rare cases

Salus' arch *Syn: Salus sign; s.u. arteriosclerotic retinopathy*

arcus arch, curve, vault

arcus aortae → *aortic arch*

arcus venosus venous arch

arginine *Syn: 2-amino-5-guanidinovaleric acid*; amino acid

arginine vasopressin *Syn: argipressin*; hormone made in the posterior lobe of the pituitary gland with vasoconstrictor action

argipressin → *arginine vasopressin*

arhythmia → *arrhythmia*

arrest standstill, stoppage

cardiac arrest *Syn: asystole, asystolia, Beau's syndrome, cardiac standstill, heart arrest, cardioplegia*; cardiovascular standstill caused by cessation of the heart muscle contraction; may be a temporary phenomenon in neurocardiogenic syncope in 1/3 of the patients; leads to the so-called flat line ECG, which is a sign of cardiac death; without immediate resuscitation, the outcome is fatal

cardiovascular arrest *Syn: circulatory arrest*; condition in which no blood circulation occurs; it can be caused by cardiac arrest [asystole] but also by ventricular fibrillation; it leads to loss of consciousness, respiratory arrest, tissue hypoxia, cyanosis, pupillary rigidity, areflexia, and brain death; **therapy**: cardiopulmonary resuscitation

circulatory arrest → *cardiovascular arrest*

heart arrest → *cardiac arrest*

reflexogenic cardiac arrest death caused by a reflex, e.g., following a blow to the carotid sinus

respiratory arrest → *apnea*

sinus arrest *Syn: sinus standstill*; cardiac standstill due to the cessation of the initiation of excitation in the sinoatrial node

arrhythmia *Syn: arhythmia, irregularity of pulse*; disturbance to the normal heart rhythm or normal rhythm formation and conduction of excitation; depending upon the site of the disturbance, **ventricular arrhythmias** [in the ventricle or arising from the ventricle, e.g., ventricular fibrillation] and **supraventricular arrhythmias** [e.g., AV-node tachycardia] can be differentiated; arrhythmias are a common associated feature and complication of myocardial infarcts; depending upon the time they develop, **early** [< 30 min after the onset of ischemia] and

late arrhythmias can be differentiated, whereby the earlier arrhythmias are responsible for the high mortality of infarcts [30%] before reaching hospital; the manifestation depends upon the extent of the infarct, the presence of collaterals and the autonomic activity; particularly in the border zone between ischemic and healthy tissues, polymorphic ventricular tachycardias may result in ventricular fibrillation; following reperfusion, dangerous arrhythmias may also arise; they result from leaching out of acidic metabolites [e.g., lactate], which had formed in the myocytes during the ischemia

continuous arrhythmia *Syn: perpetual arrhythmia*; arrhythmia of the heartbeat without recognizable fundamental frequency; mostly occurs in atrial fibrillation, which causes beat-to-beat variation in the diastolic filling of the ventricle; the ventricle can beat slowly [**bradyarrhythmia**] or quickly [**tachyarrhythmia**]

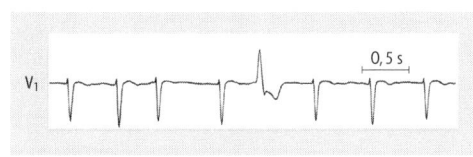

Continuous arrhythmia. Atrial fibrillation in V_1

perpetual arrhythmia → *continuous arrhythmia*
sinus arrhythmia arrhythmia arising in the sinoatrial node; physiologic as **respiratory arrhythmia**, pathologic in, for example, sinoatrial node syndrome or mitral valve prolapse syndrome
arrhythmic *Syn: rhythmless*; without rhythm
arrhythmogenic causing or promoting arrhythmia
arrhythmokinesis formation/development of disturbances of the heart rhythm
arterectomy → *arteriectomy*
arterenol → *noradrenalin*
arteri- combining form denoting relation to an artery or arteries
arteria → *artery*
  arteria axillaris → *axillary artery*
  arteria basilaris → *basilar artery*
  arteria brachialis → *brachial artery*
  arteriae bronchiales → *bronchial arteries*

arterial

arteria carotis communis → *common carotid artery*
arteria carotis externa → *external carotid artery*
arteria carotis interna → *internal carotid artery*
arteria coronaria → *coronary artery*
arteria coronaria dextra → *right coronary artery of heart*
arteria coronaria sinistra → *left coronary artery of heart*
arteria femoralis → *femoral artery*
arteria pulmonalis dextra *Syn:* *right pulmonary artery*; artery arising from the pulmonary trunk to the right lung
arteria pulmonalis sinistra *Syn:* *left pulmonary artery*; artery arising from the pulmonary trunk to the left lung
arteria radialis → *radial artery*
arteria renalis → *renal artery*
arteria splenica → *splenic artery*
arteria subclavia → *subclavian artery*
arteria ulnaris → *ulnar artery*
arteria vertebralis → *vertebral artery*
arterial *Syn:* *arterious*; relating to arteries
arterialization 1. s.u. Ebstein's anomaly **2.** → *vascularization*
arteriectasia → *arteriectasis*
arteriectasis *Syn:* arterial ectasia, arteriectasia; diffuse dilatation of an artery
arteriectomy *Syn:* *arterectomy*; operative (partial) excision of an artery
arterio- combining form denoting relation to an artery or arteries
arteriocapillary relating to or associated with arteries and capillaries
arteriogenesis the formation of arteries during the embryonic period, or as new vessel formation
arteriogram X-ray contrast image of arteries and their branches
arteriographic relating to arteriography
arteriography X-ray contrast demonstration of arteries and their branches

catheter arteriography arteriography with contrast agent injection via a catheter

occlusion arteriography rarely used procedure in which an artery is occluded with a balloon catheter or similar, so that contrast agent is concentrated in front of the site of occlusion

pulmonary arteriography → *pulmonary angiography*

selective arteriography demonstration of a specific artery or the territory it supplies using a catheter to selectively inject contrast agent

arteriola → *arteriole*

arteriolar relating to arterioles

arteriole *Syn: arteriola, precapillary artery*; small arteries; arterioles have the same wall structure as muscular arteries, although they are substantially weaker; lying at the end of the arterial tree, it is the job of the arterioles to regulate the perfusion of downstream capillaries and the blood pressure; narrowing of the arterioles leads to increased resistance in the circulation [which is why they are also known as **resistance vessels**]; relaxation of the arterioles, e.g., in allergic reactions, leads to a fall in the blood pressure, because large amounts of blood flow into the capillaries and veins

  silver-wire arterioles *Syn: silver-wire reflexes, silver-wire vessels*; narrowed, thread-like retinal arteries in hypertensive retinopathy

arteriolitic relating to or caused by arteriolitis

arteriolitis inflammation of the arterioles

  necrotizing arteriolitis → *arteriolonecrosis*

arteriology study of the structure and diseases of the arteries

arteriolonecrosis *Syn: arteriolar necrosis, necrotizing arteriolitis*; inflammation leading to necrosis of the arteriolar wall; arteriolonecrosis of the meninges and brain can mimic pneumococcal meningitis

arteriolonecrotic relating to or caused by arteriolonecrosis

arteriolosclerosis *Syn: arteriolar sclerosis*; damage to the arteriolar wall with fibrotic change and sclerosis; usually part of a generalized arteriosclerosis; leads to the pattern of red granular atrophy in the kidney

arteriolosclerotic relating to arteriolosclerosis

arteriomyomatosis hyperplasia or hypertrophy of the arterial musculature leading to thickening of the wall

arterionecrosis necrosis of the arterial wall

arterionecrotic relating to or caused by arterionecrosis

arterionephrosclerosis *Syn: arterial nephrosclerosis, senile nephrosclerosis*; age-related, slowly progressive sclerosis of the renal blood vessels

arteriopathy (non-inflammatory) arterial disease

  hypertensive arteriopathy arteriopathy caused by arterial hypertension

  plexogenic pulmonary arteriopathy → *Ayerza's syndrome*

arteriorenal relating to arteries and kidney(s)

arteriorrhaphy suture of an artery after its operative or traumatic opening

arteriorrhexis rupture of an artery; tearing of an artery

arteriosclerosis most common systemic arterial disease with fibrous changes in the intima and media, which lead to hardening, thickening, loss of elasticity, and narrowing of the lumen; the most important risk factors are high blood pressure, nicotine abuse, obesity, lack of exercise, metabolic disorders [diabetes mellitus, hyperlipoproteinemia]; the connection between arteriosclerosis [predominantly of the coronary vessels] and primary and secondary disturbances of fat metabolism is of great clinical importance; all disorders that lead to elevation of the LDL-cholesterol level also lead to an exponential increase in coronary heart diseases and myocardial infarcts; hypertension, smoking and diabetes mellitus lead to a further increase in the risk; HDL deficiency is also a significant risk factor, whereas elevated HDL levels are protective

cerebral arteriosclerosis arteriosclerosis affecting the brain arteries predominantly; leads to dizziness, impaired (mental) performance, and possibly dementia; associated with an increased risk of stroke

coronary arteriosclerosis *Syn: coronary artery sclerosis, coronary sclerosis*; arteriosclerosis of the coronary vessels; the most common cause of coronary stenosis

hyaline arteriosclerosis arteriosclerosis with hyaline thickening of the vessel wall

hyperplastic arteriosclerosis arteriosclerosis with hyperplasia of the artery wall

hypertensive arteriosclerosis arteriosclerosis in the setting of high blood pressure

infantile arteriosclerosis rare form of arteriosclerosis, which is already apparent in childhood, in the setting of metabolic diseases [disorders of lipid metabolism]

intimal arteriosclerosis arteriosclerosis affecting the intima primarily

Mönckeberg's arteriosclerosis → *Mönckeberg's sclerosis*

nodose arteriosclerosis → *nodular arteriosclerosis*

nodular arteriosclerosis *Syn: nodose arteriosclerosis*; arteriosclerosis with atherosclerotic plaques in the vessel wall

presenile arteriosclerosis premature, usually unexplained, arteriosclerosis

senile arteriosclerosis age-related arteriosclerosis; favored by the risk factors mentioned

arteriosclerotic relating to or caused by arteriosclerosis

arteriospasm *Syn: spasm of an artery*; spastic narrowing of the arteries

arteritis

during direct stimulation or vasomotor influences, e.g., in Raynaud's phenomenon

arteriospastic pertaining to or causing arterial spasm

arteriostenosis *Syn: hemadostenosis*; luminal narrowing of an artery; can in extreme cases lead to occlusion of the artery; the most common cause is arteriosclerosis

arteriotomy operative opening of arteries

arteriotony → *blood pressure*

arterious → *arterial*

arteriovenous relating to or associated with an artery or arteries and vein(s)

arteritic relating to or caused by arteritis

arteritis inflammation of an artery or its wall; can affect the entire wall, or just parts of it

brachiocephalic arteritis *Syn: Martorell's syndrome, pulseless disease, reversed coarctation, Takayasu's arteritis, Takayasu's syndrome, Takayasu's disease*; inflammation of the brachiocephalic trunk where it arises from the aorta; the disease affects mainly women under 40 years of age and leads to fever, weight loss, night sweats, joint pains, fatigue, and stenosis of the aortic branches, which leads to its description as the pulseless disease; the most commonly affected are the subclavian artery [90%], common carotid [45%], vertebral [25%]; **therapy**: corticosteroids, cyclophosphamide, anticoagulants, possibly surgical intervention [endarterectomy]

coronary arteritis → *coronaritis*

cranial arteritis → *Horton's arteritis*

giant-cell arteritis → *Horton's arteritis*

granulomatous arteritis → *Horton's arteritis*

Horton's arteritis *Syn: cranial arteritis, giant-cell arteritis, granulomatous arteritis, Horton's disease, temporal arteritis, Horton's syndrome*; subacute granulomatous inflammation affecting predominantly older patients, which involves mainly the large and medium-sized arteries, particularly the carotid arteries; the etiology is unclear; there is, however, an association with viral infections or immunization that suggests an autoimmune process; about half of patients also suffer from polymyalgia rheumatica; **clinical**: giant cell arteritis has three stages: the **prodromal stage** lasts weeks to months and is characterized by non-specific general symptoms [low grade fever, fatigue, weight loss] and gradually increasing and persistent headaches; when the **acute stage** begins, there is sudden worsening of the headaches; the arteries in the temple [**superficial temporal arteries**] become visible and palpable; they are tender and pulseless; in more than 50% of cases, other cranial arteries are also affected and involvement of the eyes can lead to bilateral transient impairment of vision or indeed permanent blindness; the muscles of mastication are painful when chewing or swallowing [**masseteric claudication**]; more rarely there may also be damage to the organs of hearing and balance, tongue necrosis, subarachnoid hemorrhage, and psychosis; most of the symptoms resolve spontaneously after some months and the **chronic stage** begins with painless, pulseless, thread-like temporal arteries; **diagnosis**: biopsy of the superficial temporal artery; **therapy**: corticosteroids; lifelong therapy may be required

localized visceral arteritis → *allergic vasculitis*

arteritis nodosa → *Kussmaul's disease*

rheumatic arteritis inflammation mostly of small arteries and arterioles in the setting of rheumatic fever

Takayasu's arteritis → *brachiocephalic arteritis*

temporal arteritis → *Horton's arteritis*

artery *Syn: arteria*; vessel that conveys blood away from the heart; in the systemic circulation, the arteries carry oxygenated blood and in the pulmonary circulation deoxygenated blood; arteries have three wall layers: an **inner coat** [**tunica intima**], a **middle coat** [**tunica media**], and an **outer coat** [**tunica adventitia**]; the tunica intima, which consists of vascular endothelium and subendothelial connective tissue, controls the exchange of substances and gas between the blood and vessel wall and forms various humoral factors [e.g., nitrogen monoxide]; the **tunica media** has the function of elastically absorbing the vessel wall ring and longitudinal tension caused by the blood pressure and pulse wave and regulating the vessel diameter; it is the thickest of the wall layers and consists, for instance, of elastic fibers, smooth muscle cells, and collagen fibers; the outermost wall layer, the **tunica adventitia**, consists primarily of elastic fibers and collagen fibers; it can absorb external longitudinal stress forces; **elastic arteries** and **muscular arteries** differ in the thickness of the different wall layers; the smaller arteries are supplied with nutrients by diffusion from the vessel lumen, whereas larger vessels have their own supply vessels [**vasa vasorum**]; fibers of the autonomic nervous system innervate the vascular smooth muscles

anastomotic atrial artery *Syn: ramus atrialis anastomoticus arteriae* *coronariae sinistrae; s.u. left coronary artery of heart*

anterior interventricular artery branch of the left coronary artery in the anterior interventricular septum

anterior mediastinal arteries → *rami mediastinales arteriae thoracicae internae*

atrioventricular nodal artery 1. → *atrioventricular nodal branch of left coronary artery* **2.** → *atrioventricular nodal branch of right coronary artery*

axillary artery continuation of the subclavian artery between the lower surface of the clavicle and the lower surface of the pectoralis major muscle; gives branches to the shoulder, chest wall, and upper arm musculature, before it becomes the brachial artery

basal artery → *basilar artery*

basilar artery *Syn: basal artery, basilar trunk*; basal artery of the brain stem; arises at the junction of the right and left vertebral arteries at the lower border of the pons

brachial artery continuation of the axillary artery; runs in the medial bicipital groove to the elbow, where it divides into the ulnar and radial arteries; distal hemorrhage can be eliminated by pressure over the humerus; its branches supply bone and muscle of the upper arm and elbow

brachiocephalic artery → *brachiocephalic trunk*

bronchial arteries *Syn: rami bronchiales aortae thoracicae, arteriae bronchiales*; bronchial branches of the thoracic aorta

cephalic artery → *common carotid artery*

common carotid artery *Syn: cephalic artery, common carotid*; vessel root of the external and internal carotid arteries; arises on the right from the brachiocephalic trunk and on the left from the aortic arch; runs behind the sternocleidomastoid muscle to the carotid trigone, where it divides at the level of the upper border of the 5. cervical vertebra into the external and internal carotid arteries; at the bifurcation point, it widens to form the carotid sinus; on the posterior wall of the bifurcation point lies the carotid body [**glomus caroticum**]

copper wire arteries typical, engorged, and tortuous retinal artery in hypertensive retinopathy

coronary artery *Syn: coronaria, coronary, coronary artery of heart*; artery supplying the heart muscle; the coronary arteries arise in the vicinity of the right or left aortic valve cusps in the aortic sinuses; variations from the normal pattern of supply are named the **left type** [pre-

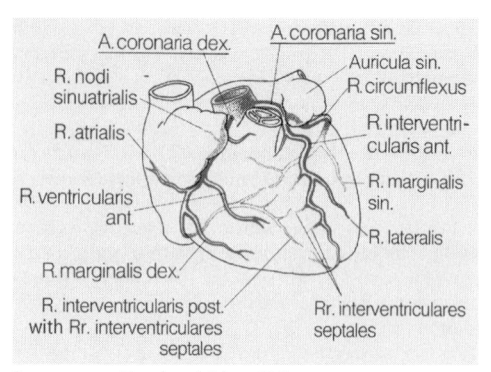

Coronary artery. Branches of right and left coronary artery

dominance of the left coronary artery] or **right type** [predominance of the right coronary artery]

coronary artery of heart →*coronary artery*

crural artery →*femoral artery*

elastic artery →*artery of elastic type*

artery of elastic type *Syn: elastic artery, elastic vessel;* the large vessels near the heart [aorta, common carotid artery, subclavian artery, pulmonary artery, pulmonary trunk] have a histologic structure, which allows them to tolerate the large pressure variations between systole and diastole [damper function]; the **intima** is relatively thick and contains, among other things, elastic fibers and collagen fibers; the **intima** is not sharply demarcated from the intima and adventitia and contains a multitude of concentrically arranged elastic fibers, which are tangled together; the **adventitia** contains nerve fibers and vasa vasorum

emulgent artery →*renal artery*

end arteries *Syn: end-arteries;* terminal branches of an artery, which do not communicate with other arteries

external carotid artery *Syn: external carotid;* arises in the carotid trigone from the common carotid artery; supplies the majority of the skull, the scalp, and scalp muscles, as well as the dura mater; runs on the stylopharyngeus muscle and under the anterior digastric muscle belly and the stylohyoid muscle to the retromolar fossa; after piercing the parotid gland it divides at the level of the angle of the mandible into its terminal branches, the maxillary artery and the superficial temporal artery; its other branches are the superior thyroid artery, lingual artery, facial artery, ascending pharyngeal artery, occipital artery, posterior auricular artery

femoral artery *Syn: crural artery*; continuation of the external iliac artery; runs beneath the inguinal ligament medial to the hip joint to the iliopectineal fossa; it enters the adductor canal behind the sartorius muscle and reaches the popliteal fossa through the adductor hiatus, where it becomes the popliteal artery; supplies the leg, hip, genital region, and deep layers of the gluteal region

gooseneck lamp arteries *Syn: trachea-like arteries*; *s.u. Mönckeberg's sclerosis*

innominate artery → *brachiocephalic trunk*

internal carotid artery *Syn: internal carotid*; arises in the carotid trigone from the common carotid artery; supplies the majority of the brain, the orbits, and the mucous membranes of the ethmoidal, frontal and paranasal sinuses; it has four segments: **pars cervicalis** from the origin to the skull base, **pars petrosa** in the carotid canal of the temporal bone, **pars cavernosa** in the carotid sulcus and cavernous sinus, and **pars cerebralis** up to the division into its terminal arteries the anterior cerebral artery and the middle cerebral artery; additional branches include the ophthalmic artery, superior hypophyseal artery, anterior choroid artery, and posterior communicating artery to the circle of Willis

left conal artery → *conus branch of left coronary artery*

left coronary artery of heart arises in the left aortic sinus above the aortic valve and runs forwards between the left auricle and the pulmonary trunk; divides into the **circumflex branch** and the **anterior interventricular branch**; the **circumflex branch** runs in the left coronary sulcus to the diaphragmatic surface [facies diaphragmatica]; through its branches [**atrial anastomotic branch, atrioventricular branches, left marginal branch, intermediate atrial branch**], it supplies parts of the left ventricle, the atrium, and the ventricular septum; the **anterior interventricular branch** runs in the anterior interventricular sulcus to the heart apex; its branches [**conus arteriosus branch, lateral branch, septal interventricular branches**] supply parts of the ventricular septum and the left ventricle

left marginal artery *Syn: ramus marginalis sinister*; *s.u. left coronary*

artery of heart
left pulmonary artery → *arteria pulmonalis sinistra*
lienal artery → *splenic artery*
muscular artery → *artery of muscular type*
artery of muscular type *Syn: muscular artery*; medium sized and small arteries in the systemic circulation show the typical structure of a muscular artery; the **intima** is relatively flat and is clearly separated from the media by an **internal elastic lamina** containing elastin fibers; the **media** consists almost exclusively of circular and spirally arranged smooth muscle fibers; it is separated by the **external elastic lamina** from the adventitia
nodal artery 1. → *sinoatrial nodal branch of left coronary artery* **2.** → *sinoatrial nodal branch of right coronary artery*
posterior interventricular artery branch of the right coronary artery in the posterior interventricular septum
posterior pericardiac arteries → *pericardiac branches of thoracic aorta*
precapillary artery → *arteriole*
pulmonary arteries arteries to the right lung [arteria pulmonalis dextra] and left lung [arteria pulmonalis sinistra] originating from the pulmonary trunk
radial artery arises from the brachial artery under the bicipital aponeurosis in the concavity of the elbow; crosses the pronator teres muscle and passes inferiorly in the channel for the radial vessels and nerve between the flexor carpi radialis muscle and the brachioradialis muscle; at the lower end of the radius, it lies so superficial that the pulse can be felt [**radial pulse**]; reaches the palm under the tendon of the extensor pollicis longus muscle, where it passes into the deep palmar space; supplies the forearm muscles on the radial side, thenar eminence, back of the hand and fingers
renal artery *Syn: emulgent artery*; substantial branch of the abdominal aorta, which divides into one anterior [**ramus anterior**] and posterior branch [**ramus posterior**] to the anterior and posterior parts of the kidneys before it reaches the renal hilum; in the kidney, each ramus further divides into 4–5 branches, which enter the renal parenchyma and become the interlobar arteries; the renal artery also gives branches to the renal capsule, the adrenal gland, and the ureter
right conal artery → *conus branch of right coronary artery*
right coronary artery of heart arises in the right aortic sinus and runs in the right coronary sulcus under the right auricle to the diaphrag-

matic surface [facies diaphragmatica]; its terminal branch [**posterior interventricular branch**] runs in the posterior interventricular sulcus to the cardiac apex; its branches [**conus arteriosus branch, sinoatrial node branch, atrial branches, atrioventricular branches, right marginal branch, intermediate atrial branch, septal interventricular branches**] supply the right atrium, the right ventricle, and parts of the ventricular septum and the left ventricle

right marginal artery *Syn: ramus marginalis dexter; s.u. right coronary artery of heart*

right pulmonary artery → *arteria pulmonalis dextra*

sinoatrial nodal artery 1. → *sinoatrial nodal branch of left coronary artery* **2.** → *sinoatrial nodal branch of right coronary artery*

sinuatrial nodal artery 1. → *sinoatrial nodal branch of left coronary artery* **2.** → *sinoatrial nodal branch of right coronary artery*

sinus node artery 1. → *sinoatrial nodal branch of left coronary artery* **2.** → *sinoatrial nodal branch of right coronary artery*

splenic artery *Syn: lienal artery*; substantial left branch of the celiac trunk; gives rise to multiple branches to the stomach and pancreas in its course along the upper border of the pancreas before dividing into multiple **rami splenici** in the splenic hilum

subclavian artery arterial branch arising from the brachiocephalic trunk on the right and the aortic arch on the left; passes through the posterior scalenus opening to the neck and onwards in the groove for the subclavian artery on the first rib; at the end of the groove, it becomes the axillary artery; the subclavian artery is involved in the supply to the chest wall, shoulder girdle, muscles of the back of the neck, neck, spinal cord, and parts of the brain

third conus artery → *conus branch of right coronary artery*

trachea-like arteries *Syn: gooseneck lamp arteries; s.u. Mönckeberg's sclerosis*

ulnar artery arises in the concavity of the elbow from the brachial artery; runs under the flexor carpi ulnaris muscle to the wrist, where the pulse can be felt near the tendon of the flexor carpi ulnaris muscle; passes under the palmar aponeurosis into the superficial palmar space; supplies the elbow joint, the superficial flexors on the ulnar side, skin on the ulnar side, hypothenar eminence and fingers

vertebral artery branch of the subclavian artery; subdivided into the **vertebral part** [before it enters the foramen transversarium of the 6. cervical vertebra], **cervical part** or **pars transversaria** [in the fo-

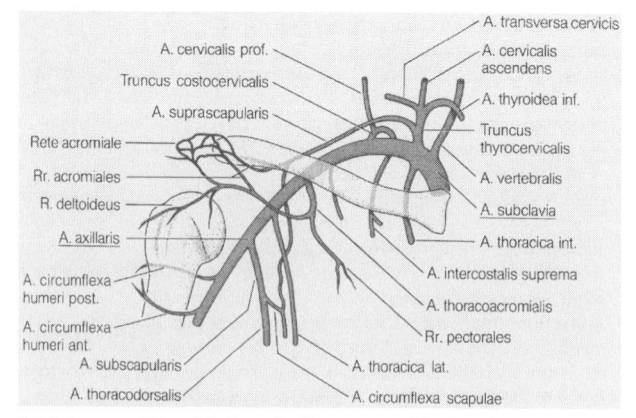

Subclavian artery. Right subclavian and axillary arteries and their branches

ramina transversaria of the cervical vertebrae], **pars atlantica** [on the posterior arch of the atlas] and **pars intracranialis** within the skull; through its branches, it supplies the neck muscles, spinal canal, spinal cord, dura mater, and parts of the cerebellum

arthritis *Syn: articular rheumatism*; inflammation of one or more joints; the inflammation can run an acute or chronic course, and may be caused by pathogens [bacteria, viruses], foreign bodies [including gouty crystals] or (auto-)immune processes; in chronic joint inflammation, which not only affects the synovial membrane but also the bone and cartilage, its distinction from arthrosis is not always easy

acute rheumatic arthritis → *rheumatic fever*

hemophilic arthritis → *bleeder's joint*

arthropathy *Syn: arthropathia, arthronosus, joint disease*; any disease or disorder of a joint

hemophilic arthropathy → *bleeder's joint*

artificial *Syn: factitious, synthetic*; not natural

ascending increasing, climbing

ascites *Syn: abdominal dropsy, hydroperitoneum, hydroperitonia*; collection of fluid in the peritoneal cavity; depending upon the cause the collection may be **inflammatory ascites** [an exudate], **non-inflam-**

matory ascites [a transudate], **chylous ascites** [lymph fluid], or **hemorrhagic ascites** [with the admixture of blood]; the most common causes are elevated capillary permeability [hypoxic, inflammatory, toxic in liver insufficiency], increased portal venous pressure [liver cirrhosis, portal vein thrombosis], reduced colloid osmotic pressure [albumin deficiency, above all in liver insufficiency or malnourishment], increased water and electrolyte retention [particularly in liver cirrhosis]; **therapy**: the treatment of the cause is the mainstay; if this is not possible, e.g., in the most common form, the **hepatic ascites** of liver cirrhosis, then the first attempt is to increase water excretion with diuretics; if the ascites is refractory to this therapy, then repeated aspiration of ascites can be considered; on occasion, it may be necessary to create a peritoneovenous shunt or transjugular intrahepatic shunt [TIPS] to drain it

ascitic relating to ascites

aseptic without the involvement of pathogens; free from infection; sterile

aspartate aminotransferase *Syn: aspartate transaminase, glutamic-oxaloacetic transaminase, serum glutamic oxaloacetic transaminase*; an aminotransferase occurring in liver, brain, and heart muscle, among others, which catalyzes the conversion of L-aspartate into oxaloacetic acid; important for the diagnosis and clinical monitoring of liver and muscle diseases, as well as of myocardial infarcts

aspartate transaminase → *aspartate aminotransferase*

asphyctic *Syn: asphyxial*; relating to or caused by asphyxia

asphygmia temporary absence of pulse; it is often wrongly equated with asphyxia

asphyxia respiratory depression or respiratory arrest [apnea] with a weak or absent pulse [asphygmia], caused by a disruption of breathing or cardiovascular function; it leads to hypoxia, hypercapnia, cyanosis, and loss of consciousness; outcome is fatal without cardiopulmonary resuscitation

asphyxial → *asphyctic*

aspirin → *acetylsalicylic acid*

assay test, analysis

direct hemagglutination-inhibition assay antibodies present in serum neutralize antigens [e.g., viral antigen], which would lead to hemagglutination; the absence of hemagglutination demonstrates the presence of specific antibodies in the test serum and can thereby provide indirect evidence of a current or previous infection

hemagglutination-inhibition assay *Syn: hemagglutination-inhibition reaction, hemagglutination-inhibition test*; serologic test to demonstrate antibodies or antigens, which are responsible for blocking hemagglutination that would normally occur

indirect hemagglutination-inhibition assay *Syn: passive hemagglutination-inhibition assay, passive hemagglutination-inhibition test*; a test serum is mixed with a specific antiserum; the antibodies in the antiserum neutralize the antigens in the test serum and thereby inhibit the agglutination of added erythrocytes

latex agglutination assay → *latex agglutination test*

latex fixation assay → *latex agglutination test*

passive hemagglutination-inhibition assay → *indirect hemagglutination-inhibition assay*

plasma renin assay → *plasma renin activity*

assisted supported, with the help of

asthenia *Syn: adynamia, lack of energy*; (general) weakness, lack of energy, frailty; inability to provide physical or mental effort; term only used sporadically nowadays

neurocirculatory asthenia *Syn: cardiophrenia, DaCosta's syndrome, disordered action of the heart, effort syndrome, irritable heart, functional cardiovascular disease, phrenocardia, soldier's heart*; symptom complex of hyperventilation, tachycardia, chest pain, and a feeling of tightness unrelated to stress, which occurs mostly in younger men; in addition to psychosomatic components, overexcitability of the respiratory centers is also being discussed as a possible cause

asthma *Syn: suffocative catarrh*; episodic dyspnea; it is usually equated with bronchial asthma

cardiac asthma *Syn: Rostan's asthma, cardial asthma, cardiasthma*; dyspnea usually occurring at night due to pulmonary congestion in left ventricular failure; in the extreme case, it can lead to heart-related acute pulmonary edema; differentiation from bronchial asthma is often difficult, because both diseases cause a similar symptomatology [extreme dyspnea, bronchospasm, paradoxical pulse, upright sitting position with arm support, diffuse rhonchi, etc.]

cardial asthma → *cardiac asthma*

Elsners asthma → *angina pectoris*

Heberden's asthma → *angina pectoris*

Rostan's asthma → *cardiac asthma*

asthmatic relating to asthma, short of breath

asthmatiform asthma-like, resembling asthma, with asthma symptoms

asthmogenic causing or inducing asthma

astringent *Syn: staltic*; hemostatic agent that acts by precipitating proteins, e.g., formaldehyde, tanning agents, metal salts

asynchronous not simultaneous, not synchronous

asystole *Syn: asystolia, Beau's syndrome, cardiac standstill*; cardiovascular standstill caused by cessation of the heart muscle contraction; may be a temporary phenomenon in neurocardiogenic syncope in 1/3 of patients; leads to the so-called flat line ECG, which is a sign of cardiac death; without immediate resuscitation, the outcome is fatal; in ventricular fibrillation, the totally uncoordinated electric activity of the heart leads to so-called **hyperdynamic cardiac arrest**

asystolia → *asystole*

asystolic relating to asystole

atelocardia incomplete development of the heart

atenolol cardioselective beta-blocker; **usage**: coronary heart disease, tachycardic disturbances of rhythm, arterial hypertension, angina pectoris, functional chest pains; **side effects**: fatigue, worsening of cardiac insufficiency, AV-block, disturbances of peripheral perfusion, bradycardia, bronchoconstriction

atherectomy operative cleaning of the arterial wall to remove atheromatous changes

athermic → *afebrile*

atheroembolism *Syn: cholesterol embolism*; embolism caused by an arterial thrombo-embolic event

atheroembolus *Syn: cholesterol embolus*; embolus formed by dislodgement of atheromatous material

atherogenic promoting the formation of atherosclerosis, leading to the formation of atheroma

atheroma plaques of atherosclerotic change occurring in the vessel wall

atheromatosis *Syn: atherosis*; description of the degenerative changes in the arterial intima in atherosclerosis

atheromatous relating to atheroma

atherosclerosis *Syn: arterial lipoidosis, atherosis, nodular sclerosis*; the changes in the vessel wall which underpin arteriosclerosis; chronic injury of the endothelium leads to the penetration of lipid-poor and fibrin-rich fluid into the intima and the formation of the initial intimal edema; local or migrated phagocytes take up the deposited lipids and cholesterol and change into foamy cells, which as a group form

lipid spots or **fatty streaks**; these changes are already found in a small percentage of 10–14 year olds; microthrombi form on the endothelial defect; the platelet factors that this releases lead to an increase in the permeability of the endothelium and worse insudation and swelling; myofibroblasts proliferate, phagocytose the insudated lipids and cholesterol and partially die as a result; the consequence of this is fibrous plaques with cholesterol crystals in the intima; the cell necrosis and the cholesterol crystals are covered with an intimal plate made of collagen and elastic fibers; together these form **atheroma**; if this breaks through to the inside and forms an ulcer in the vessel wall, it is described as an **atheromatous plaque**; it can calcify or ossify [arterial calcification], but can also be the point of origin of emboli, thromboses, ulcers, stenoses, and aneurysms; the **risk factors** for atherosclerosis include age, gender, hypertension, diabetes mellitus, adiposity, hyperlipidemia, smoking, and lack of exercise

atherosclerotic relating to or caused by atherosclerosis

atherosis 1. →*atheromatosis* **2.** →*atherosclerosis*

atonic without tone/tension, flaccid; feeble

atopic →*ectopic*

ATPase *Syn: adenosine triphosphatase*; enzyme that catalyzes the hydrolysis of ATP to ADP, releasing energy that is used in the cell

  sodium-potassium-ATPase →Na^+-K^+-*ATPase*

atransferrinemia congenital [autosomal dominant] or acquired deficiency of transferrin; leads to iron deficiency anemia and siderosis of internal organs [liver, spleen, pancreas, kidney, heart muscle]

atresia congenital absence or closure of an opening

  pulmonary atresia congenital absence of the pulmonary valve – i.e., the right ventricle has no connection to the pulmonary artery; there are two types: **pulmonary atresia with ventricular septal defect** and **pulmonary atresia without ventricular septal defect**; pulmonary atresia with ventricular septal defect [2–3% of all congenital heart defects] is generally regarded as an extreme variant of the tetralogy of Fallot and called **pseudotruncus arteriosus**; in both forms, pulmonary blood flow occurs either via a patent ductus arteriosus or aortopulmonary collaterals

  tricuspid atresia *Syn: tricuspid valve atresia*; congenital absence of the tricuspid valve [approx. 3% of all congenital heart defects]; due to the absence of a connection between the right atrium and ventricle, infants will only survive if there is a coexistent atrial septal and ventricu-

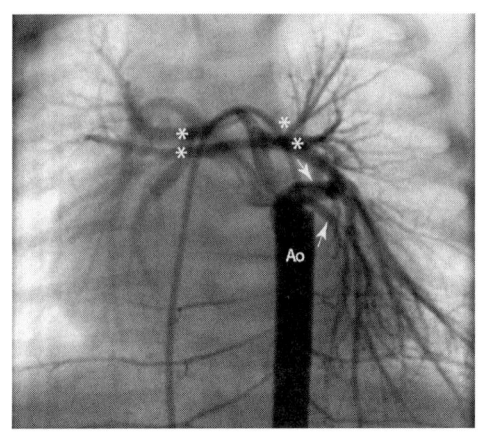

Pulmonary atresia. Angiography. Ao = aorta

lar septal defect, or if the ductus arteriosus remains patent; the great vessels can arise normally [**ventriculoarterial concordance**] or transposed [**ventriculoarterial discordance**] from the respective ventricles; often, the artery arising from the right ventricle is also narrowed or hypoplastic [pulmonary stenosis or hypoplastic pulmonary artery or aortic isthmus stenosis or hypoplastic aorta as appropriate]; the size of the right ventricle depends upon the size of the ventricular septal defect; the smaller the defect, and therefore the corresponding shunt volume, the smaller the ventricle [hypoplastic right ventricle]; **clinical**: directly after birth, cyanosis develops due to the right-to-left shunting at atrial level; **diagnosis**: echocardiography, cardiac catheterization, chest X-ray; **therapy**: anatomic correction is not possible; initially, formation of an aortopulmonary shunt, which is later replaced by a cavopulmonary shunt [Glenn operation]; this connects the superior vena cava with the right pulmonary artery; after the 2. year of life, a **Fontan operation** can be performed, which either connects the right atrium or the two venae cavae with the pulmonary arteries [also called **separation of the circulations** or **total cavopulmonary connection**]
tricuspid valve atresia → *tricuspid atresia*

atri- combining form denoting relation to an atrium
atrial *Syn: auricular*; relating to an atrium
atrial natriuretic peptide *Syn: atrial natriuretic factor, atrial natriuretic hormone, atriopeptide, atriopeptin*; originally only the **atrial natriuretic peptide** formed in the myocytes of the left atrium [atriopeptin], known nowadays as **natriuretic peptide type A**, was recognized; in addition there is now **natriuretic peptide type B** made predominantly in the ventricular myocardium [brain natriuretic peptide, BNP] as well as **natriuretic peptide type C** made in the endothelial cells; natriuretic peptides produce vasodilatation of the arteries and veins including the coronary vessels, increase the excretion of sodium in the kidneys, act as diuretics, and suppress the renin-angiotensin-aldosterone system
atrio- combining form denoting relation to an atrium
atriomegaly enlargement of the right or left cardiac atrium
atrionector → *Keith-Flack's node*
atriopeptide → *atrial natriuretic peptide*
atriopeptin → *atrial natriuretic peptide*
atrioseptoplasty plastic procedure to close an atrial septal defect
atrioseptostomy operative division of the atrial septum
atriotomy operative opening of the atrium
atrioventricular *Syn: ventriculoatrial*; relating to an atrium and a ventricle
atrium 1. chamber, vestibule, vestibulum 2. atrium cordis
  atrium cordis atrium of heart, cardiac atrium, atrium, antechamber
  atrium cordis dextrum → *right atrium*
  atrium cordis sinistrum → *left atrium*
  left atrium receives oxygen-rich blood from the pulmonary veins and pumps it during diastole through the mitral valve into the left ventricle; the wall is relatively thin and smooth, with only the posteriorly placed auricle containing muscle ridges [musculi pectinati]
  right atrium receives the venous blood coming from the systemic circulation and pumps it through the tricuspid valve into the right ventricle during diastole; the region between the openings of the inferior and superior venae cavae, in which the blood from the two great veins mixes, is called the **sinus of the vena cava**; the cardiac veins open into the ostium of the coronary sinus; the heart muscle wall starts at the crista terminalis, which is characterized by pectinate muscle ridges [musculi pectinati]; the diaphragm between the two atria [interatrial septum] contains the fossa ovalis, which is bordered by the limbus of the fossa ovalis; on the anterior surface of the atrium lies a blind sac,

the right auricle

atrophia → *atrophy*

atrophy *Syn: atrophia*; tissue or organ regression, degeneration; divided into **homologous atrophy** [reduction in the size of the cells with constant cell number] and **numerical atrophy** [reduction in the cell number]; in many cases, however, there is a mixed form with reduction of both the cell number and size; if a whole organ is affected [e.g., skeleton], this is **generalized** or **universal atrophy**, whereas **local atrophy** only affects circumscribed areas of a tissue

brown atrophy brown pigmentation mainly affecting the heart and liver in senile atrophy

congestive atrophy → *stasis atrophy*

cyanotic atrophy of liver → *cardiac cirrhosis*

myocardial atrophy atrophy of the heart musculature

stasis atrophy *Syn: congestive atrophy*; parenchymal regression of an organ in chronic venous engorgement

vascular atrophy atrophy due to impaired vascular supply

white atrophy superficial, painful capillary inflammation due to venous insufficiency; mostly occurs around the knuckles on the top of the foot

atropine *Syn: d/l-hyoscyamine, tropine tropate*; poisonous alkaloid with parasympatholytic action that occurs in the nightshade family, such as **belladonna** [Atropa belladonna], **white jimson weed** [Datura stramonium], and **henbane** [Hyoscyamus niger]

atropinism *Syn: atropism*; characterized by skin reddening, dry skin, dry mouth, disturbances of micturition, fever [central hyperthermia], mydriasis, tachycardia, agitation, and hallucinations; **therapy**: elimination of poisons [stomach pumping, activated charcoal], cooling, β-blockers, physostigmine

atropism → *atropinism*

attack *Syn: episode, ictus*; sudden or brief event

transient ischemic attack *s.u. cerebrovascular accident*

auricle ear-shaped appendage

left auricle blind sac at the root of the pulmonary trunk arising from the left atrium

right auricle blind sac on the anterior wall of the right atrium that surrounds the aortic root

auricular relating to an auricle or to the ear

auscultation listening for sounds within the body using the ear, ear trumpet, or stethoscope

cardiac auscultation auscultation of the heart sounds and heart murmurs; there are 4 standard auscultation points: **aortic valve** 2. intercostal space in the right parasternal region, **pulmonary valve** 2. intercostal space in the left parasternal region, **mitral valve** cardiac apex, **tricuspid valve** start of the 5. rib in the right parasternal region

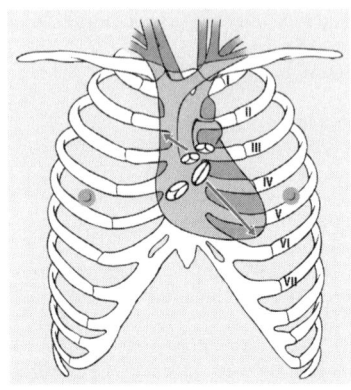

Cardiac auscultation. Standard auscultation points

auscultatory relating to auscultation, determined or determinable by auscultation
auto- combining form denoting relation to self
autoagglutination agglutination of blood corpuscles by autogenous serum
autoagglutinin agglutinin directed against autogenous blood corpuscles
  platelet autoagglutinin *Syn: autothromboagglutinin*; autoagglutinin against blood platelets
autoanalyzer *Syn: analysor, analyzer*; apparatus for automatically analyzing blood, tissue, or urine samples, etc.
autogeneic → *autologous*
autogenous **1.** arising from within **2.** produced in the organism itself **3.** → *autologous*
autohemagglutination agglutination of autogenous blood corpuscles
autohemagglutinin agglutinin against autogenous blood corpuscles
autohemolysis hemolysis of autogenous blood corpuscles, e.g., by autoan-

tibodies

autohemolytic relating to autohemolysis

autohemotransfusion → *autotransfusion*

autoinfusion relative increase in the blood volume in the systemic circulation caused by elevation or bandaging of the legs in the treatment of shock

autologous *Syn: autogeneic, autogenous*; derived from the same person

autonomic → *autonomous*

autonomical → *autonomous*

autonomous *Syn: autonomic, autonomical*; independent, self-sufficient (functional); self-directed; vegetative

autopathic → *idiopathic*

autoprothrombin prothrombin derivatives made during the formation of thrombin
  autoprothrombin C → *factor X*
  autoprothrombin I → *factor VII*
  autoprothrombin II → *factor IX*

autorhythmia *Syn: autorhythmicity*; ability to produce rhythmic excitation or stimuli; autorhythmia is the basis for the cardiac and respiratory rhythm

autorhythmicity → *autorhythmia*

autothromboagglutinin autoagglutinin against blood platelets [thrombocytes]

autotransfusion *Syn: autohemotransfusion*; transfusion of the patient's own blood; the blood can be removed pre-operatively [**autologous blood donation**] or is collected during the intervention and returned to the patient after cleaning

avalvular *Syn: nonvalvular*; without valve(s), valveless

avascular without blood vessels

av-bundle → *atrioventricular bundle*

avirulent non-virulent, not infective

AV-node → *Aschoff-Tawara's node*

axis the line about which a rotating body turns
  costocervical axis → *costocervical trunk*
  costocervical arterial axis → *costocervical trunk*
  thyroid axis → *thyrocervical trunk*

azidocillin semisynthetic oral penicillin; **indications**: gram-positive microorganisms, Haemophilus influenzae, Bordetella pertussis

azlocillin acylaminopenicillin with a broad action spectrum against gram-positive and gram-negative pathogens

azosemide furosemide derivative; loop diuretic

B

baby an infant or very young child

blue baby description of infants with bluish discoloration due to congenital heart defects with right-to-left shunting or methemoglobinemia

bacampicillin broad-spectrum penicillin derived from ampicillin; it is converted into ampicillin in the body after oral administration

bacillus a genus of gram-positive, usually motile, rod-shaped bacteria of the family Bacillaceae

influenza bacillus → *Haemophilus influenzae*

Pfeiffer's bacillus → *Haemophilus influenzae*

backflow the blood flowing backwards into the atrium or ventricle during systole or diastole in valve insufficiency

bacteremia → *bacteriemia*

bacterial *Syn: bacteriogenic, bacteriogenous, bacteritic*; relating to or caused by bacteria

bactericidal destructive to bacteria

bactericide an agent that kills bacteria, antibiotic with bactericidal action

bacteriemia *Syn: bacteremia*; transient appearance of bacteria in the blood

bacteriogenic *Syn: bacteriogenous, bacteritic*; caused by bacteria, bacterial

bacteriogenous → *bacteriogenic*

bacteriostasis inhibition of bacterial growth, e.g., using antibiotics; since the bacteria are not killed but rather only prevented from multiplying, they can start to reproduce again following a fall in the antibiotic concentration; the resistance of the body is therefore a decisive factor in the killing and elimination of pathogens

bacteriostat → *bacteriostatic*

bacteriostatic 1. an agent with bacteriostatic properties **2.** relating to or causing bacterial stasis, inhibiting the growth of bacteria

bacteritic → *bacteriogenic*

balance equilibrium

electrolyte balance totality of metabolism of the electrolytes present in the body; since unbound electrolytes can only occur in dissolved form, electrolyte balance and water balance are intimately connected; the most important inorganic electrolytes in the body are Na^+, K^+, Ca^{2+}, Mg^{2+}, Cl^-, HCO_3^-, SO_4^{2-} and phosphate ions; protein anions play an important role in the maintenance of a constant blood pH and colloid osmotic pressure of the blood plasma; inside the cells, K^+ and phosphate ions are the most common, in the extracellular space Na^+ and Cl^- predominate; electrolytes contribute significantly to the colloid osmotic pressure of the blood plasma and the cells; in the blood serum there is **electroneutrality**, i.e., the sum of anions and cations is equal; if the concentration of one or more electrolytes increases or reduces, the body must ensure that the equilibrium is restored; deviations from equilibrium also cause changes in the pH value of the blood plasma; if the anion concentration falls, the pH value rises and vice versa; an increase in the cation total elevates the pH value, a reduction drops the pH value; **disturbances** of electrolyte homeostasis are usually combined with disturbances of water balance and acid-base balance, since there is a direct connection between action and effect; the clinical features of disturbed electrolyte balance depend upon the type and cause of the disturbance; in addition to isolated disturbances [e.g., hypokalemia] there are disturbances that affect several electrolytes [e.g., hyperaldosteronism] or all of them simultaneously [e.g., electrolyte losses in massive bleeding]

balanced equalized, equilibrated, in equilibrium

ballistocardiogram graphic demonstration produced by ballistocardiography

ballistocardiograph equipment for ballistocardiography

ballistocardiographic relating to ballistocardiography

ballistocardiography recording and depiction of the ballistic forces of the heart and aorta

band → *ligamentum*

  atrioventricular band → *atrioventricular bundle*
  auriculoventricular band → *atrioventricular bundle*
  His' band → *atrioventricular bundle*
  moderator band → *septomarginal trabecula*
  septomarginal band → *septomarginal trabecula*

banding operative reduction of a vessel, usually the pulmonary artery

barrier any natural obstacle, a limit or boundary of any kind

blood-brain barrier *Syn: blood-cerebral barrier, Held's limitting membrane, hematoencephalic barrier*; selective barrier between blood vessels and the brain, which only allows certain substances [lipophilic substances, small molecules] through and which protects the brain tissue from harmful substances [including medications]; poisonings, various bacterial toxins, high fever, hypoxia, and tumors can all breach the blood-brain barrier

blood-cerebral barrier → *blood-brain barrier*

blood-cerebrospinal fluid barrier → *blood-CSF barrier*

blood-CSF barrier *Syn: blood-cerebrospinal fluid barrier*; selective barrier between the blood vessels and the fluid compartments, which only allows certain substances to pass

hematoencephalic barrier → *blood-brain barrier*

Bartonella Gram-negative, aerobic, partially flagellated, polymorphic bacteria of the **Bartonellaceae** family; contains at least 4 forms pathogenic to humans

Bartonella elizabethae has been identified as a cause of endocarditis

Bartonella quintana pathogen which causes five-day fever and was formerly called Rickettsia quintana or Rochalimaea quintana; can cause bacillary angiomatosis or peliosis like Bartonella henselae and has also been identified as the cause of endocarditis

base *Syn: basis*; lower surface or area of an organ

base of heart the upper, broad end of the heart from which the great vessels enter/leave

basis → *base*

basis cordis → *base of heart*

bathmotropic changing the excitation threshold of the heart muscle

bathmotropism change in the excitation threshold of the heart muscle, bathmotropic action

bathycardia *Syn: Wenckebach's disease, drop heart, cardioptosia, cardioptosis*; low-lying heart, mostly in combination with enteroptosis

batroxobin enzyme [protease] made by the poisonous snake Bothrops atrox; formerly used as a hemostyptic; nowadays only used to determine the reptilase time

beat stroke or blow; heart beat

apex beat *Syn: apex impulse, apical impulse*; tapping of the heart against the chest wall felt over the cardiac apex

cardiac beat → *cardiac cycle*

coupled beat *Syn:* *paired beat, coupled pulse, coupled rhythm, bigeminal pulse, bigeminus; s.u. bigeminy*

ectopic beat formation of excitation outside the sinoatrial node if the sinoatrial node fails or as an additional excitation, which can lead to extrasystoles, disturbances of rhythm, etc.

escape beat →*escaped beat*

escaped beat *Syn:* *escape beat, escape contraction, escaped contraction;* extrasystole occurring when the sinoatrial node malfunctions

paired beat *Syn:* *coupled pulse, coupled rhythm, bigeminal pulse, bigeminus, coupled beat; s.u. bigeminy*

parasystolic beat →*parasystolic rhythm*

premature beat →*extrasystole*

premature atrial beat →*atrial extrasystole*

premature ventricular beat →*ventricular extrasystole*

bemetizide saluretic; **usage**: hypertension, edema; **side effects**: hypokalemia, elevation of the blood sugar and uric acid levels

bencyclane vasodilator; **usage**: peripheral and central hypoperfusion states, thrombo-prophylaxis, migraine

bendrofluazide →*bendroflumethiazide*

bendroflumethiazide *Syn:* *bendrofluazide, benzydroflumethiazide;* saluretic; **usage**: hypertension, edema, renal diseases; **side effects**: hypokalemia, elevation of the blood sugar and uric acid levels

benzazoline direct α-sympatholytic, vasodilator; **usage**: peripheral disturbances of perfusion, disturbances of perfusion in the eye

benzodiazepines *Syn:* *benzodiazepine derivatives;* psychoactive drugs from the tranquilizer group, with antianxiety, sedative, anticonvulsant, and muscle-relaxing activity; **indications**: 1. **tranquilizer, anxiolytic, antidepressant**: for example, alprazolam, bromazepam, chlordiazepoxide, clobazam, clonazepam, diazepam, lorazepam, prazepam 2. **hypnotic**: for example, flunitrazepam, flurazepam, loprazolam, lorazepam, nitrazepam, temazepam 3. **anticonvulsant, antiepileptic**: for example, clobazam, diazepam, clonazepam, nitrazepam 4. **muscle relaxant**: for example, tetrazepam, diazepam, nitrazepam; benzodiazepines protect the limbic system from external effects and suppress the effect of the limbic system on the reticular formation; they are absorbed rapidly and well after oral administration; their binding to plasma proteins varies [diazepam up to 90%]; benzodiazepines are metabolized in the liver, in part with the formation of metabolites with a long duration of action; **side effects**: apathy, fatigue, loss of appetite, accommodation disorders, inhibition of the respiratory and vasomotor center [only with i.v. administration]; paradoxical effects with, for example, agitation and fits of rage can occur in older patients; all benzodiazepines have a risk of tolerance development and dependence; sometimes, there is a partial cross-dependence with alcohol and barbiturates

benzydroflumethiazide → *bendroflumethiazide*

benzylpenicillin → *penicillin G*

benzathine benzylpenicillin → *benzylpenicillin benzathine*

benzylpenicillin benzathine *Syn: benzathine benzylpenicillin, penicillin G benzathine*; depot form of benzylpenicillin

beta-blocker *Syn: beta-receptor blocker, β-adrenoceptor blocker, beta-adrenoceptor blocker, β-blocker, β-sympatholytic*; the β-receptor blocking drugs; blockade of the $β_1$-receptors reduces the heart rate and contractility, as well as conductivity, and reduces renin release from the kidney; $β_2$-blockade inhibits glycogen breakdown in the muscles and the liver; **indications**: beta-blockers are the agent of choice in hypertension; they are also used for the prophylaxis of angina pectoris, reinfarction, and migraines; **side effects**: airway obstruction, peripheral circulatory disturbance, allergic reactions

beta-hemolysis *Syn: β-hemolysis*; total hemolysis of the erythrocytes following bacterial growth on blood agar

beta-hemolytic → *β-hemolytic*

betaine *Syn: glycine betaine, glycyl betaine, lycine, oxyneurine*; used as a lipotropic substance in liver disease, arteriosclerosis, and coronary arteriosclerosis

beta-lactamase *Syn: β-lactamase*; enzyme that opens the β-lactam ring and thereby inactivates beta-lactam antibiotics

penicillin beta-lactamase → *penicillinase*

betaquinine → *quinidine*

bi- combining form denoting relation to life or living organisms

bicarbonate *Syn: dicarbonate, supercarbonate*; acidic salt of carbonic acid, e.g., sodium bicarbonate [$NaHCO_3$]

standard bicarbonate the bicarbonate concentration in the blood plasma, when the measurement is carried out under standardized conditions [total oxygen saturation of the hemoglobin, 37 °C, CO_2 partial pressure of 40 mmHg]; normal value: 24 mmol/l; increased in metabolic alkalosis, lowered in metabolic acidosis

bicarbonatemia *Syn: hyperbicarbonatemia*; elevation of the bicarbonate concentration in the blood

bicuspid *Syn: bicuspidate;* (*heart valve*) with two cusps; (*tooth*) with two tubercles
bicuspidate → *bicuspid*
bifurcatio *Syn: bifurcation;* branching, forking, fork, division into two
  bifurcatio aortae → *bifurcation of aorta*
  bifurcatio carotidis → *carotid bifurcation*
  bifurcatio trunci pulmonalis → *bifurcation of pulmonary trunk*
bifurcation → *bifurcatio*
  bifurcation of aorta division of the abdominal aorta into right and left common iliac arteries at the level of the 4. lumbar vertebra
  carotid bifurcation division of the common carotid artery into the internal and external carotid arteries at the level of the upper border of the 5. cervical vertebra in the carotid triangle
  bifurcation of pulmonary trunk *Syn: bifurcatio trunci pulmonalis;* division of the pulmonary trunk into the right and left pulmonary arteries
bigemini → *bigeminy*
bigeminus *Syn: coupled beat, paired beat, coupled pulse, coupled rhythm, bigeminal pulse; s.u. bigeminy*
bigeminy *Syn: bigemini, pairing, twinning;* disturbance of the heart rhythm with extrasystoles following every heartbeat and double pulse [bigeminus]
bio- combining form denoting relation to life or living organisms
bioamine *Syn: biogenic amine;* natural amine important for metabolism, which occurs in plants or animals
bioavailability speed and extent to which the therapeutically active ingredient of a medication is released, absorbed, and made available at its site of action
  absolute bioavailability the portion of a dose which is available
  relative bioavailability bioavailability of a drug from one pharmaceutical in comparison to its bioavailability from a different pharmaceutical
biocidal lethal to plants or animals, acting as a biocide
biocompatibility tolerability/compatibility of foreign substances with the body tissues
biocompatible tolerated by body tissues/compatible; not damaging to the tissues
biodegradability biologic biodegradability; substances, which cannot be degraded biologically, tend to be bioaccumulated within the food

chain [e.g., pesticides]

bioelectricity electricity generated in living tissues

bioequivalence concordance of the bioavailability of two preparations of a single agent

bioequivalent with identical bioequivalence

biofeedback visualization of physiologic parameters in the setting of psychotherapy, which are then consciously altered by relaxation; a clinical application of operant conditioning; the most important **indications** for its use are migraine, tension headache, cardiac neurosis, stutter, and cervicalgia

biomarkers substances found in blood, other body fluids, or tissues that can be objectively measured and evaluated as a sign of a normal or pathological process, or of a condition or disease; biomarkers may be used to see how well the body responds to a specific pharmacological intervention for a disease or condition

biopsy removal of tissue from the living body by puncture or excision

bioptic relating to biopsy

biorhythm *Syn: biological rhythm, body rhythm*; rhythmic fluctuations of various bodily functions caused by external [day-night alternation] or internal factors [biologic clock]

biorhythmic relating to biorhythm

biotelemetric relating to biotelemetry

biotelemetry *Syn: radiotelemetry*; generally wireless transmission of measurements, e.g., ECG, for remote diagnosis or remote monitoring

biventricular relating to both ventricles

bleeding loss of blood from a ruptured or injured vessel

    arterial bleeding *Syn: arterial hemorrhage*; bleeding from an artery; bright spurting blood

    petechial bleeding →*petechia*

    venous bleeding *Syn: phleborrhagia, venous hemorrhage*; bleeding from a vein; welling, dark red blood

block 1. →*heart block* **2.** blocking or occlusion of a vessel

    3-in-1 block inguinal block of the femoral, lateral femoral cutaneous, and obturator nerves; used in operations on the upper ventral thigh and for analgesia in femoral fractures

    air block →*air-block syndrome*

    arborization block heart block due to a disturbance of the conduction of excitation in the divisions of the Tawara branches

    atrioventricular block →*a-v block*

atrioventricular heart block →*a-v block*

a-v block *Syn: atrioventricular block, atrioventricular heart block*; prolongation of the atrioventricular conduction time; first degree AV block, second degree AV block, and third degree AV block are described, as well as higher degree blocks; the **cause** may be functional influences [medication, autonomic nervous system], disease of the conduction system, coronary heart disease, myocarditis, dilated cardiomyopathy, and the like; the **clinical symptoms** depend upon the degree of block and the ventricular rate resulting from the disturbance; the spectrum ranges from an asymptomatic course through reduced exercise capacity to Stokes-Adams attacks; **therapy**: symptomatic AV block usually requires implantation of a pacemaker

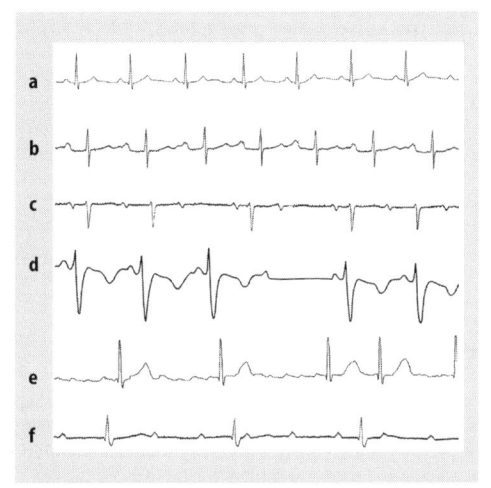

a-v block. **a** normal conduction; **b** first degree a-v block; **c** type 1 second degree a-v block [Wenckebach type]; **d** type 2 second degree a-v block [Mobitz type]; **e** bradyarrhythmia in atrial fibrillation; **f** third degree a-v block

bifascicular block *s.u. intraventricular block*
bundle-branch block *Syn: bundle-branch heart block, interventricular block, interventricular heart block*; corresponding to the branching of

block

the ventricular excitation conduction system into right, left anterior and left posterior branches, conduction delays or conduction block in one or more of the conduction pathways can give rise to typical features of block in the ECG; the term "block" is not totally correct, since the surface ECG cannot differentiate between delayed conduction and a total block of conduction; in **right bundle branch block** [RBB], there is conduction slowing or block in the right Tawara branch; the isolated occurrence of right bundle branch block is not prognostically relevant; if there is a simultaneous underlying cardiac disease [coronary heart disease, cor pulmonale] the prognosis is determined by that; in **left bundle branch block** [LBB], there is generally a severe disturbance of the intraventricular spread of excitation, which is caused by marked slowing or interruption of the left Tawara branch; the presence of complete left bundle branch block virtually always indicates a cardiac disease and is therefore prognostically less favorable than a RBB; the left branch consists, at least functionally, of anterior and posterior branches; an isolated slowing of conduction or block in only one of these branches is described as **left anterior** [LAH] or **left posterior hemiblock** [LPH]; **multiple blocks**: in bifascicular block, **two Tawara branches** are affected: left anterior and left posterior hemiblock [LAH + LPH], left anterior hemiblock and right bundle branch block [LAH + RBB] or left posterior hemiblock and right bundle branch block [LPH + RBB]; **trifascicular block** affects all three branches simultaneously; it results in functional 3. degree AV-block

bundle-branch heart block → *bundle-branch block*

depolarization block muscle relaxation by a depolarizing blocker

first degree atrioventricular block → *first degree a-v block*

first degree a-v block *Syn: delayed conduction, first degree atrioventricular block, first degree heart block*; all excitatory impulses are transmitted from the atrium to the ventricle, although with a conduction delay [PQ interval > 0.2 s]; most commonly, the delay occurs in the AV-node, but sometimes intra-atrial or intraventricular conduction disturbances can be the cause

first degree heart block → *first degree a-v block*

focal block heart block confined to a relatively small region

heart block disturbance to or interruption of the normal conduction of excitation in the heart; depending upon localization, **atrioventricular block** [block to conduction from the atrium to the ventricle], intra-atrial block and intra-ventricular block can be differentiated; the block to conduction can be transient [e.g., in vagotonia] or permanent; it is important to differentiate between partial, which leads to prolongation of the conduction time and perhaps to loss of individual systoles, and complete block

higher degree blocks *s.u. a-v block*

high grade a-v block *s.u. second a-v block*

interventricular block → *bundle-branch block*

interventricular heart block → *bundle-branch block*

intra-atrial block block of the excitatory impulse within the atrium

intraventricular block blockage of the excitatory impulse in the ventricular myocardium; according to the concept of trifascicular intraventricular conduction of excitation suggested by von Rosenbaum et al., one can differentiate based on changes in the QRS-complex in the standard leads between **monofascicular**, **bifascicular**, and **trifascicular block**; the **monofascicular blocks** include **right bundle branch block** [RBB], **left anterior hemiblock** [LAH], and **left posterior hemiblock** [LPH]; a **bifascicular block** is due to a combination of two monofascicular blocks [RBB and LAH; RBB and LPH; LAH and LPH = left bundle branch block, LBB]

left bundle-branch block blockage or slowing of the conduction of excitation in the left Tawara branch

monofascicular block *s.u. intraventricular block*

right bundle-branch block *Syn: right bundle-branch heart block*; blockage or slowing of the conduction of excitation in the right Tawara branch

right bundle-branch heart block → *right bundle-branch block*

S-A block interruption of the conduction of excitation from the sinoatrial node to the atrium

second a-v block not all excitatory impulses are conducted; in **type 1 second degree AV-block** [Wenckebach type], the PQ interval increases from beat to beat until an atrial impulse is eventually blocked; thereafter the rhythm repeats; in **type 2 second degree AV-block** [Mobitz type], there are fixed sudden losses of conduction of excitation; the PQ interval before and after the dropped beat is identical; in **higher degrees of block** [4:1, 5:1 conduction], the cause may be either type 1 or type 2 second degree AV-block

sinoatrial block → *sinuatrial block*

sinuatrial block *Syn: S-A block, sinoatrial block, sinuauricular block,*

blockade

sinus block; interruption of the conduction of excitation from the sino-atrial node to the atrium

sinuauricular block → *sinuatrial block*

sinus block → *sinuatrial block*

sympathetic block blockade of part of the sympathetic chain [**cervical, thoracic, lumbar sympathetic block**] using local anesthetic agents

third a-v block complete interruption of the conduction of excitation with atrioventricular dissociation and the appearance of an escape rhythm [e.g., AV rhythm]; in congenital complete heart block, the cause is usually in the AV node, in acquired forms in the His-Purkinje system

trifascicular block *s.u. intraventricular block*

vena caval block blockage of the inferior vena cava from the outside [**vena cava clip**] or the inside [**vena cava filter**] as prophylaxis against embolism

Wilson's block most common form of right bundle branch block

blockade blocking or occlusion of a vessel

alpha blockade *Syn: alpha-adrenergic blockade*; blockade of the alpha receptors

alpha-adrenergic blockade → *alpha blockade*

blocker *Syn: blocking agent, blocking drug*; the action of one substance to block the effect of another; blocking substance

β-adrenoceptor blocker → *beta-blocker*

β-blocker → *beta-blocker*

beta-adrenoceptor blocker → *beta-blocker*

beta-receptor blocker → *beta-blocker*

calcium channel blocker → *calcium antagonist*

ECE blockers *Syn: ECE inhibitors; s.u. endothelins*

potassium channel blockers substances that block the influx of potassium ions through potassium channels

blood liquid tissue consisting of cells [corpuscles] and plasma; cells constitute approximately 44–46% of the volume and plasma the rest; the most important functions of the blood are the transport of respiratory gases [oxygen, carbon dioxide], nutrients, metabolites, hormones, and vitamins, thermoregulation, and defense [specific and nonspecific defense]; the blood makes up approximately 6–8% of the body's mass, i.e., an adult has about 4–6 l of blood [normovolemia], of which about 85% is found in the venous system and only about 15% in the arterial system; a reduction of the blood volume is called **hypovolemia**, and an increase **hypervolemia**; blood has a relative viscosity of about 4.5 [3.5–5.4] in comparison with water; the viscosity increases with a rising hematocrit

arterial blood *Syn: oxygenated blood*; blood flowing in the arteries; it is oxygenated in the systemic circulation and deoxygenated in the pulmonary circulation

banked blood *Syn: banked human blood*; donor blood treated with stabilizers, which can be used as **whole blood** or as special preparations [**plasma, red cell concentrate**]

banked human blood → *banked blood*

citrated blood blood prevented from clotting by the addition of citrate

defibrinated blood blood that is free of fibrin and does not coagulate

deoxygenated blood → *venous blood*

fresh blood batch of whole blood, which is no older than three days

mixed blood arterial and venous mixed blood

oxalated blood blood prevented from clotting by the addition of oxalate

oxygenated blood → *arterial blood*

venous blood *Syn: deoxygenated blood*; blood flowing in the veins; it is oxygenated in the pulmonary circulation and deoxygenated in the systemic circulation

whole blood *s.u. banked blood*

bloodletting *Syn: bleeding*; artificial opening of a blood vessel for sampling blood; hardly performed nowadays for therapeutic purposes

B-lymphocytes *Syn: B cells, thymus-independent lymphocytes*; the cells of the immune system originally form in the bone marrow, then mature in the lymphatic tissues; they migrate via the blood from the bone marrow to the secondary lymphatic organs [spleen, lymph nodes]; after exposure to antigens, they can transform into cells that make antibodies [plasma cells] or **B-memory cells;** the plasma cells make specific antibodies targeted against the antigen, whereas the memory cells produce the immune response on second exposure to the antigen

BNP → *brain natriuretic peptide*

body principal mass of a structure

  adrenal body → *adrenal gland*

  Anichkov's body → *Anichkov's myocyte*

  Anitschkow's body → *Anichkov's myocyte*

  carotid body *Syn: carotid gland, carotid glomus, intercarotid body*;

parasympathetic paraganglion at the carotid bifurcation; detects changes in oxygen partial pressure and pH

chromaffin body → *paraganglion*

glomiform body *Syn: glomiform gland, glomus, glomus body, glomus organ*; small tufts of vessels embedded in the skin; probably important for skin perfusion and thermoregulation

glomus body → *glomiform body*

intercarotid body → *carotid glomus*

jugular body → *jugular paraganglion*

pheochrome body → *paraganglion*

tympanic body → *jugular paraganglion*

brachial relating to the arm

brachycardia → *bradycardia*

brady- combining form denoting relation to slow

bradyarrhythmia slow, total arrhythmia of the heart

bradycardia *Syn: brachycardia, bradyrhythmia, oligocardia*; excessively slow pulse [pulse rate less than 60/min] due to dysfunction of the triggering of excitation [**sinus bradycardia**] or disruption of the conduction of excitation [2. degree SA block, 1. and 2. degree AV block]; may also occur in performance athletes, hypothyroidism, and hypothermia; **clinical**: impaired performance, dizziness, Stokes-Adams attacks, angina pectoris, cardiac insufficiency, bradyarrhythmia; **therapy**: medical management using sympathomimetics [orciprenaline] or vagolytics [atropine]; if this does not adequately increase the rate, or if the patient has a sinoatrial node syndrome, then implantation of a pacemaker is indicated

sinoatrial bradycardia → *sinus bradycardia*

sinus bradycardia *Syn: sinoatrial bradycardia*; bradycardia arising in the sinoatrial node; e.g., in sinoatrial node syndrome

bradycardiac *Syn: bradycardic*; relating to bradycardia

bradycardic → *bradycardiac*

bradycrotic reducing the pulse, slowing the pulse

bradydiastole slowed diastole

bradydiastolic relating to bradydiastole

bradykinin a tissue hormone from the kinin family; it causes the contraction of the smooth muscles of vessels, bronchi, uterus, and intestine, lowers blood pressure, and increases capillary permeability

bradykininogen → *kallidin*

bradyrhythmia → *bradycardia*

bradysphygmia *Syn: slowness of the pulse*; slowing of the pulse, reduced pulse rate in bradycardia

brain natriuretic peptide *Syn: B-type natriuretic peptide*; polypeptide produced mainly in the ventricular muscle cells and released in response to excessive stretching of the myocardium; binds to and activates atrial natriuretic factor receptors [NPRA, NPRB]; decreases systemic vascular resistance and central venous pressure thus increasing cardiac output and natriuresis, leading to a decreased blood volume

branch division, twig

    anterior interventricular branch *Syn: ramus interventricularis anterior; s.u. left coronary artery of heart*

    atrial branches of left coronary artery *Syn: rami atriales arteriae coronariae sinistrae; s.u. left coronary artery of heart*

    atrial branches of right coronary artery *Syn: rami atriales arteriae coronariae dextrae; s.u. right coronary artery of heart*

    atrioventricular branches of left coronary artery *Syn: rami atrioventriculares arteriae coronariae sinistrae; s.u. left coronary artery of heart*

    atrioventricular nodal branch of left coronary artery *Syn: atrioventricular nodal artery*; branch of the left coronary artery to the atrioventricular node

    atrioventricular nodal branch of right coronary artery *Syn: atrioventricular nodal artery*; branch of the right coronary artery to the atrioventricular node

    atrioventricular branches of right coronary artery *Syn: rami atrioventriculares arteriae coronariae dextrae; s.u. right coronary artery of heart*

    branch of av-bundle → *right and left bundle branch*

    bronchial branches of thoracic aorta → *bronchial arteries*

    bundle branch → *right and left bundle branch*

    carotid sinus branch of glossopharyngeal nerve → *Hering's sinus nerve*

    circumflex branch of left coronary artery *Syn: ramus circumflexus arteriae coronariae sinistrae; s.u. left coronary artery of heart*

    conus branch of left coronary artery *Syn: left conal artery, left conus artery, left conus branch of left coronary artery*; branch of the left coronary artery to the conus arteriosus

    conus branch of right coronary artery *Syn: right conal artery, right conus artery, right conus branch of right coronary artery, third conus artery*; branch of the right coronary artery to the conus arteriosus

intermediate atrial branch of left coronary artery *Syn: ramus atrialis intermedius arteriae coronariae sinistrae; s.u. left coronary artery of heart*

intermediate atrial branch of right coronary artery *Syn: ramus atrialis intermedius arteriae coronariae dextrae; s.u. right coronary artery of heart*

lateral branch of anterior interventricular branch of left coronary artery *Syn: ramus lateralis interventricularis anterior arteriae coronariae sinistrae; s.u. left coronary artery of heart*

left branch of av-bundle → *left bundle branch*

left bundle branch *Syn: left branch of av-bundle, left leg of av-bundle*; left branch of the excitation conduction system of the heart; arises from the bundle of His and runs subendocardially in the ventricular septum in the left ventricle; branches into **rami subendocardiales**, which terminate as the Purkinje fibers

left conus branch of left coronary artery → *conus branch of left coronary artery*

pericardiac branch of phrenic nerve *s.u. nervus phrenicus*

pericardiac branches of thoracic aorta *Syn: posterior pericardiac arteries*; pericardial branches of the thoracic aorta

phrenicoabdominal branches of phrenic nerve *s.u. nervus phrenicus*

posterior interventricular branch of right coronary artery *Syn: ramus interventricularis posterior arteriae coronariae dextrae; s.u. right coronary artery of heart*

right bundle branch *Syn: right branch of av bundle, right leg of av-bundle*; right limb of the excitation conduction system of the heart; arises from the bundle of His and passes subendocardially into the right ventricular portion of the interventricular septum; divides into the **rami subendocardiales**, which terminate in the Purkinje fibers

right conus branch of right coronary artery → *conus branch of right coronary artery*

right branch of av bundle → *right bundle branch*

sinoatrial nodal branch of left coronary artery *Syn: nodal artery, sinoatrial nodal artery, sinuatrial nodal artery, sinus node artery*; branch of the left coronary artery to the sinoatrial node

sinoatrial nodal branch of right coronary artery *Syn: nodal artery, sinoatrial nodal artery, sinuatrial nodal artery, sinus node artery*; branch of the right coronary artery to the sinoatrial node

thoracic cardiac branches of vagus nerve thoracic cardiac branches of

the vagus nerve
breathing *Syn: respiration*; the gas exchange consisting of **internal** and **external respiration** in the body

amphoric breathing →*amphoric respiration*

auxiliary breathing *Syn: auxiliary respiration*; forced breathing with use of the accessory respiratory muscles

bronchial breathing *Syn: bronchial murmur, bronchial rales, bronchial respiration, bronchial breath sound*; normal breath sound over the bronchi, which can be heard during inhalation and exhalation; it is louder and sharper than vesicular breathing and has a higher frequency range with clearly evident high tones; it has a deeper tone over the trachea and for this reason is called **tracheal breathing**; pure bronchial breathing is not audible above the chest wall, because the high frequencies are filtered out by air-containing lung tissue; however, during infiltration of lung tissue, atelectasis, or shifting of the large bronchi closer to the chest wall [bronchiectasis], bronchial breathing is audible on auscultation

bronchovesicular breathing *Syn: rude respiration, transitional respiration, bronchovesicular respiration, harsh respiration, bronchovesicular breath sound*; bronchial breath sound with a strong vesicular overtone

cavernous breathing →*amphoric respiration*

chest breathing *Syn: thoracic breathing, costal breathing, costal respiration*; shallow type of breathing in which only the chest (thoracic) muscles are used

Cheyne-Stokes breathing →*Cheyne-Stokes respiration*

costal breathing →*chest breathing*

diaphragmatic breathing →*diaphragmatic respiration*

harsh breathing nonspecific term for loud vesicular respiration or mixed type of respiration [bronchovesicular or vesiculobronchial breathing], e.g., in infiltration or emphysema, but also in emotional excitement or physical exertion

labored breathing →*dyspnea*

periodic breathing →*Cheyne-Stokes respiration*

puerile breathing →*puerile respiration*

vesicular breathing *Syn: vesicular breath sounds, vesicular murmur, vesicular respiration*; normal breath sound over the peripheral lung sections, created by the turbulence of the air stream in the small air passages; it is quiet, of low frequency, and can be heard during inspiration and at the start of expiration over the entire lung; it is heard most clearly over the inferior lobe of the lung

breathlessness → *dyspnea*

bridge bridge-like structure

Gaskell's bridge → *atrioventricular bundle*

brittle → *fragile*

bruit sound, murmur, noise

bruit de diable *Syn: jugular bruit, humming-top murmur, nun's murmur, venous hum*; flow murmur over the jugular vein, e.g., in anemia or hyperthyroidism; quiet, low-frequency soughing or buzzing on the right or left side above the midpoint of the clavicle; physiologic in children and adolescents

jugular bruit → *bruit de diable*

systolic bruit → *systolic murmur*

Traube's bruit → *gallop*

B-scan *s.u. sonography*

B-type natriuretic peptide → *brain natriuretic peptide*

bubbling *s.a. moist rales*

deep bubbling *s.u. moist rales*

bucardia → *bovine heart*

buffer shield, cushion, bumper

bicarbonate buffer the buffer system in the blood consisting of bicarbonate [HCO_3^-] and carbonic acid [H_2CO_3]; important for acid-base balance

phosphate buffer aqueous solution of primary and secondary phosphate, with primary phosphate [$H_2PO_4^-$] acting as an acid and secondary phosphate [HPO_4^{2-}] acting as a base; buffers in the range of pH 6–8; the concentration in the blood is so low that the buffering capacity is small

protein buffer → *proteinate buffer system*

proteinate buffer → *proteinate buffer system*

bulb any round, enlarged part

bulb of aorta → *aortic bulb*

aortic bulb *Syn: arterial bulb, bulb of aorta*; dilated initial part of the ascending aorta; site of origin of the coronary arteries

arterial bulb → *aortic bulb*

bulb of heart precursor of the right ventricle during embryonic development

inferior bulb of jugular vein enlargement of the internal jugular vein before its junction with the subclavian vein

superior bulb of jugular vein enlargement of the internal jugular vein where it lies in the jugular fossa

bulboatrial relating to bulbus cordis and atrium

bulbus → *bulb*

  bulbus aortae → *aortic bulb*

  carotid bulbus → *carotid sinus*

  bulbus cordis → *bulb of heart*

  bulbus inferior venae jugularis → *inferior bulb of jugular vein*

  bulbus superior venae jugularis → *superior bulb of jugular vein*

bunazosin α_1-receptor blocker; **usage**: essential hypertension

bundle an aggregation of fibers, such as nerve or muscle fibers

  atrioventricular bundle *Syn:* atrioventricular band, atrioventricular trunk, auriculoventricular band, av-bundle, bundle of Stanley Kent, bundle of His, Gaskell's bridge, His' band, Kent-His bundle, ventriculonector; fiber bundle of the excitation conduction system of the heart emerging from the atrioventricular node; divides in the ventricular septum into the Tawara branches

  Bachmann's bundle accessory conduction bundle between the two heart chambers

  bundle of His → *atrioventricular bundle*

  Kent's bundle accessory conduction bundle from the right atrium to the right ventricle; leads to disturbances of the conduction of excitation [Wolff-Parkinson-White syndrome]

  Kent-His bundle → *atrioventricular bundle*

  pectinate bundles → *pectinate muscles*

  bundle of Stanley Kent → *atrioventricular bundle*

buthiazide *Syn:* thiabutazide; saluretic; **indications**: edema in cardiac insufficiency, renal insufficiency; **side effects**: hypokalemia, elevation of blood sugar and uric acid levels

buttonhole hole, slit, loop

  mitral buttonhole → *fishmouth stenosis*

bypass *Syn:* shunt; surgically created, temporary or permanent bypassing of vessels or sections of the intestine

  anatomical bypass bypass that follows the normal anatomical course; e.g., aortofemoral bypass

  aortocoronary bypass *Syn:* coronary artery bypass, coronary bypass; operative connection of the aorta and coronary artery(ies) to bypass a stenosis; depending upon the number of stenosed vessels, a **single**, double, or **triple bypass** may be performed; the great saphenous vein, internal thoracic artery, gastroepiploic artery, or radial artery may all be used as the graft; the so-called **MIDCAB technique** [**m**inimally **i**nvasive **d**irect **c**oronary **a**rtery **b**ypass] permits anastomosis in the beating heart; the newest development in this area is **TECAB technique** [**t**otal **e**ndoscopic **c**oronary **a**rtery **b**ypass]; this involves the operator steering the working arms of a telemanipulator

aortofemoral bypass operative joining of the abdominal aorta and the femoral artery

cardiopulmonary bypass basic principle of blood flow diversion during heart surgery with extracorporeal circulation; the venous blood is taken out of the body through cannulas in the right atrium or the two vena cavas and after oxygenation conveyed back into the aorta; in a **partial cardiopulmonary bypass**, blood still flows in the heart and is pumped into the aorta; in a **total cardiopulmonary bypass**, all of venous blood is drained using the heart-lung machine

coronary bypass → *aortocoronary bypass*

coronary artery bypass → *aortocoronary bypass*

cross-leg bypass operative joining of the common iliac artery of one side to the femoral or common iliac artery of the other side to improve perfusion

double bypass *s.u. aortocoronary bypass*

extra-anatomic bypass bypass that does not follow the normal anatomical course, or joins structures that are not normally directly connected

femorofemoral bypass operative joining of the femoral artery on one side of the body with the femoral artery on the other side in order to improve perfusion

femoropopliteal bypass operative joining of the femoral artery and popliteal artery to circumvent a stenosis

in-situ bypass a bypass that lies at practically the same position as the bypassed vessel; achieved by using a neighboring vessel

left heart bypass extracorporeal blood circulation in which blood is pumped through a heart-lung machine from the left atrium to the left femoral artery or common iliac artery; mainly used in interventions on the thoracic aorta

single bypass *s.u. aortocoronary bypass*

triple bypass *s.u. aortocoronary bypass*

venous bypass bypass using a segment of a vein

C

calcemia → *hypercalcemia*

calci- combining form denoting relation to calcium or calcium salts

calcification hardening of tissue by deposition of lime or other insoluble calcium salts

    Mönckeberg's calcification → *Mönckeberg's sclerosis*

    Mönckeberg's medial calcification → *Mönckeberg's sclerosis*

callicrein → *kallikrein*

canal narrow tubular passage or channel

    canal of Arantius → *ductus venosus*

    arterial canal → *ductus arteriosus*

    atrioventricular canal connection between the primitive atrium and the primitive ventricle during embryonic development; the atrioventricular valves later develop from it

    canal of Cuvier → *ductus venosus*

    pulmoaortic canal → *ductus arteriosus*

    Theile's canal → *transverse sinus of pericardium*

Candida *Syn: Monilia, Oidium*; a genus of yeast-like imperfect fungi with many species pathogenic to humans; they cause superficial and deep skin and mucosal mycoses, organ mycoses, catheter-associated infections, and septic clinical pictures; the most important species by far is Candida albicans; Candida glabrata, Candida krusei, Candida parapsilosis, and Candida tropicalis play a minor clinical role

    Candida albicans *Syn: thrush fungus, Saccharomyces albicans, Saccharomyces anginae, Zymonema albicans*; most frequent causative agent of fungal infections; it occurs worldwide as the causative agent of superficial and deep mycoses of skin and mucosa, organ mycoses, catheter-associated infections, and septic clinical pictures; promoting factors for an infection are HIV infection, immunosuppression, antibiotic therapy and chemotherapy, intravasal catheter, burns, and blood diseases; **diagnosis**: detection of the causative agent in blood, cerebrospinal fluid, urine, or biopsy material by culturing and microscopy; **ther-**

apy: in superficial infections, nystatin, amphotericin B, clotrimazole, or miconazole topically; in systemic involvement, amphotericin B [possibly together with flucytosine, fluconazole, ketoconazole] orally

candidiasis Syn: *Candida mycosis, thrush, thrush mycosis, moniliasis, moniliosis, oidomycosis, oidosis, candidosis*; localized or systemic mycosis caused by Candida species [usually Candida albicans]

disseminated candidiasis → *Candida sepsis*

endocardial candidiasis endocarditis caused by Candida albicans, which usually occurs on previously damaged or artificial heart valves; runs a subacute course with fever, lassitude, cardiac insufficiency, sometimes embolism

capacity storage ability or capability

O_2-binding capacity → *oxygen-binding capacity*

oxygen-binding capacity Syn: *O_2-binding capacity*; **1.** the **maximum oxygen-binding capacity** of hemoglobin is 1.39 ml of O_2/g of hemoglobin at 15°C and an oxygen partial pressure of 200 mmHg **2.** the **maximum oxygen-binding capacity** of the blood is 0.21 l of O_2/l of blood at 15°C and an oxygen partial pressure of 200 mmHg

capillarectasia congenital or acquired dilatation of capillaries

capillarioscopy → *capillaroscopy*

capillaritic relating to or marked by capillaritis

capillaritis inflammation of a capillary or changes in the capillaries in the region of inflammation

capillaroscopy Syn: *capillarioscopy, microangioscopy*; direct observation of surface capillaries with a capillary microscope

capillary Syn: *capillary vessel*; the smallest blood vessels, which lie between the arterial and venous sides of the circulation; they subserve the exchange of substances and gas between the tissues and the blood, or the blood and atmospheric air; the structure of capillaries is organ-specific, but all are in principle muscle-free endothelial tubes whose wall is strengthened by a basal membrane and pericytes; the endothelium consists of flat cells, between which there are occasional holes named **pores**; **fenestrations** are areas in which the cell body barely contains any cytoplasm and therefore only consists of cell membranes; pores and fenestrations make substance exchange with the environment easier

capsule case, envelope, or covering

adrenal capsule → *adrenal gland*

capsule of heart → *pericardial sac*

suprarenal capsule → *adrenal gland*

captopril ACE-antagonist; **usage:** hypertension, severe cardiac insufficiency

carazolol beta-blocker; **usage:** hypertension

carbapenems beta-lactam antibiotics with a very broad spectrum of action; barely susceptible to β-lactamase; e.g., imipenem

carbon dioxide *Syn: carbonic anhydride;* colorless, noncombustible gas, which below -70 °C has the form of carbon dioxide snow or dry ice; it is heavier than air; it is the anhydride of carbonic acid; in the human body it forms as the end product of the oxidation of carbon-containing compounds; it can be reused in part for biosynthesis, but for the most part is exhaled via the lungs or excreted as urea via the kidneys; it is part of the bicarbonate buffer system of the blood; carbon dioxide can be dissolved physically in the blood or be transported in a chemically bound form [bicarbonate]; arterial [or more aptly oxygenated] blood has a carbon dioxide partial pressure of 40 mmHg; if the partial pressure rises [hypercapnia], a reflex increase in the tidal volume and respiration rate occurs; under physiological conditions, the so-called CO_2 **ventilation response** is the most effective and major breathing drive; the proportion of carbon dioxide in air is about 0.03% [0.2 mmHg], in the alveolar gas mixture 5.6% [40 mmHg], and in exhaled air 4% [29 mmHg]; if the proportion of carbon dioxide in the breathing air rises above 8–10%, headache, dyspnea, tinnitus, and an increase in blood pressure occur; a further increase leads to loss of consciousness or coma [hypoventilation coma or carbon dioxide narcosis] and death [above 12%]

carbonic anhydride → *carbon dioxide*

carbon monoxide *Syn: sweet gas;* colorless, odorless, flammable gas; extremely poisonous; the toxicity relates to hemoglobin's 300-fold higher affinity for carbon monoxide than oxygen; this means that even small amounts of carbon monoxide produce major reductions in the oxygen carrying capacity of the blood; in addition, carbon monoxide also blocks myoglobin and other iron-containing proteins

carcinomatosis *Syn: carcinosis;* diffuse invasion of the entire body, an organ, or a body cavity with carcinoma metastases

pericardial carcinomatosis *Syn: carcinous pericarditis;* carcinosis of the pericardial sac leading to (hemorrhagic) effusion and possibly pericardial tamponade

cardenolides glycosides containing a simple unsaturated γ-lactone ring, active on the heart

cardia- combining form denoting relation to the heart

cardiac 1. imprecise generic term for substances that act on the heart; these include, among others, cardiac glycosides and antiarrhythmics as well as herbal agents [arnica] **2.** relating to the heart

cardiagra → *angina pectoris*

cardialgia → *cardiodynia*

cardiasthma → *cardiac asthma*

cardiectasis *Syn: dilation of heart*; dilatation of the heart chambers or the whole heart; occurs both as a physiologic adaptation to high levels of exertion [athlete's heart] as well as pathologically in chronic volume or pressure overload [e.g., aortic insufficiency] as well as in cardiomyopathy

cardioangiology *Syn: cardiovasology*; field of internal medicine, which relates to the diagnosis and treatment of diseases of the heart and vessels

cardioaortic relating to aorta and heart

Cardiobacterium hominis *s.u. HACEK group*

cardiocele → *ectocardia*

cardiocentesis *Syn: cardiopuncture, paracentesis of heart*; puncture of a ventricle to remove blood or for injection of medications

cardiocinetic → *cardiokinetic*

cardiocirrhosis → *cardiac cirrhosis*

cardiodiaphragmatic relating to diaphragm and heart

cardiodynia *Syn: cardialgia*; non-specific description of pain in the heart or its vicinity, e.g., in angina pectoris; radiation into the left arm, shoulder, hand, or into the lower jaw is typical of organic heart pain; differentiation from psychogenic pain [cardiac neurosis] is often difficult

cardiogenesis pre- and postnatal heart development

cardiogenic 1. of cardiac origin **2.** relating to cardiogenesis

cardiogram X-ray contrast imaging of the heart chambers

  apex cardiogram → *apexcardiogram*

  esophageal cardiogram ECG recording from electrodes in the esophagus

cardiograph apparatus for cardiography

cardiographic relating to cardiography

cardiography 1. generic term for procedures for demonstrating or recording the structure or function of the heart **2.** X-ray contrast demonstration of the heart chambers; mostly in the form of angiocardiography

ultrasonic cardiography ultrasound examination; non-invasive technique in which electrical energy is converted into sound waves with a frequency of 2–10 MHz; absorption, reflection, and refraction of the sound waves in the tissues generate specific images that are displayed on a screen; three different processes are used in clinical practice: M-mode, 2-D echocardiography [B-mode imaging], and Doppler sonography; echocardiography is predominantly used to assess the pericardium, myocardium, endocardium, and heart valves

cardiohepatic relating to liver and heart

cardiohepatomegaly enlargement of the heart and liver

cardioinhibitory inhibiting the activity of the heart

cardiokinetic *Syn: cardiocinetic;* **1.** an agent with cardiokinetic properties **2.** stimulating the activity of the heart

cardiokymographic relating to cardiokymography

cardiokymography recording of the heart movements with an electrokymograph

cardiolipin → *diphosphatidylglycerol*

cardiology field of internal medicine relating to the diagnosis and treatment of the heart

cardiolysis operative freeing of the heart, mobilization of the heart

cardiomegalia → *cardiomegaly*

cardiomegaly *Syn: cardiomegalia, megacardia, megalocardia;* non-specific description of heart enlargement in hypertrophy, hyperplasia, cardiomyopathy, etc.

cardiomuscular relating to the cardiac muscle

cardiomyopathy *Syn: myocardiopathy;* generic term for diseases of the heart muscle, which lead to impairment of cardiac function; previously, this included heart diseases, which are not caused by congenital or acquired heart defects, diseases of the pericardium, arterial or pulmonary hypertension, or coronary arteriosclerosis and which lead to hypertrophy of the myocardium; the division into **primary** and **secondary cardiomyopathies** is no longer used; the currently applicable classification differentiates **dilated, hypertrophic, restrictive, specific,** and **unclassified cardiomyopathies**; in addition, **arrhythmogenic right ventricular cardiomyopathy** is a separate entity; the **clinical picture** is, in all types, one of increasing cardiac insufficiency and enlargement of the heart; **therapy**: varies depending upon the type; often a heart transplant is eventually required

alcoholic cardiomyopathy dilated cardiomyopathy caused by chronic alcohol intake

arrhythmogenic right ventricular cardiomyopathy autosomal dominant disease with incomplete penetration; mainly affects young men and leads to an increasing replacement of heart muscle tissue by fat and connective tissue; begins in the right ventricle and later also involves the left ventricle; **clinical**: right heart hypertrophy with ventricular and supraventricular tachycardias and syncopes; rarely, there may be sudden cardiac death [3% of all unexpected deaths in performance athletes]; **therapy**: symptomatic treatment of the right cardiac insufficiency, heart transplantation

dilated cardiomyopathy generic term for cardiomyopathies, which lead to enlargement of the ventricle, reduction of the left ventricular ejection fraction, and increasing impairment of cardiac function; these include both idiopathic and familial, inflammatory, toxic [alcohol toxicity cardiomyopathy], and other forms of specific cardiomyopathies

hypertensive cardiomyopathy cardiomyopathy in arterial hypertension, which leads to an unexplained impairment of function

hypertrophic cardiomyopathy cardiomyopathy with hypertrophy predominantly of the left ventricle and the ventricular septum; can occur with [hypertrophic obstructive cardiomyopathy] or without obstruction to the outflow tract [hypertrophic non-obstructive cardiomyopathy]; has a familial clustering; 50% are inherited in autosomal dominant fashion; **clinical**: angina pectoris, air hunger, transient alterations in consciousness up to syncope

hypertrophic nonobstructive cardiomyopathy hypertrophic cardiomyopathy without impairment of outflow

hypertrophic obstructive cardiomyopathy hypertrophic cardiomyopathy with impairment of outflow

inflammatory cardiomyopathy in principle, a chronic myocarditis with dilatation of the ventricle and progressive dysfunction; usually caused by chronic viral or autoimmune myocarditis

metabolic cardiomyopathy specific cardiomyopathy in endocrine diseases [diabetes mellitus, hyperthyroidism, pheochromocytoma], storage disorders, or neuromuscular diseases

primary cardiomyopathy cardiomyopathy without identifiable cause; most commonly a dilated or hypertrophic cardiomyopathy

restrictive cardiomyopathy cardiomyopathy due to an impairment in the compliance of the ventricle; mostly a secondary cardiomyopathy, such as, e.g., in endomyocardial fibrosis, amyloidosis, sarcoidosis, hemochromatosis, or Löffler's endocarditis; the **therapy** consists of treating the underlying cause; the cardiac insufficiency can sometimes be improved by digitalis and diuretics

secondary cardiomyopathy *s.u. cardiomyopathy*

thyroid cardiomyopathy *Syn: cardiothyrotoxicosis, thyrocardiac disease, thyrotoxic heart disease*; damage to the heart caused by untreated hyperthyroidism

cardionatrin → *atrial natriuretic peptide*

cardionecrosis → *myocardial necrosis*

cardionephric → *cardiorenal*

cardioneural *Syn: neurocardiac*; relating to both heart and nervous system

cardioneurosis → *cardiac neurosis*

cardiopathic relating to or characterized by disease of the heart

cardiopathy *Syn: heart disease, heart disorder, cardiopathia*; any disease or disorder of the heart

arteriosclerotic cardiopathy cardiopathy caused by arteriosclerosis of the heart vessels

cardiopericarditic relating to or marked by cardiopericarditis

cardiopericarditis simultaneous inflammation of the heart (muscle) and pericardium

cardiophobia pathologic fear of a heart attack due to a real or imagined heart disease

cardiophobic relating to or marked by cardiophobia

cardiophrenia → *neurocirculatory asthenia*

cardioplegia (artificially induced) cardiac standstill

cardioplegic relating to cardioplegia

cardioptosia → *bathycardia*

cardioptosis → *bathycardia*

cardiopulmonary *Syn: pneumocardial*; relating to or associated with the heart and lung(s)

cardiopuncture → *cardiocentesis*

cardiorenal *Syn: nephrocardiac, cardionephric*; relating to heart and kidney(s)

cardiorespiratory relating to the heart and respiration

cardiorrhaphy *Syn: myocardiorrhaphy*; suturing of the heart wall or muscles after traumatic or operative division or incision

cardiorrhexis → *rupture of the myocardial wall*
cardiosclerosis fibrosis and hardening of the heart muscle tissue leading to cardiac insufficiency
cardiosclerotic relating to or marked by cardiosclerosis
cardioselective with selective action on the heart
cardiothyrotoxicosis → *thyroid cardiomyopathy*
cardiotomy opening of the ventricles or atria
cardiotonic 1. agent with cardiotonic properties **2.** strengthening the action of the heart
cardiotoxic damaging the heart, causing heart damage
cardiovalvotomy → *valvotomy*
cardiovalvulotomy → *valvotomy*
cardiovascular *Syn: vasculocardiac*; relating to heart and circulation or blood vessels
cardiovasology → *cardioangiology*
cardioversion *Syn: electroversion*; normalization of the heart rhythm with medication or electric current; defibrillation, ventricular fibrillation
    electric cardioversion process related to electro-defibrillation used to treat atrial fibrillation and atrial flutter; the DC shock is triggered from the P-wave of the ECG and restores the normal sinus rhythm; mostly used intraoperatively or on the intensive care unit
cardioverter → *defibrillator*
    implantable cardioverter-defibrillator ICD is predominantly used in the treatment of non-persistent ventricular tachycardia
carditic relating to or marked by carditis
carditis inflammation of the heart; generic term for endocarditis, myocarditis, pericarditis, and pancarditis
carotid *Syn: carotid artery*; either of the two large arteries that carry blood to the head
    common carotid → *common carotid artery*
    external carotid → *external carotid artery*
    internal carotid → *internal carotid artery*
carteolol beta-blocker; **usage**: hypertension
carvedilol highly potent non-selective 3rd generation beta-blocker and alpha-blocker; reduces the systolic and diastolic blood pressures at rest and during exercise as well as the heart rate; improves left ventricular contractility by reducing the afterload; **usage**: arterial hypertension, coronary heart disease, cardiac insufficiency
catarrh inflammation of a mucous membrane, usually with increased

discharge of mucus or exudate

suffocative catarrh →*asthma*

catheter a flexible or rigid hollow tube used to drain fluids from body cavities or to distend body passages

angiographic catheter catheter for (selective) angiography

balloon catheter *Syn: balloon-tipped catheter*; tube with an inflatable terminal balloon

balloon-tipped catheter →*balloon catheter*

central venous catheter *Syn: central line*; catheter mostly introduced via the arm or jugular vein, which is placed in the superior or inferior vena cava; allows one to measure the central venous pressure, infuse hyperosmolar solutions [e.g., in high calorie infusions], administer intravenous drugs, which might damage peripheral veins [e.g., cytostatics], inject cardioactive drugs, and sample central venous blood

flow-directed catheter catheter that is floated toward the heart by the blood flow after introduction into a vein; flotation catheters can remain in the body for several days; they are mainly used for blood sampling, intracardiac pressure measurement, and ECG recording

left heart catheter *s.u. cardiac catheterization*

pulmonary artery catheter is introduced through the jugular veins and superior vena cava into the right atrium and then threaded through the bloodstream into the right or left pulmonary artery; it permits the measurement of several circulatory parameters, such as wedge pressure, central venous pressure, and cardiac output, as well as the drawing of central venous blood

right heart catheter *s.u. cardiac catheterization*

Swan-Ganz catheter double lumen balloon flotation catheter, which is used to measure the pulmonary artery pressure and the pressure in the right atrium

venous catheter *Syn: venous line*; catheter inserted into a vein

catheterization *Syn: catheterism*; introduction of a catheter into the body

cardiac catheterization introduction of a thin catheter into the heart chambers after puncture of a vein [**right heart catheterization**] or artery [**left heart catheterization**] for direct pressure measurement, removal of samples, injection of contrast agents, etc.

cavitas *Syn: cavum*; cavity, hollow space, space

cavitas pericardiaca →*pericardial cavity*

cavity a hollow place

chest cavity *Syn: thoracic cavity, pectoral cavity*; the space within the thorax that contains the chest organs [lung, heart]; it is separated below from the abdominal cavity by the diaphragm; the mediastinum divides the chest cavity into a left and right half for the two lungs, and a central area for the heart, thymus, esophagus, and vascular trunks

mediastinal cavity → *mediastinum*

pericardial cavity cleft between the epicardium and the pericardium filled with serous fluid [**liquor pericardii**]

thoracic cavity → *chest cavity*

cefacetrile i.m. or i.v. cephalosporin

cefaclor oral cephalosporin

cefadroxil oral cephalosporin

cefalexin *Syn: cephalexin*; oral cephalosporin

cefalotin i.m. or i.v. cephalosporin

cefamandole i.m. or i.v. cephalosporin used only in rare cases

cefazedone second-generation cephalosporin

cefazolin i.v. cephalosporin

cefepime cephalosporin with a broad action spectrum, effective primarily against gram-positive causative agents

cefixime oral cephalosporin

cefmenoxime oral cephalosporin

cefoperazone third-generation cephalosporin

cefotaxime i.v. cephalosporin

cefotetan second-generation cephalosporin

cefotiam i.v. cephalosporin

cefoxitin i.v. cephalosporin

cefsulodin cephalosporin effective only against Pseudomonas aeruginosa

ceftazidime i.v. cephalosporin

ceftizoxime i.v. cephalosporin

ceftriaxone i.v. cephalosporin

cefuroxime i.v. cephalosporin

cell smallest unit of living tissue, consisting of a nucleus, cytoplasm and a cell membrane

Abbé-Zeiss counting cell → *Thoma-Zeiss counting cell*

adventitial cells *Syn: pericapillary cells, pericytes, perithelial cells*; macrophages in the blood vessel wall

Anichkov's cell → *Anichkov's myocyte*

Anitschkow's cell → *Anichkov's myocyte*

B cells → *B-lymphocytes*

blood cells *Syn: blood corpuscles, hemocytes*; umbrella term for cells present in blood, i.e., **red blood cells** [erythrocytes], **white blood cells** [leukocytes], and **platelets**, and their precursors

blood mast cells basophilic granulocytes containing heparin and histamine in the granules

carrier cell → *phagocyte*

caterpillar cell → *Anichkov's myocyte*

commited stem cell *s.u. blood formation*

foam cells *Syn: xanthoma cells*; *s.u. xanthoma*

heart-disease cells → *heart-failure cells*

heart-lesion cells → *heart-failure cells*

heart-failure cells *Syn: heart-disease cells, heart-lesion cells, siderophages, siderophores*; alveolar macrophages laden with hemosiderin and occurring in the sputum in heart-related pulmonary congestion

heart muscle cell *Syn: myocardial cell*; *s.u. cardiac muscle*

helmet cell *Syn: schistocyte, schizocyte*; small, malformed erythrocytes; arise by splitting off other erythrocytes or are remnants of erythrocytes, from which portions have been cleaved; found predominantly as a result of mechanical damage [artificial heart valves], anemia, and hemolysis

hemopoietic stem cell *Syn: hematoblast, hematocytoblast, hemoblast, hemocytoblast, stem cell*; pluripotent stem cells in the bone marrow

lymphatic stem cell *s.u. blood formation*

muscle cell *Syn: myocyte*; *s.u. muscle tissue*

myeloic stem cell *s.u. blood formation*

myocardial cell *Syn: heart muscle cell*; *s.u. cardiac muscle*

packed blood cells *Syn: packed human blood cells*; concentrates of individual constituent cell types derived from whole blood, e.g., **red cell concentrate, thrombocyte concentrate, leukocyte concentrate**

packed human blood cells → *packed blood cells*

packed human red cells → *packed red cells*

packed red cells *Syn: packed human red cells*; there are various erythrocyte concentrates that differ in their residual content of leukocytes, thrombocytes, and plasma as well as in the additives used in them; **filtered erythrocyte concentrates** contain practically no more leukocytes and thrombocytes [**leukocyte free erythrocyte concentrate**], whereas **leukocyte depleted erythrocyte concentrates** still contain a certain number of leukocytes; **washed erythrocyte concentrates** are made by triple flotation in physiologic salt solutions; they are used in patients with protein hypersensitivity

pericapillary cells → *adventitial cells*
perithelial cells → *adventitial cells*
pluripotent stem cell *s.u. blood formation*
precursor cell *Syn: precursor, progenitor; s.u. blood formation*
red blood cells → *erythrocytes*
Rouget's cells *Syn: capillary pericytes, spider cells*; adventitial cells of the blood capillaries
spider cells → *Rouget's cells*
stem cells *Syn: hematoblasts, hematocytoblasts, hemoblasts, hemocytoblasts, hemopoietic stem cells*; pluripotent cells, from which [mostly under the influence of specific growth factors] differentiated cells, e.g., parenchymal cells, are derived
Thoma-Zeiss counting cell *Syn: Abbé-Zeiss apparatus, Abbé-Zeiss counting cell, Abbé-Zeiss counting chamber, Thoma-Zeiss counting chamber, Thoma-Zeiss hemocytometer*; counting chamber for red blood corpuscles
vasofactive cell → *angioblast*
vasoformative cell → *angioblast*
white blood cells → *leukocytes*
xanthoma cells *Syn: foam cells; s.u. xanthoma*

central aortic pressure blood pressure within the aorta; considered to be a stronger indicator of cardiovascular risk in hypertensive patients than blood pressure in peripheral arteries, such as brachial blood pressure

cephalexin → *cefalexin*

cephalosporin β-lactam antibiotic, related to penicillin, with bactericidal activity against gram-positive and gram-negative bacteria in the growth phase; cephalosporins are usually subdivided into **first-generation cephalosporins**, **second-generation cephalosporins**, and **third-generation cephalosporins** [also **broad-spectrum cephalosporins**]; **first-generation cephalosporins** [e.g., cefazolin] exhibit good activity against gram-positive and gram-negative microorganisms, and are resistant to penicillinase-producing staphylococci; **second-generation cephalosporins** [e.g., cefamandole, cefuroxime, cefotiam] are largely β-lactamase-resistant; they are more effective against, e.g., Escherichia coli, Enterobacteriaceae, Haemophilus influenzae, and Neisseria gonorrhoeae than the first-generation cephalosporins but less effective against gram-positive cocci; **third-generation cephalosporins** [e.g., cefotaxime, ceftriaxone, ceftizoxime] have a lower activity than first- and second-generation cephalosporins but are much more resistant to β-lactamase; **side effects:** allergic reactions [caution: cross-reaction in penicillin allergy!], gastrointestinal symptoms, hepatic dysfunction, nephrotoxicity; **contraindications:** allergy to cephalosporins

cephalosporinase enzyme cleaving the β-lactam ring of cephalosporins

cephradine oral cephalosporin

cerebrocardiac relating to brain and heart

cerebrovascular relating to the blood vessels of the brain

cessation arrest, standstill

   cessation of breathing → *apnea*

chain a series of objects connected one after the other

   respiratory chain *Syn: cytochrome system*; multi-enzyme system localized in the mitochondria of the cells, which oxidizes hydrogen with oxygen in stages to make water; the energy this produces is released as heat or stored in high-energy bonds [ATP, ADP]

chamber a compartment or enclosed space

   Abbé-Zeiss counting chamber → *Thoma-Zeiss counting cell*

   climate chamber chamber in which the temperature, air pressure, and humidity can be set to predefined values; it is used, for example, for the treatment of bronchial asthma and other allergic diseases

   pressure chamber chamber for treatment with air or oxygen under increased pressure

   Thoma-Zeiss counting chamber → *Thoma-Zeiss counting cell*

chemo- combining form denoting relation to chemistry or a chemical

chemoceptor → *chemoreceptor*

chemoprophylaxis *Syn: chemical prophylaxis*; prophylaxis against infection using chemotherapeutic agents

chemoreception reception of chemical stimuli by specific receptors

chemoreceptive sensitive to or perceiving chemical stimuli

chemoreceptor *Syn: chemoceptor*; receptor especially adapted to chemical stimuli; **arterial** and **central chemoreceptors** play an important role in the control of respiration; they monitor the CO_2 and O_2 partial pressure and the blood pH and adjust the respiratory minute volume to requirements

chemoreflex reflex initiated by stimulation of a chemoreceptor, e.g., respiratory reflex

chemoresistance resistance of bacteria to chemotherapeutic agents

chemosensitive susceptible to changes in chemical composition

chemosensitivity susceptibility to changes in chemical composition

chemosensor sensor sensitive to chemical stimuli

chemosuppression prophylactic prescription of antibiotics during the incubation period in order to suppress the illness or weaken its course

chemotherapeutic relating to chemotherapy, by means of chemotherapy

chlorthalidone saluretic

cholesteremia → *hypercholesterolemia*

cholesterin → *cholesterol*

cholesterinemia → *hypercholesterolemia*

cholesterinosis → *cholesterolosis*

cholesterinuria → *cholesteroluria*

cholesterol *Syn:* cholesterin; steroid alcohol occurring in free and esterified forms in the body; building block for steroid hormones and bile acids; excreted in the bile and mostly then reabsorbed [**enterohepatic circulation**]; the majority of the daily requirement of approx. 1 g is made in the body [**endogenous cholesterol**], the rest is taken in through the diet [animal fat, **exogenous cholesterol**] and is transported from the intestines to the liver by chylomicrons; from the liver, cholesterol is transported in low-density lipoproteins to the peripheral tissues; excess cholesterol is transported back to the liver by high-density lipoproteins, where it is metabolized to bile acids and excreted; since cholesterol is a basic constituent of all animal cell membranes, it is assumed that all cells can synthesize cholesterol; disorders of cholesterol metabolism can lead to hypo- or hypercholesterolemia; primary hypocholesterolemia is relatively common and clinically silent; it does, however, protect the patient from coronary heart disease; primary and secondary hypercholesterolemia are significantly more common [20–25% of the population has elevated serum cholesterol values] and they play a significant role in causing disease and [indirectly] death

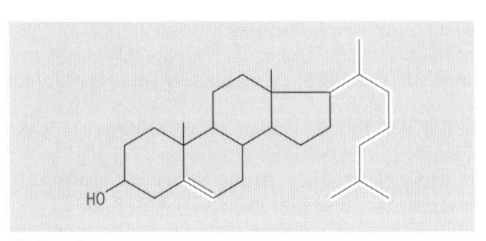

Cholesterol

cholesterolase *Syn: cholesterol esterase*; enzyme formed in the pancreas, which breaks down cholesterol ester into cholesterol and fatty acids, making it absorbable

cholesterolemia → *hypercholesterolemia*

cholesterol ester ester of cholesterol and higher fatty acids occurring in the body

cholesterol esterase → *cholesterolase*

cholesterolosis *Syn: cholesterinosis, cholesterosis*; deposition of cholesterol in the tissues

cholesteroluria *Syn: cholesterinuria*; cholesterol excretion in the urine

cholesterosis → *cholesterolosis*

choline *Syn: sinkaline*; a natural amine

   choline phosphoglyceride → *phosphatidylcholine*

choline phosphatidyl → *phosphatidylcholine*

chromone → *coumarin*

chromones → *coumarins*

chronotropic influencing the time course; (*heart*) influencing the beat frequency

chylomicron *Syn: lipomicron*; lipoprotein particles made in the intestinal mucosa for transporting triglycerides in the blood

chylomicronemia → *hyperchylomicronemia*

chylopericarditic relating to or marked by chylopericarditis

chylopericarditis pericardial inflammation [pericarditis] due to a chylous effusion

chylopericardium chylous effusion in the pericardium

cicletanine diuretic, antihypertensive

cineangiocardiography cineradiography of the heart and great blood vessels

cineangiography cineradiography of contrast-filled blood vessels

cinecardiography cineradiography of the heart

cinedensitometry method of determining the sequence of movements in vessels or the heart using photoelectric measurement of the changes in darkening of cine X-ray films

cinephlebography phlebography with serial imaging

ciprofloxacin gyrase inhibitor; **indications**: urinary tract infections, respiratory tract infections, bacterial prostatitis, bacterial bone and joint inflammations, and nosocomial infections; **side effects**: gastrointestinal symptoms, CNS disorders, dizziness, seizures

circadian (spread) over the whole day, lasting or encompassing about

24 hours

circle *Syn: circulus, ring*; circular or ring-shaped formation

arterial circle arterial anastomotic ring

arterial circle of cerebrum *Syn: circle of Willis*; anastomosis between the basilar and internal carotid arteries at the base of the brain

circle of Willis → *arterial circle of cerebrum*

circulation *Syn: circulatory system, blood circulation*; the blood circulation in the body or the cardiovascular system as a functional unity of the heart and blood vessels; the compartment of the circulation that takes blood from the right ventricle to the lungs and back to the left ventricle is called the **lesser circulation** or **pulmonary circulation**; it contains deoxygenated blood in the first compartment [right ventricle – lungs] and oxygenated blood in the second compartment [lungs – left ventricle]; the **greater circulation** or **systemic circulation** takes oxygenated blood from the left ventricle to the body's peripheral areas and deoxygenated blood from the periphery back to right ventricle; the heart is situated as the pump between the two circulatory compartments; both circulatory compartments have arteries, arterioles, capillaries, venules, and veins; in contrast to the systemic circulation, the arteries of the pulmonary circulation carry deoxygenated blood and the veins, oxygenated blood

blood circulation → *circulation*

collateral circulation *Syn: compensatory circulation*; bypass circulation developing in the setting of disturbed perfusion, which uses naturally present collateral vessels [**preformed collaterals**]; the development of a collateral circulation in the coronary area is important, since the coronary arteries are functional end-arteries; the more extensive the collateral circulation is [**degree of collateralization**], the longer a narrowing of the coronary arteries can be compensated for and the smaller the infarct volume is during acute myocardial infarction; the speed of development of collaterals in man is not known; in animal experiments, it is improved by physical training and certain drugs [dipyridamide, hexobendine]; it has not yet been possible to confirm these findings in man

compensatory circulation → *collateral circulation*

extracorporeal circulation blood diversion, e.g., during open heart surgery

fetal circulation in the fetal circulation, the oxygenated [arterial] blood flows from the placenta through the umbilical vein and the ductus venosus into the inferior vena cava, where it mixes in part with the venous blood from the systemic circulation; most of the arterial blood flows through the oval foramen into the left atrium and is pumped through the left chamber into the aorta; the rest is circulated as mixed blood through the right ventricle into the pulmonary artery; a portion reaches the lungs and the rest flows through the arterial duct into the aorta, which thereby takes mixed blood to the body's peripheral areas; but the brain of the fetus receives oxygenated blood; after birth, there is an increase in the resistance in the systemic circulation and, with the development of the lungs, a decline in the pressure in the pulmonary circulation; the increase in pressure in the left atrium closes the oval foramen and the blood is pumped out of the right atrium through the right ventricle into the pulmonary circulation; the ductus venosus and arteriosus are obliterated by the loss of the umbilical vein flow or the rise in arterial oxygen partial pressure

greater circulation *Syn: systemic circulation, major circulation*; *s.u. circulation*

lesser circulation →*pulmonary circulation*

major circulation →*greater circulation*

minor circulation →*pulmonary circulation*

pulmonary circulation *Syn: lesser circulation, minor circulation*; *s.u. circulation*

systemic circulation *s.u. circulation*

circulatory relating to the circulation

circulus circle, ring, circular or ring-shaped formation

circulus arteriosus →*arterial circle*

circulus arteriosus cerebri →*arterial circle of cerebrum*

circulus vasculosus vascular circle

circumvascular *Syn: perivascular*; situated or occurring around a vessel

circumventricular situated or occurring around a ventricle

cirrhose cardiaque →*cardiac cirrhosis*

cirrhosis *Syn: fibroid induration, granular induration*; chronic interstitial inflammation of any tissue or organ

cardiac cirrhosis *Syn: cardiac liver, cardiocirrhosis, congestive cirrhosis, congestive cirrhosis of liver, pseudocirrhosis, cyanotic atrophy of liver, stasis cirrhosis, stasis cirrhosis of liver*; engorgement of the liver caused by right heart insufficiency with distension of the periportal septa; no cirrhosis in the pathologic/anatomic sense

congestive cirrhosis →*cardiac cirrhosis*

congestive cirrhosis of liver → *cardiac cirrhosis*
stasis cirrhosis → *cardiac cirrhosis*
stasis cirrhosis of liver → *cardiac cirrhosis*

classification the act, process, or result of classifying
  Fontaine's classification *s.u. chronic arterial occlusive disease*
  Lown classification classification of the tachycardic ventricular arrhythmias based on an ECG trace
  Stanford classification *s.u. aortic dissection*

claudication limping, lameness
  intermittent claudication *Syn: angina cruris, Charcot's syndrome, intermittent claudication of the leg*; severe calf pain caused by impaired peripheral arterial perfusion, which forces the patient to limp temporarily or else to stand still; corresponds to stage II of chronic peripheral arterial occlusive disease; if the claudication can be tolerated by the patient, it is called stage IIa, if it cannot be tolerated for personal or professional reasons, then stage IIb; this differentiation is important for therapy, since stage IIa can be managed conservatively [removal of risk factors, systematic vessel training, medical prophylaxis against progression], whereas stage IIb usually requires surgical intervention [percutaneous transluminal angioplasty, stent implantation, bypass]
  intermittent claudication of the leg → *intermittent claudication*
  jaw claudication *Syn: masseteric claudication*; *s.u. Horton's arteritis*
  masseteric claudication *Syn: jaw claudication*; *s.u. Horton's arteritis*

clavulanic acid substance formed by **Streptomyces clavuligerus**, which works as a powerful, irreversible inhibitor of β-lactamase and thus increases the susceptibility of bacteria to β-lactam antibiotics

cleft a space or opening made by cleavage; split, fissure
  synaptic cleft *Syn: synaptic gap*; *s.u. chemical synapse*

click high-frequency additional heart sound, e.g., appearing as an **early systolic click** or **ejection click** at the start of the ejection phase, and as a **late systolic click**, predominantly in mitral valve prolapse syndrome
  ejection click heart sound at the start of the ejection phase

clindamycin oral and i.v. macrolide antibiotic; **indications**: infections with gram-positive and gram-negative causative agent [Actinomyces, Borrelia, Clostridium, Corynebacterium, Staphylococcus, Streptococcus, Chlamydia]; **side effects**: antibiotic-associated enterocolitis, gastrointestinal symptoms, leukopenia, elevation of GOT, alkaline phosphatase, and bilirubin

clip a device that grips and holds tightly

vena caval clip *s.u. vena caval block*

clipping *s.u. intracranial aneurysm*

clock an instrument for measuring and recording time

biological clock internal timekeeper, which synchronizes the circadian rhythms of the body

clonidine peripheral and central α_2-sympathomimetic, antihypertensive; **usage**: hypertension, hypertensive crisis, migraine prophylaxis, eye drops for glaucoma, alcohol withdrawal delirium; **side effects**: dry mouth, drowsiness, color vision, disturbances of accommodation

clonospasm → *clonus*

clonus *Syn: clonic spasm, clonospasm*; rhythmic cramping muscle contraction

clopamide saluretic; **usage**: edema, hypertension

clopidogrel ADP-antagonist, inhibitor of thrombocyte aggregation; **usage**: acute myocardial infarction, usually in combination with acetylsalicylic acid

clot 1. → *blood clot* **2.** → *thrombus*

bacon-rind clot *Syn: chicken fat clot, chicken fat thrombus*; yellow-white cadaveric clot consisting of fibrin, blood platelets, and leukocytes

blood clot *Syn: clot, coagulation, coagulum, crassamentum, cruor*; fibrin net containing entrapped erythrocytes, leukocytes and thrombocytes, which forms during blood clotting

chicken fat clot → *bacon-rind clot*

fibrin clot *Syn: fibrin coagulum*; net-like coagulum forming during blood clotting; also a description for fibrin layering in fibrinous inflammation

mixed clot combination thrombus consisting of a white head and a red tail

postmortem clot intravascular blood clotting occurring after death; mostly red, moist-slick, rubbery, elastic, and flabby

washed clot *Syn: conglutination-agglutination thrombus, laminated thrombus, mixed thrombus, pale thrombus, white clot, plain thrombus, white thrombus*; thrombus arising on the injured vessel wall, which is covered on the outside by a grey-white layer of leukocytes

white clot → *washed clot*

clotting → *blood coagulation*

blood clotting → *blood coagulation*

cloxacillin penicillinase-resistant, bactericidal antibiotic; it is effective against gram-positive and gram-negative microorganisms

coagulability the quality [mainly of the blood] of being coagulable

coagulable able to clot

coagulant 1. clot forming agent **2.** promoting coagulation

coagulase enzyme formed by Staphylococcus aureus, among others, which binds to prothrombin and directly catalyzes the formation of fibrin from fibrinogen; thereby promotes the formation of a fibrin capsule in infections

coagulation 1. clotting **2.** → *blood coagulation*

blood coagulation *Syn: blood clotting, clotting, coagulation*; blood clotting is the second step in the staunching of bleeding and is therefore also known as **secondary hemostasis**; in 1905, Paul Morawitz had already described a classical schema for blood clotting, which is still valid today; over time, however, it has become clear that there are two different mechanisms of activation of the so-called clotting cascade, one the **intrinsic pathway** or **intravascular system**, which is activated within minutes, and an **extrinsic pathway** or **extravascular system**, which is active within seconds of a tissue injury; factor X forms the final common pathway of the extrinsic and intrinsic pathways; its active form [factor Xa] together with factor V, calcium ions, and phospholipids forms a complex called prothrombin kinase, which catalyzes the conversion of prothrombin to thrombin; thrombin itself catalyzes the formation of fibrin monomers from fibrinogen; the soluble fibrin monomers align themselves under the influence of electrostatic forces to make fibrin polymers; in the presence of factor XIIIa and Ca ions, the monomers are linked by covalent bonds and insoluble fibrin polymers are formed

diffuse intravascular coagulation → *disseminated intravascular coagulation*

disseminated intravascular coagulation *Syn: consumption coagulopathy, diffuse intravascular coagulation, disseminated intravascular coagulation syndrome*; in consumptive coagulopathy, intravascular activation of blood clotting leads to increased formation of fibrin thrombi, which leads to microthrombosis; at the same time, there is a reactive increase in fibrinolysis and thereby an increased consumption of clotting factors, fibrinolysis factors, and thrombocytes, which leads to an increased bleeding tendency; disseminated intravascular coagulation is not a disease as such, rather only the consequence of an underlying disease [e.g., sepsis, septic abortion]; it can, however, lead to life-threatening organ failure due to thrombosis of the microcirculation and massive bleeding; it can be divided into three phases: in the **initial phase** or **activation phase** consists of a compensated hypercoagulability with formation of fibrin thrombi; during the **early consumption phase**, a deficiency of clotting factors with disturbance of hemostasis and/or microcirculation develops due to thrombosis; the **late consumption phase** shows the complete picture of reactive hyperfibrinolysis and clotting disturbance with bleeding; **diagnosis:** determination of the clotting parameters [Quick, PTT, fibrinogen, bleeding time, thrombin time, D-dimers, AT-III]; **therapy:** treatment of the hematologic disturbance, intensive medical management of shock, and treatment of the underlying cause

coagulator apparatus for thermocoagulation, e.g., **coagulation electrodes**

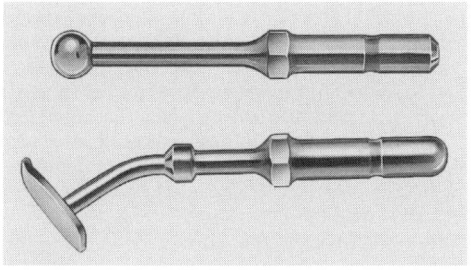

Coagulators

coagulo- combining form denoting relation to clotting or coagulation

coagulopathy congenital or acquired disturbance of blood clotting; disturbances that lead to a bleeding tendency are described as **minus coagulopathies**, disturbances with an increased clotting tendency are correspondingly described as **plus coagulopathies**
  consumption coagulopathy → *disseminated intravascular coagulation*
  deficiency coagulopathy coagulopathy due to an inborn deficiency of one or more clotting factors, e.g., afibrinogenemia, hemophilia A
  dilution coagulopathy increased bleeding tendency caused by an increase in the fluid content of the blood

coagulum → *blood clot*

fibrin coagulum → *fibrin clot*

coarctation narrowing, constriction

adult type aortic coarctation stenosis distal to the opening of the ductus arteriosus leads, despite the formation of a collateral blood supply, to underperfusion of the lower half of the body and to an increase in the blood pressure above the stenosis; in the long term, this leads to left ventricular hypertrophy and subsequent cardiac insufficiency; the **therapy** of choice is resection of the stenosis with end-to-end anastomosis; balloon dilatation with stent implantation is increasingly used and shows good long-term results

coarctation of aorta → *aortic isthmus stenosis*

aortic coarctation → *aortic isthmus stenosis*

infantile type aortic coarctation form of stenosis of the aorta before the origin of the ductus arteriosus, which becomes clinically manifest in infancy; the patent ductus leads to a right-to-left shunt with cyanosis of the lower half of the body, (usually) pulmonary hypertension and prerenal renal failure; the **diagnosis** is based upon the clinical picture, blood pressure, and pulse differences between the upper and lower extremities, auscultation [pansystolic flow murmur in the left parasternal region], ECG [right ventricular strain], echocardiography [among other factors, determination of the degree of stenosis]; **therapy**: maintenance of patency of the ductus of Botallo by infusion of prostaglandin E_1; balloon dilatation of the stenosis; later stent implantation to prevent restenosis

reversed coarctation → *brachiocephalic arteritis*

coat a layer that covers a surface

adventitial coat → *adventitia*

buffy coat layer consisting of leukocytes and thrombocytes at the boundary layer between plasma and erythrocytes in preserved blood

external coat → *tunica externa*

serous coat of serous pericard the serosa of the serous pericardium coated in serous fluid [**liquor pericardii**] filling the **pericardial cavity**

coefficient a constant number that serves as a measure of some property or characteristic

erythrocyte color coefficient → *mean corpuscular hemoglobin*

coeur heart

coeur en sabot → *wooden-shoe heart*

cofactor 1. one of two or more contributing factors **2.** any of various organic or inorganic substances necessary to the function of an enzyme

platelet cofactor 1. →*factor VIII* **2.** →*factor IX*
cofactor of thromboplastin →*accelerator globulin*
cofactor V →*factor VII*

collapse 1. (*physical or psychologic*) breakdown **2.** collapse of an organ or part of an organ **3.** →*cardiovascular collapse*

cardiovascular collapse *Syn: circulatory collapse*; collapse with or without loss of consciousness due to transient circulatory insufficiency

collateral a side branch, as of a blood vessel or nerve

preformed collaterals *s.u. collateral circulation*

column *Syn: columna*; any column-like structure

fleshy columns of heart →*muscular trabeculae of heart*

combination a result or product of combining

single pill combination the combination of two or more therapeutic agents in one pill

commissure 1. a connecting band of nerve fibers **2.** the point or surface where two parts, such as the cardiac valves, join or form a connection

commissure of cardiac valves commissure at the boundaries between the side walls and the semilunar cusps of the aortic or pulmonary valve

commissure of semilunar valves of aortic valve commissure at the junction of the semilunar cusps of the aortic valve with the side wall

commissure of semilunar valves of pulmonary valve commissure at the junction of the semilunar cusps of the pulmonary valve with the side wall

commissurorrhaphy tightening of the heart valve commissures

commissurotomy division of the heart valve commissures in valve stenosis; in **open commissurotomy**, the access is via the aorta [in aortic valve stenosis] or the pulmonary arteries [in pulmonary stenosis]; the division can be performed with a finger **digital commissurotomy** or with a special **commissurotomy**; **closed commissurotomy** uses dilatators [**Brock dilatation**], **transventricular commissurotomy**, or balloon catheters [**balloon valvuloplasty**]

Brock commissurotomy *Syn: closed commissurotomy*; *s.u. commissurotomy*

closed commissurotomy *Syn: Brock commissurotomy*; *s.u. commissurotomy*

transventricular commissurotomy *s.u. commissurotomy*

communicable →*contagious*

complex an entity made up of different parts

Eisenmenger's complex → *Eisenmenger's tetralogy*
Lutembacher's complex → *Lutembacher's disease*
prothrombin complex factors II, VII, IX, and X made in the liver
QRS complex ventricular complex in the electrocardiogram
symptom complex pattern of complaints consisting of several distinct symptoms; syndrome
VACTERL complex *s.u. VATER complex*
VATER complex complex severe malformation syndrome with Vertebral defects, Anal atresia, Tracheoesophageal fistula with Esophageal atresia and dysplasia of the kidneys [Renal] and Radius; if there are also malformations of the heart [Cor] and Limbs, it is called **VACTERL association**; in the so-called **VACTERL association plus** there is also a hydrocephalus

component constituent part; element; ingredient
component A of prothrombin → *accelerator globulin*
plasma thromboplastin component → *factor IX*
thromboplastic plasma component → *factor VIII*

concealed → *masked*

concentrate a concentrated form of something
leukocyte concentrate *s.u. packed red cells*
platelet concentrate thrombocyte-rich plasma obtained from fresh blood

concentration the amount of a specified substance in a unit amount of another substance
blood concentration → *blood level*
mean corpuscular hemoglobin concentration calculated from the hemoglobin concentration of the blood divided by the hematocrit; in **hypochromic anemias** the value is less than the normal [20–22 mmol/l], in **hyperchromic anemias**, it is greater than the normal value
plasma renin concentration *Syn: renin mass*; a direct measure of the level of the renin in the plasma; determines the concentration of renin molecules, both active and inactive, whereas plasma renin activity measures the enzymatic activity of activated renin only; expressed in pg/ml or ng/l

concretio → *concretion*

concretion *Syn: concretio*; coalescence or adhesion of organs or parts of organs
pericardial concretion adhesion of the layers of pericardial sac in

constrictive pericarditis; leads to a restriction of diastolic ventricular filling, which can no longer be matched to load but rather remains more or less constant; this means that the cardiac output can only be increased by increasing the heart rate, leading in the late stages to compensatory tachycardia even at rest

conduction the carrying of sound waves, electrons, heat, or nerve impulses by a nerve or other tissue

delayed conduction →*first degree a-v block*

cone *Syn: conus*; any cone-shaped structure

arterial cone *Syn: infundibulum, infundibulum of heart, pulmonary cone*; funnel-shaped transitional region between the right ventricle and the pulmonary trunk

pulmonary cone →*arterial cone*

congestion blood congestion; blood plethora; hyperemia

active congestion *Syn: active hyperemia, arterial hyperemia*; hyperemia due to dilatation of the arteries or arterioles

fluxionary congestion hyperemia due to increased blood flow

functional congestion hyperemia due to dilatation of all vessels

hypostatic congestion hyperemia due to hypostasis

inflow congestion *Syn: venous congestion*; venous inflow congestion with impedance of blood flow in the right half of the heart; the congestion causes swelling of the veins in the area of the head, neck, thorax, and the upper extremities; **clinically** remarkable are swelling of neck veins, headache, feeling of pressure, and nosebleeds; apart from heart failure, narrowing of the lumen of the superior vena cava due to internal or external factors [mediastinal or bronchial tumors] is the most frequent cause

upper venous congestion back-damming of blood in the systemic circulation [and sometimes the pulmonary circulation] due to a variety of causes [right heart insufficiency, left heart insufficiency, superior vena cava syndrome] with visible engorgement and distension of the neck veins, plethora or cyanosis, liver enlargement among others

venous congestion *Syn: venous hyperemia*; **1.** hyperemia due to impairment of venous outflow **2.** →*inflow congestion*

congestive relating to or characterized by congestion

conglutination clumping of red blood corpuscles induced by conglutinins

conglutinins proteins that bind to complement and lead to aggregation of red blood corpuscles by fixed antibodies

connection the state of being connected; anything that connects
  total cavopulmonary connection *s.u. tricuspid atresia*
conquinine → *quinidine*
constriction stenosis, stricture
  aortic constriction → *aortic isthmus*
contagious *Syn: communicable*; (directly) transmissible, infective
contaminated polluted, poisoned
continued → *continuous*
continuous *Syn: continued, steady, uninterrupted*; persistent, continued, ongoing, continuous, incessant
contracted *Syn: shortened*; abbreviated; narrowed
contractible → *contractile*
contractile *Syn: contractible*; capable of contraction
contraction a shortening or tensing of a part or organ, especially of a muscle or muscle tissue
  atrial premature contraction → *atrial extrasystole*
  escape contraction → *escaped beat*
  escaped contraction → *escaped beat*
  premature contraction → *extrasystole*
  premature atrial contraction → *atrial extrasystole*
  premature ventricular contraction → *ventricular extrasystole*
contraindicated not usable, not recommended for use
contusion bruise
  cardiac contusion injury to the heart caused by blunt force trauma to the chest wall, which can lead to disturbances of rhythm, changes in the ECG, heart valve avulsion, or heart muscle rupture
convertin → *factor VII*
cor → *heart*
  cor biloculare heart malformation with absence of the atrial and ventricular septum, i.e., the heart consists of one atrium and one ventricle and a conjoined atrioventricular valve
  cor bovinum → *bovine heart*
  cor pendulum → *pendulous heart*
  cor pulmonale acute [**cor pulmonale acutum**] or chronic [**cor pulmonale chronicum**] overload of the right ventricle
  acute cor pulmonale *Syn: acute cor pulmonale*; acute overload of the right ventricle due to an increase in systolic blood pressure in the pulmonary artery by more than 30 mmHg or in the mean pressure by more than 20 mmHg; the most frequent cause by far [more than 95%]

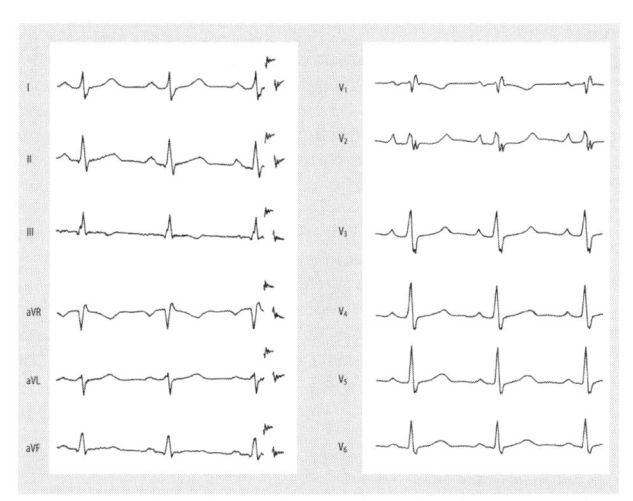

Acute cor pulmonale. ECG showing typical $S_I Q_{III}$-type [S wave in lead I and Q wave in lead III]

is a pulmonary embolism; other causes are status asthmaticus, tension pneumothorax, and severe hypoxic states of different origin; **clinical picture**: acute dyspnea, tachypnea, pleural pain, cough, palpitations, angina symptoms, accentuated second heart sound; **diagnosis**: clinical examination, ECG [$S_I Q_{III}$-**type**: S wave in lead I and Q wave in lead III], blood gas analysis, echocardiography, lung scintigraphy, chest CT; **therapy**: analgesics, oxygen, admission to intensive care unit; dobutamine in right ventricular failure; treatment of the pulmonary embolism [thrombolysis, thrombectomy]

chronic cor pulmonale right ventricular hypertrophy due to diseases affecting either the structure or function of the lungs; ultimately, pulmonary hypertension due to changes in the lungs is the cause of chronic cor pulmonale; right ventricular failure in left-sided heart failure or valve disease is not included in this definition; pulmonary hypertension has numerous causes; three groups can be differentiated: **1.** extensive damage to the lung parenchyma in, e.g., tuberculosis, chronic bronchitis, pneumoconiosis, fibrosis, bronchiectasis, or bronchial asthma causes the so-called **parenchymal heart and lung disease 2.** obstruction of pulmonary vessels by recurrent microemboli, primary pulmonary sclerosis, angiitis, or medications causes **vascular cor pulmonale 3.** extrapulmonary diseases leading to restriction of lung function, for example, funnel chest, kyphoscoliosis, pleural thickening, and poliomyelitis; **clinical picture**: initially, the symptoms of the underlying diseases are most prominent; signs of a right ventricular failure appear later [rapid exhaustion, decline in functional capacity, exertional dyspnea, tachycardia, edema, epigastric symptoms, congested jugular veins, accentuated second heart sound]; **diagnosis**: ECG: vertical heart to right axis deviation, $S_I S_{II} S_{III}$-type [S wave in I, II, and III], P pulmonale, possibly incomplete right bundle-branch block, chest X-ray, echocardiography, right-heart catheter; **therapy**: treatment of the primary illness, oxygen therapy, vasodilators [calcium antagonists, ACE inhibitors], diuretics, digitalis

parenchymal cor pulmonale *Syn: parenchymal heart and lung disease; s.u. chronic cor pulmonale*

vascular cor pulmonale *s.u. chronic cor pulmonale*

cor villosum → *hairy heart*

cord band, bundle, fascicle, tract, strand, fillet

tendinous cords of heart tendinous bands of the papillary muscles of the right and left ventricles, which attach to the margins of the atrioventricular valves and prevent them from folding back during systole

corona crown

corona phlebectatica *s.u. chronic venous insufficiency*

coronaria → *coronary artery*

coronarism 1. → *angina pectoris* **2.** → *coronary insufficiency*

coronaritic relating to or marked by coronaritis

coronaritis *Syn: coronary arteritis*; inflammation of the coronary arteries, e.g., in rheumatic arthritis; can lead to coronary insufficiency, angina pectoris, and cardiac insufficiency

coronary 1. → *coronary artery* **2.** → *coronary occlusion* **3.** relating to a coronary artery

corpuscle small body

blood corpuscles → *blood cells*

red corpuscles → *erythrocytes*

white blood corpuscles → *leukocytes*

cothromboplastin → *factor VII*

co-trimoxazole combination of the antibiotics trimethoprim and sulfamethoxazole; it is effective against gram-positive and gram-negative causative agents, especially Salmonella, Shigella, Klebsiella, Escherichia coli, Proteus, enterococci, pneumococci, and Haemophilus; **indications**: respiratory tract infections, infections of the kidneys and efferent urinary tract, sexually transmitted diseases, Pneumocystis carinii pneumonia

coumarin *Syn: chromone, cumarin*; glycoside used in the synthesis of anticoagulants [coumarin derivatives] and antibiotics [novobiocin], which occurs in many plants [woodruff, stone clover, tonka beans]

coumarins *Syn: chromones, coumarin derivatives, cumarins*; inhibitors of blood clotting derived from coumarin [anticoagulants]; inhibit the formation of vitamin K-dependent clotting factors due to their structural similarity to vitamin K

count enumeration, numerical computation

  blood count *Syn: hemogram*; quantitative determination of blood components and their graphic or tabular presentation

  complete blood count *Syn: full blood count*; counting of red and white blood cells and platelets and determination of hemoglobin

  differential count *Syn: differential blood count, hemogram*; blood picture with enumeration of the various types of leukocyte

  differential blood count → *differential count*

  erythrocyte count → *red blood count*

  full blood count → *complete blood count*

  red blood count *Syn: erythrocyte count, erythrocyte number, red cell count*; determination of the number of erythrocytes in a defined blood volume; previously performed in counting chambers; nowadays automated analyzers are used, which measure the scattering of laser light by the blood corpuscles or changes in the electric conductivity; the normal value for the erythrocyte count for men is 4.5–6.2×10^{12}/l and for women 4.2–5.4×10^{12}/l

  red cell count → *red blood count*

  Stansfeld-Webb count determination of the cell count in mid-stream urine by counting in a counting chamber; if there are more than 5 erythrocytes per ml, this is referred to as hematuria; if there are more than 5 leukocytes per ml, this is referred to as leukocyturia

  white blood cell count *Syn: differential white blood count, white blood count, white cell count*; counting of white blood cells [leukocytes]

  white cell count → *white blood cell count*

counterpulsation technique for reducing the workload on the heart by

lowering systemic blood pressure just before or during expulsion of blood from the ventricle and by raising blood pressure during diastole
intra-aortic balloon counterpulsation method of increasing the diastolic blood pressure, improving the coronary perfusion, reducing the systolic blood pressure, and increasing the cardiac minute volume; **principle**: a balloon catheter is passed retrogradely [usually via the femoral artery] into the descending aorta; using ECG-guidance, the balloon is inflated during diastole and deflated in systole; used, among other **indications**, in heart operations, hypotension due to acute heart failure [infarction, papillary muscle rupture], and cardiogenic shock

coxsackievirus *Syn: Coxsackie virus, C virus*; picornaviruses divided into two subgroups, **coxsackie A** [with 23 serotypes] and **coxsackie B** [with 6 serotypes], found worldwide; they cause, for example, herpangina, respiratory tract infections, summer flu, myocarditis, viral meningitis, and viral encephalitis; transmission occurs as a droplet or contact infection, with a more frequent occurrence of the infections in the summer season

crackles → *rales*

crackling → *crepitation*

   fine crackling *s.u. moist rales*

crassamentum → *blood clot*

creatine kinase *Syn: creatine phosphokinase, creatine phosphotransferase*; intracellular enzyme, which catalyzes the reversible reaction of creatine and ATP to form creatine phosphate and ADP; occurs in three isoforms: CK-BB [**brain type**], CK-MM [**skeletal muscle type**], and CK-MB [**heart muscle type**]; CK-MB is used in the diagnosis and subsequent monitoring of myocardial infarction

creatine phosphokinase → *creatine kinase*

creatine phosphotransferase → *creatine kinase*

crepitation *Syn: crepitus, crepitant rale, crackling*; crackling heard on auscultation over the lung or pleura

crest ridge

   infundibuloventricular crest → *supraventricular crest*

   supravalvular crest supravalvular ridge above the pulmonary valve [valve of the pulmonary trunk] or the aortic valve

   supraventricular crest *Syn: infundibuloventricular crest*; supraventricular muscle ridge in the right heart chamber, which divides the inflow and outflow tracts

   terminal crest of right atrium ridge on the inside of the right atrium

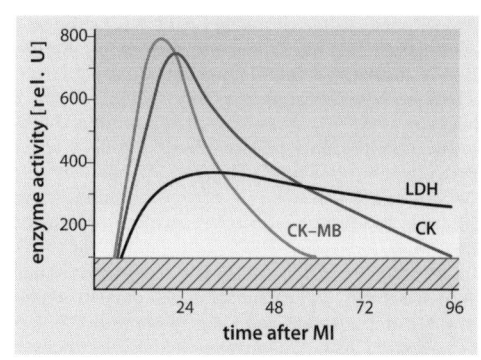

Creatine kinase. Plasma levels of lactate dehydrogenase [LDH], creatine kinase [CK], and creatine kinase heart muscle type [CK-MB] after myocardial infarction

from which the heart muscle arises

crisis a crucial or decisive point or situation; a turning point

addisonian crisis *Syn: acute adrenocortical insufficiency, adrenal crisis*; acute adrenal crisis developing from chronic adrenal insufficiency with signs of hypovolemic shock with marked hypotension, tachycardia, vomiting, and diarrhea, anergy, and loss of consciousness, which can progress to coma; **therapy**: urgent infusion of NaCl and glucose solution [2–4 l/24 h]; high doses of glucocorticoids i.v.

adrenal crisis → *addisonian crisis*

cerebral crisis → *cerebrovascular accident*

hypertensive crisis very sudden increase in the blood pressure to systolic values in excess of 200 mmHg or diastolic values in excess of 120 mmHg; as long as there is no discernible organ damage, this is referred to as a hypertensive crisis, whereas if there is organ damage and the situation is life-threatening, and demands immediate reduction of blood pressure, then this is a **hypertensive emergency**; the most common causes are essential, renovascular or renal parenchymatous hypertension, eclampsia, hyperthyroidism, pheochromocytoma, intracerebral bleeding, and sudden cessation of antihypertensives; **clinical**: headache, dizziness, confusion, visual disturbances, reduction of conscious level to the point of coma, dyspnea, angina pectoris, oliguria, or anuria; **therapy**: immediate, but not abrupt reduction of the blood pressure; oral administration of nifedipine, nitrendipine, or nitroglycerine, i.v. injection of clonidine, dihydralazine, urapidil

salt-depletion crisis → *salt-depletion syndrome*

crista (bone) crest, ridge

crista supravalvularis → *supravalvular crest*
crista supraventricularis → *supraventricular crest*
crista terminalis atrii dextri → *terminal crest of right atrium*

criterion a standard, rule, or test on which a judgment or decision can be based

Jones' criteria criteria for the diagnosis of rheumatic fever; **5 main criteria** [carditis, polyarthritis, chorea, subcutaneous nodes, erythema annulare] and **6 sub-criteria** [fever, joint pains, prolonged P-R interval in the ECG, increased ESR, C-reactive protein or leukocytosis, evidence of previous infection with β-hemolytic streptococci, history of rheumatic fever] are recognized; in addition, there may be accompanying symptoms such as weight loss, sweats, pallor, anemia, mild fatigue, etc.; the presence of 2 main criteria or 1 main criterion and 2 sub-criteria make the diagnosis likely

cross-resistance resistance of a pathogen to an antibiotic and other, usually related, antibiotics [e.g., against penicillin and cephalosporin]

cruor → *blood clot*

crus leg, limb

crus dextrum fasciculi atrioventricularis → *right bundle branch*
crus sinistrum fasciculi atrioventricularis → *left bundle branch*

culture the growing of microorganisms, tissue cells, or other living matter in a specially prepared nutrient medium

blood culture *Syn: hemoculture*; method of directly growing bacteria from blood; blood cultures must be taken before the start of antimicrobial therapy, otherwise results will be unreliable; even in sepsis, only approx. 20% of cultures yield a positive result; i.e., a positive blood culture has a high predictive value, but a negative culture by no means excludes an infection

cumarin → *coumarin*
cumarins → *coumarins*

curative *Syn: remediable, remedial, sanative, sanatory, therapeutical, therapeutic*; curing, targeted at cure, promoting cure

current a flow of electric charge

action current *Syn: nerve-action current*; current caused by potential changes in the membrane of a nerve or muscle; basis of the electrical currents recorded by electrocardiography, electromyography, electroneurography, electroencephalography, etc.

nerve-action current →*action current*

curve nonangular deviation from a straight line; graphic representation of a value

carotid pulse curve recording of the pulse waveform of the common carotid artery

oxygen dissociation curve *Syn: oxygen-hemoglobin dissociation curve, oxyhemoglobin dissociation curve*; graphic representation of the relationship between oxygen partial pressure in the blood and the proportion of oxyhemoglobin with respect to total hemoglobin; it is influenced, for example, by pH, CO_2 partial pressure, and temperature

oxygen-hemoglobin dissociation curve →*oxygen dissociation curve*

oxyhemoglobin dissociation curve →*oxygen dissociation curve*

pulse curve *Syn: sphygmogram*; trace obtained by sphygmography

cusp *Syn: cuspis*; lappet

anterior cusp of left atrioventricular valve anterior cusp of the mitral valve [left atrioventricular valve]

anterior cusp of right atrioventricular valve anterior cusp of the tricuspid valve [right atrioventricular valve]

cusps of commissures two small cusps, which form the lateral portion of the posterior cusp of the mitral valve

medial cusp →*septal cusp*

posterior cusp of left atrioventricular valve posterior cusp of the mitral valve [left atrioventricular valve]

posterior cusp of right atrioventricular valve posterior cusp of the tricuspid valve [right atrioventricular valve]

semilunar cusp *Syn: flap valve, semilunar valve*; semilunar valves, which together form the aortic valve and pulmonary valve; the valves are rich in collagen fibers and are covered on their upper and lower surfaces with endothelium; they sit like epaulettes on the wall with their free edges pointing upwards; on the upper edge there are semilunar strengthening strips [**lunulae valvularum semilunarium**], which consist of sickle-shaped inclusions of collagen fibers and nodular thickenings in the middle [**noduli valvularum semilunarium**]; during systole they lie flat against the wall and allow the blood to stream out of the ventricle; at the beginning of diastole they are filled by blood flowing backwards and this closes the orifice

septal cusp *Syn: medial cusp*; septal cusp of the tricuspid valve [right atrioventricular valve]

cuspis → *cusp*

cuspis anterior valvae atrioventricularis dextrae anterior cusp of the tricuspid valve [right atrioventricular valve]

cuspis anterior valvae atrioventricularis sinistri anterior cusp of the mitral valve [left atrioventricular valve]

cuspides commissurales valvae atrioventricularis sinistri → *cusps of commissures*

cuspis posterior valvae atrioventricularis dextrae posterior cusp of the tricuspid valve [right atrioventricular valve]

cuspis posterior valvae atrioventricularis sinistri posterior cusp of the mitral valve [left atrioventricular valve]

cuspis septalis valvae atrioventricularis dextrae septal cusp of the tricuspid valve [right atrioventricular valve]

cyanochroic → *cyanotic*

cyanochrous → *cyanotic*

cyanoderma → *cyanosis*

cyanosed → *cyanotic*

cyanosis *Syn: cyanoderma*; bluish, livid discoloration of skin and mucous membranes caused by a decline in the blood oxygen saturation; cyanosis of the oral mucosa, tongue, and conjuctiva occurs in **central cyanosis**; it is due to a cardiac or pulmonary right-to-left shunt; **peripheral cyanosis** occurs during reduced perfusion in heart failure or peripheral vasospasms and affects the nose, lips, earlobes, and fingertips

pulmonary cyanosis cyanosis due to impairment/reduction of alveolar gas exchange in the lung in lung disease or hypoventilation

shunt cyanosis cyanosis caused by a right-to-left shunt

cyanotic *Syn: cyanochroic, cyanochrous, cyanosed*; relating to, affected with, or characterized or caused by cyanosis

cycle an interval of time during which a characteristic, often regularly repeated event or sequence of events occurs

cardiac cycle *Syn: cardiac beat, heartbeat*; the rhythmically repeating process of muscle contraction [systole] and ejection of blood into the systemic and pulmonary circulation and muscle relaxation [diastole] with filling of the ventricles; both during diastole and systole, phases of activity can be separated from one another, in which either a pressure change at constant volume or a volume change at constant pressure occurs; during systole, one can define the: **1. contraction phase**: with the start of systole, the contraction of the myocardial fibers leads to deformation of the ventricle, an increase in pressure, and immediate closure of the atrioventricular valve; since the volume does not change during this phase, it is called isovolumetric contraction; the contraction phase can be subdivided into **deformation period** [start of the QRS-complex to the 1. heart sound] and **pressure increase period** [start of 1. sound to start of ejection] **2. ejection phase**: as soon as the pressure in the ventricle exceeds the diastolic pressure in the aorta or pulmonary artery, the semilunar valves open and the blood flows out of the ventricle into the vessel; the ventricular pressure initially increases further then falls toward the end of systole; during this time, the volume falls from the **end-diastolic volume** of approx. 140 ml to the **residual volume** of approx. 50 ml, i.e., the **stroke volume** amounts to approx. 90 ml and the **ejection fraction** 0.64; the ejection phase ends with closure of the semilunar valves; diastole is subdivided into: **1. relaxation phase**: isovolumetric relaxation of the heart muscle fibers leads to a fall in pressure in the ventricles; as soon as the pressure reaches nearly 0 mmHg, the atrioventricular valves open and filling of the ventricle begins **2. filling phase**: the filling proceeds quickly at first [**rapid filling phase**] but slows toward the end of diastole [**diastasis**]; atrial contraction plays hardly any role when the heart rhythm is normal, since ventricle filling is almost complete; at higher heart rates, diastole is more significantly shortened than systole and thus atrial contraction contributes significantly more to filling

cymarin *Syn:* k-*strophanthin-α*; cardioactive glycoside with positive inotropic action

cyst a closed cavity lined by epithelium
    aneurysmal bone cyst → *aneurysmal giant cell tumor*
    hemangiomatous bone cyst → *aneurysmal giant cell tumor*
    hemorrhagic bone cyst → *aneurysmal giant cell tumor*

cythemolysis → *hemolysis*

cytometry the counting of cells, especially blood cells
    flow cytometry continuous measurement of cells or particles, which are suspended in a solution and flow through a measuring apparatus [particle counter, flow cytometer]; the counted or measured impulses can be displayed graphically or numerically

cytopenia reduction in one type of cell in the blood; if two cell types are affected, this is called **bi-cytopenia**, if three cell types **tri-cytopenia**

D

d/l-hyoscyamine *Syn: daturine, hyoscyamine*; very poisonous alkaloid with parasympatholytic action that occurs in the nightshade family, such as **belladonna** [Atropa belladonna], **white jimson weed** [Datura stramonium], and **black henbane** [Hyoscyamus niger]

daturine → *d/l-hyoscyamine*

dearterialization conversion of arterial blood into venous blood by utilization of oxygen

death the act of dying; the end of life

    cardiac death death due to cardiac standstill

    sudden cardiac death cardiac death occurring within a few seconds; the most common causes are coronary heart disease, acute myocardial infarction, myocarditis, tachycardia, heart block, and acute cor pulmonale following pulmonary embolism

decompensated unbalanced, decompensated

defect shortcoming, fault, imperfection, deficiency

    aortic valve defects generic term for aortic insufficiency and aortic valvular stenosis

    atrial septal defect *Syn: atrioseptal defect*; congenital heart defect with formation of holes in the septum between the two atria; approx. 11% of all congenital heart defects; often occurs in trisomy 21; subdivided, depending upon the position, into: **1. superior** or **upper sinus venosus defect**: in the upper part of the septum in the region of the opening of the superior pulmonary vein and superior vena cava **2. atrial septal defect of secundum type** [ASD II]: in the central region of the fossa ovalis **3. atrial septal defect of primum type** [ASD I]: in the lower part, near the tricuspid valve **4. coronary sinus defect**: in the region of the coronary sinus and **5. inferior** or **lower sinus venosus defect**: deep down in the septum in the region of the opening of the inferior pulmonary vein and inferior vena cava; independent of the level, every atrial septal defect leads to a left-to-right shunt at atrial level and thereby to volume loading of the right ventricle; pulmonary hypertension with shunt reversal and cyanosis develops only after decades; **clinical**: in childhood there are hardly any symptoms [only in the primum type], at most an increased tendency to infections; later, reduced load capacity and supraventricular disturbances of rhythm [atrial fibrillation/flutter] develop; **diagnosis**: wide and fixed splitting of the 2. heart sound on **auscultation**; functional flow murmur over the pulmonary valve [systolic, 2.-3. intercostal space on the left] and tricuspid valve [muted diastolic]; in the **ECG** signs of right-sided hypertrophy and disturbances of the spread of excitation in the right ventricle; the **X-ray** is unremarkable; in the **echocardiogram** the defect and the enlargement of the right ventricle are visible; a **cardiac catheterization study** is now only indicated if there is a suspicion of malposition of the opening of the pulmonary veins; **therapy**: operative closure by interventional closure [e.g., Amplatzer system], direct suture or sewing of an onlay patch

atrioseptal defect → *atrial septal defect*

atrioventricular canal defect if the AV-canal does not close or only does so incompletely, this results in the formation of an endocardial cushion defect; the clinical symptomatology depends upon the type of disturbance [**partial atrioventricular canal**, **complete atrioventricular canal**] and the associated defects [atrial septal defect, valve malformation]; mostly a left-to-right shunt forms, which leads to pulmonary and arterial hypertension and in the long term to shunt reversal [Eisenmenger reaction]

coronary sinus defect *s.u. atrial septal defect*

endocardial cushion defect cardiac defect caused by a developmental disturbance to the endocardial cushion, an embryonic precursor of the heart valves; declares itself as ostium primum defect or as a persistent atrioventricular canal

equal pressure defect *s.u. ventricular septal defect*

heart defect *Syn: organic heart defect, vitium*; generic term for congenital or acquired malformations of the heart or heart valves; heart defects with narrowing of the heart valves or outflow tracts can lead to pressure loading and cardiac hypertrophy; in heart valve insufficiency or defects with left-to-right shunting, there is volume loading that eventually causes dilatation of the chambers [cardiac dilatation]; it has proved useful to divide heart defects into two groups: **1. heart and vessel abnormalities without shunting**: this includes, among others, congenital and acquired heart valve abnormalities, transposition of the great vessels, aortic isthmus stenosis, aortic arch anomalies 2. **heart and vessel defects with left-to-right shunting**: e.g., persistent ductus arteriosus, atrial septal defect, ventricular septal defect, atrioventricular septal defect 3. **heart and vessel defects with right-to-left shunting**: e.g., Fallot's tetralogy, trilogy, pentalogy, pulmonary atresia with ventricular septal defect, tricuspid atresia

inferior sinus venosus defect *Syn: lower sinus venosus defect; s.u. atrial septal defect*

inflow defect *Syn: inlet defect; s.u. ventricular septal defect*

inlet defect *Syn: inflow defect; s.u. ventricular septal defect*

lower sinus venosus defect *Syn: inferior sinus venosus defect; s.u. atrial septal defect*

mitral valve defect generic term for mitral insufficiency and mitral stenosis

muscular ventricular septal defect *s.u. ventricular septal defect*

non-pressure-separating defect *s.u. ventricular septal defect*

organic heart defect →*heart defect*

ostium primum defect atrial septal defect type one

ostium secundum defect atrial septal defect of secundum type

outflow defect *Syn: outlet defect; s.u. ventricular septal defect*

outlet defect *Syn: outflow defect; s.u. ventricular septal defect*

perimembranous ventricular septal defect *s.u. ventricular septal defect*

pressure-separating defect *s.u. ventricular septal defect*

septal defect defect in the septum between the atria [atrial septal defect] or the ventricles [ventricular septal defect]

superior sinus venosus defect *Syn: upper sinus venosus defect; s.u. atrial septal defect*

Swiss cheese defect *s.u. ventricular septal defect*

upper sinus venosus defect *Syn: superior sinus venosus defect; s.u. atrial septal defect*

valvular defect *Syn: vitium*; congenital or acquired malformation of a heart valve, which can lead to inability to close [**heart valve insufficiency**] or narrowing [**heart valve stenosis**]

ventricular septal defect congenital or acquired defect of the ventricular septum; congenital ventricular septal defects are found alone or in combination with other anomalies in approx. 30% of all congenital heart defects; divided, depending upon the position, into: **perimembranous ventricular septal defects** [immediately below the aortic valve or septal cusp of the tricuspid valve, approx. 70%], **muscular ventricular septal defects** [in the muscular part of the septum, approx. 10%], **inflow defects** [in the inflow tract between or below the AV-valves, approx. 10%] and **outflow defects** [in the right ventricular outflow tract]; muscular defects can be multiple and can have appearances called **Swiss cheese defect;** the size of the defect and its influence on the hemodynamics are important for prognosis and therapy; in small defects, a pressure differential between the two ventricles remains after birth [**pressure-separating defect**], whereas in large defects the pressures in the two ventricles equalize, leading to a left-to-right shunt [**non-pressure-separating** or **equal pressure defect**]; the left-to-right shunt leads to pulmonary recirculation, left ventricular volume loading, and corresponding symptoms [see below]; in pressure-separating defects, a left-to-right shunt also develops, although it is mostly hemodynamically insignificant; **clinical**: small defects are hemodynamically insignificant and are asymptomatic; however, on auscultation a loud [2/6–4/6], harsh systolic murmur is heard in the left parasternal region in the 3.-4. intercostal space; this defect, called the maladie de Roger, mostly sits in the muscular septum and closes spontaneously in 90% of cases; in large defects, dyspnea, sweating, growth arrest, recurrent respiratory tract infections, and very poor suckling develop; on auscultation, a pansystolic, spindle-shaped murmur is heard in the 3.-4. left parasternal intercostal spaces, with wide radiation; **diagnosis**: history, examination, ECG, echocardiography, cardiac catheterization; **therapy**: 70–80% of the defects close spontaneously within 6 months; if closure does not occur, then operative closure is required [e.g., transatrial/transventricular/transarterial suture with an artificial or pericardial patch]

defibrillation pharmaceutical, mechanical, or electrical treatment of ventricular fibrillation

electric defibrillation *Syn: electrodefibrillation*; emergency measure for the treatment of ventricular fibrillation or flutter; in **external electrodefibrillation**, two large surface area electrodes are placed on the chest wall and a DC pulse [1–4 ms, 50–400 Joules] is applied; the goal is to depolarize all the non-refractory heart muscle fibers at the same time and thereby to synchronize them; after a brief pause, the normal heart rhythm may restart; in **direct** or **internal electrodefibrillation**, the electrodes are applied directly to the heart; the field strength is then 10–50 Joules

defibrillator *Syn: cardioverter*; apparatus for electrical defibrillation; **implantable cardioverter/defibrillators** [ICD] are mainly used to treat non-sustained ventricular tachycardias; early defibrillation by **automated external defibrillators** [AED] is the only treatment option for patients in cardiac standstill, which can interrupt ventricular fibrillation and pulseless ventricular tachycardia; the longer the defibrillation is delayed, the worse the survival chances for the patient

defibrinated fibrin free, without fibrin

defibrination removal of fibrin from the blood

deficiency → *deficit*

    antithrombin III deficiency deficiency of antithrombin III leading to deranged blood clotting and an increased tendency to thrombosis

    apolipoprotein C-II deficiency → *type V familial hyperlipoproteinemia*

    C1-INH deficiency *Syn: C1 inhibitor deficiency, hereditary angioneurotic edema, hereditary angioedema; s.u. angioedema*

    C1 inhibitor deficiency *Syn: hereditary angioneurotic edema, C1-INH deficiency, hereditary angioedema; s.u. angioedema*

    factor I deficiency 1. → *afibrinogenemia* **2.** → *hypofibrinogenemia*

    factor II deficiency *Syn: hypoprothrombinemia, prothrombinopenia*; inherited [rare] or acquired [liver insufficiency, vitamin K deficiency] deficiency of blood clotting factor II [prothrombin] with an increased bleeding tendency; the transient **hypoprothrombinemia of the newborn** is related to immature liver cells or vitamin K deficiency

    factor V deficiency *Syn: hypoproaccelerinemia, Owren's disease, parahemophilia*; rare, autosomal recessive deficiency of blood clotting factor; leads to an increased bleeding tendency if the levels drop below 10–20%; **therapy**: replacement therapy with fresh plasma

    factor VII deficiency *Syn: hypoproconvertinemia*; inherited [phenotypically autosomal recessive, genotypically autosomal codominant] deficiency of blood clotting factor VII; leads to an increased tendency to bleed similar to hemophilia

    factor IX deficiency → *Christmas disease*

    factor XI deficiency *Syn: hemophilia C, PTA deficiency*; inherited bleeding tendency caused by autosomal recessive deficiency of factor XI

    factor XII deficiency → *Hageman factor deficiency*

    factor XIII deficiency autosomal recessive deficiency of blood clotting factor XIII; can lead to disturbances of wound healing and secondary hemorrhage

factor X deficiency rare, autosomal recessive deficiency of blood clotting factor X; leads to mild symptoms of hemophilia

familial LCAT deficiency →*idiopathic LCAT deficiency*

familial lecithin-cholesterol acyltransferase deficiency →*idiopathic LCAT deficiency*

familial lipoprotein lipase deficiency 1. →*hyperchylomicronemia* **2.** →*type V familial hyperlipoproteinemia*

familial LPL deficiency 1. →*hyperchylomicronemia* **2.** →*type V familial hyperlipoproteinemia*

deficiency of fibrinogen 1. →*afibrinogenemia* **2.** →*hypofibrinogenemia*

Hageman factor deficiency *Syn: factor XII deficiency, Hageman syndrome*; autosomal recessive deficiency of factor XII; clinically silent

11β-hydroxylase deficiency clinical course suggestive of the adrenogenital syndrome due to a 21-hydroxylase defect but without salt wasting syndrome; there is also hypertension due to an excess of desoxycorticosterone

17α-hydroxylase deficiency the external genitalia of girl is unremarkable, but in boys there can be an intersex condition at birth; hypertension, hypernatremia, hypokalemia, and hypokalemic alkalosis are clinically important

idiopathic LCAT deficiency *Syn: familial LCAT deficiency, familial lecithin-cholesterol acyltransferase deficiency, Norum-Gjone disease*; autosomal recessive enzymopathy, which upsets the retrograde transport of cholesterol; leads to, among others, hemolytic anemia due to disruption of the erythrocyte membrane, proteinuria, kidney disease, and corneal opacification due to lipid deposition; the free cholesterol in the serum is elevated; **therapy**: low cholesterol diet

oxygen deficiency →*hypoxia*

PTA deficiency *Syn: factor XI deficiency, hemophilia C*; autosomal recessively inherited deficiency of factor XI with an inherited bleeding tendency

deficit *Syn: deficiency, shortage, shortfall*; deficiency, lack; (functional) inadequacy, insufficiency

base deficit deficiency of buffer bases in the blood

prolonged reversible ischemic neurologic deficit *s.u. cerebrovascular accident*

pulse deficit difference between heart rate and pulse rate, e.g., in ven-

tricular fibrillation
reversible ischemic neurologic deficit *s.u. cerebrovascular accident*
deformity malformation, distortion, disfigurement
buttonhole deformity → *fishmouth stenosis*
degeneration morphologically evident deterioration of cells, tissues, or organs, which proceeds with a reduction in functional ability; wasting, atrophy, regression
Abercombie's degeneration → *amyloidosis*
amyloid degeneration → *amyloidosis*
atheromatous degeneration *Syn: atheroma*; plaque-like atherosclerotic changes occurring in the vessel wall
bacony degeneration → *amyloidosis*
cellulose degeneration → *amyloidosis*
chitinous degeneration → *amyloidosis*
hyaloid degeneration → *amyloidosis*
lardaceous degeneration → *amyloidosis*
Mönckeberg's degeneration → *Mönckeberg's sclerosis*
mucoid medial degeneration → *Erdheim-Gsell medial necrosis*
Virchow's degeneration → *amyloidosis*
waxy degeneration → *amyloidosis*
degree of collateralization *Syn: degree of collateral circulation; s.u. collateral circulation*
degree of collateral circulation *Syn: degree of collateralization; s.u. collateral circulation*
dehydration 1. removal of water; dehydration therapy **2.** water deficiency of the body with or without salt deficiency
hypertonic dehydration dehydration due to loss of water without simultaneous loss of NaCl; the causes are mostly insufficient intake of water or excessive loss of water in diarrhea, fever, hyperthermia, or ADH deficiency
hypotonic dehydration *Syn: hypotonic hypohydration*; dehydration mainly caused by NaCl losses with reduced osmolality; leads to reduction in the extracellular space and expansion of the intracellular space
isotonic dehydration dehydration with normal osmolality in the extra- and intracellular fluid; occurs due to a deficiency of water and NaCl, e.g., in vomiting, diarrhea, massive sweating, burns, aldosterone deficiency, or osmotic diuresis
deliquium → *syncope*

demi- combining form denoting relation to one half

depression → *fovea*

  ST segment depression location of the ST segment in the electrocardiogram below the (isoelectric) null line

derivative a substance produced from another substance either directly or by modification

  benzodiazepine derivatives → *benzodiazepines*

  coumarin derivatives agents derived from coumarin that inhibit blood clotting [anticoagulants]; they inhibit the formation of vitamin K-dependent clotting factors as a result of their structural similarity to vitamin K

descendent → *descending*

descending *Syn: descendent*; decreasing, with a downward trend

desmopressin derivative of antidiuretic hormone, which leads to an increase in the concentration of factor VIII and von Willebrand factor in the blood

desobliteration restoration of the patency of occluded vessels, e.g., by coring it out

devascularization prevention of perfusion caused by operative interventions or traumatic/pathologic processes

deviation departure from a standard or norm

  deviation to the left *Syn: leftward shift, skeocytosis*; increased occurrence of immature granulocyte precursors in the peripheral blood; referred to as **reactive left shift** in, e.g., acute infections and strenuous physical exertion, and as **pathologic left shift** in the leukemias and lymphomas

  left axis deviation *Syn: left type*; *s.u. electrocardiogram*

  right axis deviation *Syn: right type*; *s.u. electrocardiogram*

dexiocardia → *dextrocardia*

dextrocardia *Syn: dexiocardia*; right-sided positioning of the heart, e.g., in situs inversus, displacement due to mediastinal displacement [**dextroposition of the heart**] or rightwards rotation [**dextroversion of the heart**]

dextrocardiogram 1. electrocardiogram of the right half of the heart 2. → *dextrogram*

dextrocardiography 1. electrocardiography of the right half of the heart 2. selective X-ray contrast demonstration of the right atrium, right ventricle, and pulmonary circulation following direct injection of contrast agent

dextrogram X-ray contrast image of the right half of the heart
dextroposition displacement to the right
   dextroposition of heart *s.u. dextrocardia*
dextroversion turning to the right, e.g., turning the gaze to the right, rotation of the heart to the right [**dextroversion of the heart**]
diacylglycerine → *diacylglycerol*
diacylglycerol *Syn: diacylglycerine, diglyceride*; glycerin esterified with 2 fatty acid molecules; intermediate product in triglyceride biosynthesis
diagnosis *Syn: diacrisis*; **1.** the act or process of identifying or determining the nature and cause of a disease or injury **2.** the decision reached from such an examination
   serum diagnosis → *serodiagnosis*
diagram a graphic representation of an object or concept
   pressure-volume diagram *Syn: PV diagram*; graphic representation of the relationship between pressure and volume in an elastic container, e.g., heart or lungs
   PV diagram → *pressure-volume diagram*
diapedesis *Syn: diapiresis, emigration, migration*; the passage of blood cells, esp. leukocytes, through the unruptured walls of vessels
   hemorrhage by diapedesis leakage of blood through pores in the capillary endothelium, e.g., in congestion, hemorrhagic diathesis
diastasis slow filling phase of the heart at the end of diastole
diastole *Syn: cardiac diastole*; the relaxation phase that follows heart contraction [systole], during which the blood flows out of the atria into the ventricles; it begins with a brief **relaxation phase** [approx. 50 ms], during which the heart valves are closed and the ventricles relax isovolumetrically; as soon as the pressure falls below the atrial pressure, the AV-valves open and the **filling phase** begins; the filling proceeds quickly at first [**rapid filling phase**] and slows toward the end of diastole [**diastasis**]
   cardiac diastole → *diastole*
diastolic relating to diastole
   early diastolic → *protodiastolic*
diathesis congenital or acquired inclination/willingness/disposition
diazoxide antihypertensive, vasodilator, increases the blood glucose level by inhibiting insulin secretion; **usage**: hypoglycemia, islet cell tumors, arterial hypertension
dicarbonate → *bicarbonate*

diclofenamide carbonic anhydrase inhibitor; **usage**: diuretic, treatment of glaucoma

dicloxacillin penicillinase-resistant penicillin

dicrotism double-peaked nature of the peripheral pulse wave, e.g., in fever, tachycardia or arteriosclerosis; can sometimes be felt as a small after-beat to a normal pulse wave

digit finger or toe

clubbed digits → *clubbed fingers*

digitalis *Syn: fairy gloves, foxglove*; class of plant, whose species [wooly foxglove, **Digitalis lanata**; crimson foxglove, **Digitalis purpurea**; yellow foxglove, **Digitalis lutea**] in part contain cardioactive glycosides

digitalism in approx. 10% of patients on digitalis therapy, signs of intoxication develop due to overdosage, reduced breakdown in liver insufficiency, or diminished excretion in renal insufficiency; the most common symptoms are disturbances of heart rhythm, bradycardia, AV-block, gastrointestinal pains, vomiting, irritability, headaches, disturbances of color vision, and nystagmus

digitaloids term for cardioactive glycosides II order, which chemically resembles the digitalis glycosides; found among others in pheasant's eye, lilies of the valley, squill, and oleander

digitalose sugar occurring in the digitalis glycosides

digitogenin digitalis glycoside

digitonin digitalis glycoside

digitoxigenin digitalis glycoside

digitoxin digitalis glycoside

digitoxose hexose occurring in the digitalis glycosides

diglyceride → *diacylglycerol*

digoxigenin digitalis glycoside

digoxin digitalis glycoside

dihydralazine *Syn: 1,4-dihydrazinophthalazuine*; direct arterial vasodilator, antihypertensive; **usage**: mild to medium severity hypertension [mostly together with β-blockers and diuretics]

1,4-dihydrazinophthalazuine → *dihydralazine*

dihydroampicillin → *epicillin*

dihydroxyfluorane → *fluorescein*

dilatation → *dilation*

dilatator → *dilator*

coronary dilatator *Syn: coronary dilator, coronary vasodilatator, coronary vasodilator*; substance that dilates the coronary vessels

dilation *Syn: dilatation*; (pathologic or artificial) expansion, stretching
  balloon dilation distention of a vessel or hollow organ using a balloon catheter
  dilation of heart → *cardiectasis*
  left heart dilation *Syn: left ventricular dilatation*; dilatation of the left ventricle as a sign of left heart insufficiency
  right heart dilation *Syn: right ventricular dilatation*; dilatation of the right ventricle as a sign of right heart insufficiency
dilator *Syn: dilatator, dilater*; **1.** a muscle that dilates a body part **2.** an instrument that dilates a body part, such as a cavity, canal, or orifice **3.** a drug that causes dilation
  coronary dilator → *coronary dilatator*
diltiazem calcium antagonist, coronary dilatator, class-IV antiarrhythmic; **usage**: coronary heart disease, unstable angina pectoris, angina pectoris attack, arterial hypertension, supraventricular tachycardia
dipeptidyl carboxypeptidase → *angiotensin converting enzyme*
diphenylhydantoin *Syn: phenytoin*; membrane stabilizing antiepileptic with anticonvulsant action; antiarrhythmic; half life of 22 h [7–42 h]; **usage**: focal seizures, grand mal epilepsy, trigeminal neuralgia, ventricular and supraventricular arrhythmias caused by digitalis; **side effects**: nystagmus, acute cerebellar ataxia, drowsiness, blurred vision, gum hypertrophy, extrapyramidal hyperkinesias, encephalopathy, polyneuropathy, disturbances of heart rhythm, bradycardia; **contraindications**: AV-block, leukopenia
diphosphatidylglycerol *Syn: cardiolipin*; phospholipid occurring in the heart
Diplococcus obsolete genus name for spherical diplobacteria, which are now assigned to other genera, e.g., Neisseria or Streptococcus
  Diplococcus lanceolatus → *Streptococcus pneumoniae*
  Diplococcus pneumoniae → *Streptococcus pneumoniae*
dipyridamole vasodilator, coronary artery dilator; inhibitor of thrombocyte aggregation; acts as a positive inotrope; **usage**: prophylaxis against thrombosis and embolism following heart attacks or cerebral ischemia and in coronary heart disease
direct renin inhibitor new class of antihypertensive agents that decrease plasma renin activity and inhibit conversion of angiotensinogen to angiotensin I within the renin-angiotensin-aldosterone system
discharge something that is discharged, released, emitted, or excreted
  systolic discharge → *stroke volume*

disease *Syn: illness, morbus*; physical, mental, or emotional change or disturbance characterized by subjective symptoms or objective signs

Abrami's disease →*hemolytic anemia*

Adams' disease →*Adams-Stokes syndrome*

Adams-Stokes disease →*Adams-Stokes syndrome*

aorticoiliac occlusive disease *Syn: Leriche's syndrome*; underperfusion of the legs caused by occlusion of the aortic bifurcation and the symptoms that this causes [leg pains, pallor, intermittent claudication]; it requires operative removal of the cause [embolus, thrombus] or bypass for atherosclerosis

arterial occlusive diseases generic term for conditions whose clinical picture is caused by impairment or reduction in the arterial perfusion; usually described therefore as **arterial occlusive diseases** or **disturbances of arterial perfusion**; most authors narrow the definition and use it only for **chronic disturbances of arterial perfusion** and regard **acute peripheral arterial occlusion** as a separate entity; other forms of arterial occlusive disease include cerebrovascular insufficiency, basilar insufficiency, coronary heart disease, and visceral arterial insufficiency

Ayerza's disease →*Ayerza's syndrome*

Bazin's disease vasculitis of the small and medium sized subcutaneous vessels with knotty swellings, mostly affecting younger women; probably associated with tuberculosis of an organ in a large majority of cases

Beau's disease →*heart failure*

Bernard-Soulier disease →*Bernard-Soulier syndrome*

Bouillaud's disease *Syn: rheumatic endocarditis, rheumatic valvulitis*; infective/allergic inflammation of the heart valves after an infection with beta-hemolytic group A streptococci; small thrombi [vegetations] form on the closing edges of the heart valves [particularly the mitral valve], which initially consist of aggregated thrombocytes and later also contain fibrin; the organization of these thrombi leads to elongated scars and thence to insufficiency and/or stenosis of the valve; in approx. 30% of cases, the thrombi break off and give rise to clinically manifest embolization, of which 2/3 affect the brain; **therapy**: removal of the streptococcal infection with penicillin; treatment of the cardiac insufficiency [ACE inhibitors, digitalis], thromboprophylaxis

Bouveret's disease →*Bouveret's syndrome*

broad-beta disease →*type III familial hyperlipoproteinemia*

Budd-Chiari disease → *Budd-Chiari syndrome*
Buerger's disease → *Winiwarter-Buerger disease*
Bürger-Grütz disease → *Bürger-Grütz syndrome*
carotid occlusive disease → *carotid stenosis*
Chiari's disease → *Budd-Chiari syndrome*
Christmas disease *Syn: factor IX deficiency, hemophilia B*; disturbance of blood clotting caused by congenital deficiency of the Christmas factor; **therapy**: lifelong replacement therapy, which generally consists of i.v. administration performed by the patient, or in children by their parents; the factor concentrates used contain highly purified factor IX

chronic arterial occlusive disease one of the most common diseases of the industrialized nations and responsible for approx. 50% of all deaths [particularly due to coronary heart disease]; common to all forms is that the disturbance of perfusion develops slowly, i.e., there is usually sufficient collateral formation to supply the oxygen demands under normal loads; by far the most common **cause** is arteriosclerosis as a result of endogenous or exogenous disturbances of fat and carbohydrate metabolism, hypertension, obesity, and lack of exercise; alcohol and nicotine use also play a role in the pathophysiology; chronic inflammatory arterial diseases [endangiitis obliterans] are the second most common cause; not all arteries or arterial segments develop stenoses or occlusions, rather there is a predilection for involvement of vessel branching points and curvatures as well as the points of origin of smaller arteries from larger vessels; depending upon localization, cerebrovascular insufficiency, coronary heart diseases, and visceral arterial insufficiency are differentiated from **peripheral arterial occlusive disease** [PAOD]; these can themselves be subdivided by area into those affecting the upper half of the body, the **shoulder girdle type** [aortic arch syndrome, subclavian steal syndrome], **upper arm type**, **underarm type**, and **digital** or **acral type**, although all except the shoulder girdle type are rare; in the lower half of the body, which is affected by disturbances of perfusion significantly more commonly, there are corresponding **pelvic type** [aortoiliac segment], **femoral type** [femoropopliteal segment], **lower leg type** [popliteocrural segment], and **digital** or **acral type** [foot and digital segment]; naturally there are combinations of these types; the **clinical picture** depends upon the localization and degree of the occlusion; a constriction of the lumen by more than 60% is required to have hemodynamic effects; typically, in the early stages, symptoms only develop during exertion; a division into **Fontaine stages** depending upon the clinical picture has proved useful: **stage I**: demonstrable stenoses or occlusions, but with no symptoms at rest or during exertion; **stage II**: pain on exertion [intermittent claudication]; if the pains are tolerated by the patient, this is **stage IIa**, if they cause personal or professional restrictions, then this is **stage IIb**; **stage III**: ischemic rest pain; **stage IV**: spontaneous tissue lesions [necrosis, gangrene, ulcers]; **diagnosis**: history and physical findings, stress test, angiography; **therapy**: in stage I, education and control of risk factors, lifestyle adjustments, on occasion prophylactic medication [e.g., with inhibitors of thrombocyte aggregation or statins]; stage IIa as for stage I plus systematic vessel training [AVK-groups]; beyond stage IIb, the stenosis is dilated [e.g., percutaneous transluminal angioplasty], a thrombectomy undertaken or a bypass performed; the perfusion can also be improved non-operatively by, e.g., thrombolysis, hemodilution, vasoactive substances [e.g., prostaglandins, naftidrofuryl, pentoxyphyllin, buflomedil] or anticoagulation; in stage IV, amputation is often the only way to relieve the patient of persistent pain and remove the risk of life-threatening sepsis

coronary artery disease → *coronary heart disease*

coronary heart disease *Syn:* *coronary artery disease*; generic term for all forms of coronary insufficiency, which are caused by a stenosing constriction of the coronary vessels, and which can lead to angina pectoris, myocardial infarctions, cardiac insufficiency, disturbances of heart rhythm or sudden cardiac death; the main risk factors include arterial hypertension, diabetes mellitus, disorders of fat metabolism, chronic cardiac insufficiency, arteriosclerosis, nicotine abuse, contraceptives, and the post-myocardial infarct state; clinically, coronary heart disease manifests mostly as angina pectoris with typical retrosternal pain and radiation into the left pectoralis muscle, to the inside of the left arm down to the little finger, into the throat, jaw, and into the upper abdomen; acute myocardial infarction and disturbances of heart rhythm are also typical manifestations; **diagnosis**: clinical features, history, ECG, echocardiography, MRI, cardiac catheterization, coronary angiography; **lab.**: blood sugar, triglycerides, total cholesterol, HDL- and LDL-cholesterol, lipoprotein-α, apolipoprotein A and B, cardiac muscle enzymes [CK, CK-MB]; **DD**: pulmonary embolism, pneumothorax, pleuritis sicca, intercostal neuralgia, aortic dissection, cardiomyopathies, perimyocarditis, reflux esophagitis, hiatus hernia, peptic ulcer disease, esophageal rupture, functional chest pains, cardiac neurosis, panic attacks; **therapy**: for the acute manifestations, the main focus is on treatment of any angina pectoris, infarct, insufficiency, or rhythm disturbance; thereafter, attention turns to the treatment of pain and removal of risk factors or trigger factors

Curschmann's disease → *frosted liver*
Degos' disease → *Degos' syndrome*
diffuse arterial disease → *panarteritis*
Döhle's disease → *luetic mesaortitis*
Döhle-Heller disease → *luetic mesaortitis*
Duroziez's disease Syn: *congenital mitral stenosis, congenital stenosis of mitral valve*; congenital mitral stenosis combined with anemia, enteroptosis, and hemorrhoids
Ebstein's disease → *Ebstein's anomaly*
Eisenmenger's disease → *Eisenmenger's tetralogy*
embolic disease → *embolism*
eosinophilic endomyocardial disease → *Löffler's endocarditis*
Fahr-Volhard disease Syn: *hyperplastic arteriolar nephrosclerosis, malignant nephrosclerosis*; rapidly progressive nephrosclerosis leading to renal insufficiency, e.g., in malignant hypertension
Fallot's disease → *Fallot's tetrad*
floating-beta disease → *type III familial hyperlipoproteinemia*
functional cardiovascular disease → *neurocirculatory asthenia*
Gaisböck's disease → *Gaisböck's syndrome*
giant platelet disease → *Bernard-Soulier syndrome*
Glanzmann's disease Syn: *constitutional thrombopathy, Glanzmann's thrombasthenia, hereditary hemorrhagic thrombasthenia, thrombasthenia, thromboasthenia*; autosomal recessive defect of the fibrinogen receptor glycoprotein IIb/IIIA on the thrombocytes; leads to a disturbance of thrombocyte adhesion and aggregation with increased bleeding tendency [petechial hemorrhages in the skin and mucous membranes]; **diagnosis**: thromboelastography, bleeding time; **therapy**: thrombocyte concentrates
Goldstein's disease → *Osler's disease*
Heberden's disease → *angina pectoris*
Heller-Döhle disease → *luetic mesaortitis*
hemoglobin disease → *hemoglobinopathy*
Horton's disease → *Horton's arteritis*
Huchard's disease Syn: *continued arterial hypertension*; early stage of

arteriosclerosis with minimal changes or symptoms

Hutinel's disease tuberculous pericarditis in childhood with development of cardiac insufficiency, liver congestion and liver cirrhosis

immune-complex diseases → *immune-complex disorders*

Kimura's disease form of angiolymphoid hyperplasia with eosinophilia prevalent in Japan

Köhlmeier-Degos disease → *Degos' syndrome*

Kussmaul's disease Syn: *Kussmaul-Meier disease, arteritis nodosa, panarteritis nodosa*; systemic inflammation of small and medium sized arteries, mainly in the calf and forearm muscles and internal organs; mainly affects middle-aged women; there is probably an underlying allergic reaction of Arthus type; in 30% of patients, HBs antigen is found; **clinical**: in addition to general symptoms [fever, fatigue, weight loss], there may also be hypertension, renal involvement with glomerulonephritis and proteinuria [70%], cardiac symptoms [angina pectoris, pericarditis, myocardial infarct; 70%], myalgias [50%], arthralgias [50%], gastrointestinal symptoms [50%], neurologic injury [juvenile apoplexy, cramps, polyneuropathy 50%], and skin manifestations [palpable cutaneous or subcutaneous nodes along the course of arteries; 40%]; **therapy**: initially glucocorticoids and/or cyclophosphamide until remission; thereafter methotrexate, azathioprine, or cyclosporin A; **prognosis**: stepwise intermittent course; rarely fulminant and fatal course within 1–2 years

Kussmaul-Meier disease → *Kussmaul's disease*

Libman-Sacks disease → *nonbacterial thrombotic endocarditis*

Löffler's disease → *Löffler's endocarditis*

Lutembacher's disease Syn: *Lutembacher's complex, Lutembacher's syndrome*; congenital atrial septal defect with mitral stenosis; **therapy**: closure of the atrial septal defect and dilatation or commissurotomy of the mitral valve; later usually valve replacement

Marfan's disease Syn: *acromacria, arachnodactylia, arachnodactyly, Marfan's syndrome*; autosomal dominant syndrome with skeletal, ocular, and cardiovascular malformations; **clinical**: long thin limbs, which are too long in relationship to the trunk, are conspicuous; long, narrow hands [madonna hands], fingers [spidery fingers], and feet; tall stature; gothic (high-arched) palate with bite anomalies [malocclusion, retrognathy, long, irregular teeth]; chicken or funnel chest; kyphosis; scoliosis; flat back; hypermobile joints; in addition, there are also eye symptoms [lens subluxation] and symptoms of cardiovascular disease [aortic dilatation or dissection]

Mondor's disease painful, recurrent thrombophlebitis of the lateral trunk veins [thoracoepigastric veins]

Morgagni's disease → *Adams-Stokes syndrome*

Moschcowitz disease → *thrombotic microangiopathy*

Moszkowicz's disease → *thrombotic microangiopathy*

Norum-Gjone disease → *idiopathic LCAT deficiency*

Ortner's disease *Syn: abdominal angina, intestinal angina*; colicky abdominal pain with symptoms of the acute abdomen due to restriction of the perfusion of the small intestine due to arteriosclerosis of the mesenteric vessels; course, prognosis, and therapy depend upon the extent and duration of the ischemia

Osler's disease *Syn: Goldstein's disease, hereditary hemorrhagic telangiectasia, Osler-Weber-Rendu disease, Rendu-Osler-Weber disease, Rendu-Osler-Weber syndrome*; autosomal dominant disease with formation of telangiectasias in the skin and mucous membranes, arteriovenous aneurysms and recurrent internal bleeding; **therapy**: symptomatic; control of bleeding, laser coagulation of the telangiectasias and aneurysms; **prognosis**: 5% of patients die from internal bleeding

Osler-Weber-Rendu disease → *Osler's disease*

Owren's disease → *factor V deficiency*

parenchymal heart and lung disease → *parenchymal cor pulmonale*

peripheral arterial occlusive disease *Syn: peripheral occlusive disease*; *s.u. chronic arterial occlusive disease*

peripheral occlusive disease *Syn: peripheral arterial occlusive disease*; *s.u. chronic arterial occlusive disease*

pulseless disease → *brachiocephalic arteritis*

Raynaud's disease idiopathic, episodic, arterial spasms, and the disturbances of perfusion that these cause, affecting the hands and feet; particularly triggered by cold and leads to painful pallor and coldness of multiple fingers or toes, followed by cyanosis and reactive hyperemia; if it persists, it can lead to trophic changes, necrosis and gangrene; in **true Raynaud's disease**, no cause can be found, while **secondary Raynaud's disease** occurs in a series of diseases [among others, progressive scleroderma, cold agglutinin disease, vibration white finger disease]; **therapy**: treatment of the cause, avoidance of cold, elimination of nicotine, on occasion systemic treatment with vasodilators [e.g., nifedipine, prostacyclin]

regurgitant disease → *valvular regurgitation*

Rendu-Osler-Weber disease → *Osler's disease*

Roger's disease *Syn: maladie de Roger*; congenital ventricular septal defect, which mostly heals spontaneously

Rougnon-Heberden disease → *angina pectoris*

stenotic valvular disease → *valvular stenosis*

Stokes-Adams disease → *Adams-Stokes syndrome*

Takayasu's disease → *brachiocephalic arteritis*

Taussig-Bing disease → *Taussig-Bing syndrome*

thyrocardiac disease → *thyroid cardiomyopathy*

thyrotoxic heart disease → *thyroid cardiomyopathy*

Virchow's disease → *amyloidosis*

von Willebrand's disease → *angiohemophilia*

Wenckebach's disease → *bathycardia*

Werlhof's disease → *idiopathic thrombocytopenic purpura*

Winiwarter-Buerger disease *Syn: Buerger's disease, thromboangiitis obliterans*; arterial occlusive condition mostly occurring in smokers [men aged 20–40 years] affecting the small and medium sized arteries of the extremities; often accompanied by phlebitis or thrombophlebitis; leads eventually to arterial occlusive disease; **therapy**: the treatment of choice is to stop smoking and this is also of critical importance to prognosis; prostacyclin i.v. over 3–4 weeks improves the symptoms; non-steroidal anti-inflammatories for the accompanying phlebitis or thrombophlebitis; on occasion, thoracic or lumbar sympathectomy

disk *Syn: disc*; any thin, flat, circular plate or object

intercalated disk straight or zigzag discs in the heart muscle

disopyramide antiarrhythmic of chinidine type; **usage**: supraventricular and ventricular tachycardia, extrasystoles

disorder a disturbance of function or structure; disease, illness

immune-complex disorders *Syn: immune-complex diseases*; illness caused by circulating immune complexes; the immune complexes are deposited in the walls of the blood vessels of various organs and lead to the development of a local type III hypersensitivity reaction; examples include certain forms of glomerulonephritis, endocarditis, and myocarditis, as well as the collagenoses

LDL-receptor disorder *Syn: familial hyperbetalipoproteinemia, familial hypercholesteremic xanthomatosis, familial hypercholesterolemia, type IIa familial hyperlipoproteinemia*; hyperlipoproteinemia with extremely high cholesterol levels and very high arteriosclerosis risk; typically includes xanthomata, xanthelasmas, and arcus lipoides cor-

dispersion

neae

post-stress disorder disturbance of circulation due to sudden relief of physical strain

dispersion the act or process of dispersing

Q-T dispersion *s.u. electrocardiogram*

dissection a pathological splitting or separation of tissue

aortic dissection *Syn: dissecting aortic aneurysm*; dissecting aneurysm of the aorta; this disease occurs at an older age [usually after 55 years of age], primarily in patients with arterial hypertension and diabetes mellitus and in smokers; Marfan syndrome and Ehlers-Danlos syndrome also have an increased risk; a ripping pain, either in the chest [ascending aorta] or between the shoulder blades [descending aorta], usually associated with an anxiety of death, is almost always typical for **acute aortic dissection**; it is clinically silent in only a small number of cases; **diagnostic procedures**: history and physical findings, anteroposterior chest X-ray, echocardiography, aortography, CT, NMR; **therapy** is determined by the **Stanford classification**; in **Stanford type A**, the ascending aorta and possibly also the descending aorta

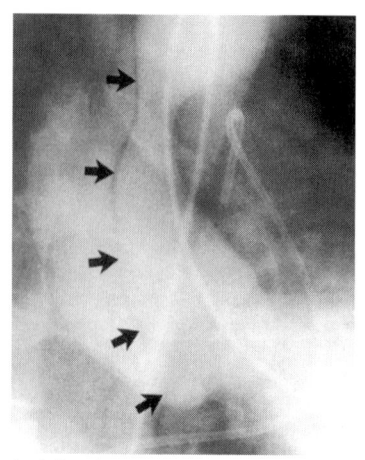

Aortic dissection

are affected, but in **Stanford type B** only the descending aorta; type A is always treated surgically; in type B, a conservative treatment is instituted first [lowering of blood pressure with β-blockers]; surgery is performed if this is unsuccessful; in type A, a partial resection with or without replacement of the aortic valve is usually performed; in type B, an attempt is made to prevent progression of dissection or an aortic rupture by insertion of a prosthesis

arterial dissection lamellar splitting of the arterial wall between the media and intima, e.g., in arteriosclerosis

dissociation incoordination of the atrial and ventricular rhythm

atrioventricular dissociation *Syn: auriculoventricular dissociation*; independent beat frequency of the atria and ventricles

auriculoventricular dissociation → *atrioventricular dissociation*

disturbance trouble, failure, breakdown, fault, defect

disturbance in conduction disturbance of the excitation conduction system of the heart that affects the heart rhythm

excitation disturbance disturbance to the normal pattern of excitation in the heart muscle tissue

disturbances in repolarization found after myocardial infarctions, in coronary stenoses, Prinzmetal angina, and other ischemic states; in the exercise ECG, they appear as (ascending, parallel, descending, synclinal) ST-depression or [rarely] ST-elevation; sometimes the ST-depression only appears after the end of the exercise

disturbance of perfusion → *impaired perfusion*

disturbance in stimulus conduction disturbance to the excitation conduction system affecting the heart rhythm

diuresis the physiological excretion of urine

water diuresis *Syn: hydrodiuresis*; increased excretion of water in excessive water intake or hyposmolarity of the blood

diuretic *Syn: evacuant, urinative, water pill*; **1.** an agent, which increases the excretion of sodium ions [**natriuretic**] or salts [**saluretic**]; the following groups are differentiated: **thiazides** and **thiazide-like substances** [hydrochlorothiazide, clopamide] prevent the reabsorption of sodium and chloride ions in the distal tubule; potassium ions are excreted increasingly; they may lead to hypokalemia and thrombophilia due to hemoconcentration **aldosterone antagonists** [spironolactone] block aldosterone receptors in tubule cells; as a result, the excretion of water and sodium and hydrogen carbonate ions is promoted and that of potassium ions reduced; there is a risk of hyperkalemia, gynecomastia, potency problems, hirsutism, and amenorrhoea **potassium-sparing diuretics** [amiloride, triamterene] prevent sodium reabsorption in tubule cells and thereby the excretion of potassium ions; **side effects**: hyperkalemia, vomiting **loop diuretics** [furosemide, ethacrynic acid] are highly potent diuretics, which inhibit the reabsorption of sodium and chloride ions in the ascending limb of Henle's loop; they are used primarily in edema and acute renal failure and may lead to hypokalemia and thrombophilia due to hemoconcentration **carbonic anhydrase inhibitors** [diclofenamide] inhibit hydrogen and sodium ion exchange in tubule cells; as a result, the excretion of potassium, sodium, and hydrogen carbonate ions is promoted and that of ammonium ions reduced; loss of bases leads to acidosis, which can influence the excretion of other drugs **osmotic diuretics** [mannitol, sorbitol] are given as an i.v. infusion and result in the excretion of water bound osmotically to them; they are used in cerebral edema and to prevent renal failure in shock **xanthine derivatives** [caffeine, theophylline] have found very little use therapeutically **2.** relating to or stimulating diuresis, promoting diuresis

high-ceiling diuretic → *loop diuretic*

loop diuretic *Syn: high-ceiling diuretic*; highly potent diuretic that inhibits the reabsorption of sodium and chloride ions in the ascending limb of Henle's loop; it is used primarily in edema and acute renal failure and potentially leads to hypokalemia and thrombophilia due to hemoconcentration

diurnal during the day, by day, daily; on a daily cycle

diverticulum circumscribed pouch or sac

pressure diverticulum → *pulsion diverticulum*

pulsion diverticulum *Syn: pressure diverticulum*; diverticulum caused by increased internal pressure and weakness of the wall

division 1. the act or process of dividing **2.** the state of being divided

thoracolumbar division of autonomic nervous system → *sympathetic nervous system*

dobutamine stimulator of the β_1-receptors in the heart; increases the contractility and stroke volume; reduces the peripheral resistance; **usage**: antihypotensive in cardiogenic shock, cardiac failure in cardiomyopathy, myocardial infarct, acute decompensated cardiac insufficiency; **side effects**: tachycardia, extrasystoles, angina pectoris, headaches, allergic reactions

dopa, decarboxylated → *dopamine*

dopamine *Syn: 3-hydroxytyramine, decarboxylated dopa*; catecholamine; intermediate product in the synthesis of adrenaline and noradrenaline which is derived from tyrosine; functions as a neurotransmitter in the putamen, corpus striatum, and caudate nucleus; inactivated by reabsorption into the nerve endings; dopamine deficiency in the putamen and caudate nucleus is the cause of Parkinson's disease; because of its action as an α_1- and β_1-sympathomimetic, dopamine is used for the i.v. treatment of cardiogenic shock, cardiovascular insufficiency, extreme hypotension, and impending renal failure

dopaminergic activated by or transmitted by dopamine, acting by releasing dopamine

dopexamine β_1-sympathomimetic; has a weaker action than dopamine; **usage**: acute cardiac insufficiency

double-diffusion in two dimensions → *Ouchterlony test*

DRI → *direct renin inhibitor*

dromogram recording of the velocity of the bloodstream using a dromograph

dromograph apparatus for flow measurement, e.g., of the bloodstream

dromotropic influencing the conduction velocity of the excitatory impulse in the heart

dromotropism *Syn: dromotropy*; action on the conduction velocity of the excitatory impulse in the heart; in **positive dromotropy**, the conduction velocity is increased, in **negative dromotropy**, it falls

dromotropy → *dromotropism*

dropsy → *hydrops*
  abdominal dropsy → *ascites*
  cardiac dropsy → *hydropericardium*

drug any substance used to treat, diagnose or prevent disease
  alpha-adrenergic receptor blocking drug → *alpha-blocker*
  alpha blocking drug → *alpha-blocker*
  blocking drug → *blocker*

duct passage, vessel
  duct of Arantius → *ductus venosus*
  arterial duct → *ductus arteriosus*
  Botallo's duct → *ductus arteriosus*

ductus duct, passage
  ductus arteriosus *Syn: arterial canal, arterial duct, Botallo's duct, pulmoaortic canal*; connection between the pulmonary trunk and the aortic arch in the fetal circulation; the wall contains smooth muscle

cells, which close the channel after birth; the **ligamentum arteriosum** is the atrophied remnant of the ductus arteriosus

ductus arteriosus apertus *Syn: patent ductus arteriosus, open Botallo's duct, persistent ductus arteriosus*; patency of the ductus arteriosus after birth; it is the most frequent congenital angiocardiopathy, which usually affects women; other cardiovascular malformations are present in about 15% of the cases [primarily atrial septal defect, atrioventricular septal defect, ventricular septal defect]; because the pressure is lower in the pulmonary circulation, a left-to-right shunt develops; the **clinical picture** depends on the width of the shunt and the shunt blood volume; small shunts remain clinically unremarkable, but with larger shunts heart failure occurs in the longterm and thereby also a decline in physical functional capacity; only extremely large shunts produce symptoms even in infancy [poor feeding, dyspnea, hepatomegaly]; auscultation reveals a continuous machinery murmur over the second-third intercostal space and the second heart sound is barely audible; the ECG is usually normal; only large shunts produce signs of a left ventricular load and hypertrophy; size and flow can be determined by Doppler sonography; the **prognosis** depends on the size of the left-to-right shunt; without treatment, the life expectancy is about 25–35 years, but 30% of patients die during childhood; **therapy**: the treatment of choice today is closure by double umbrella occluder, coil, or spirals, which are positioned through a catheter

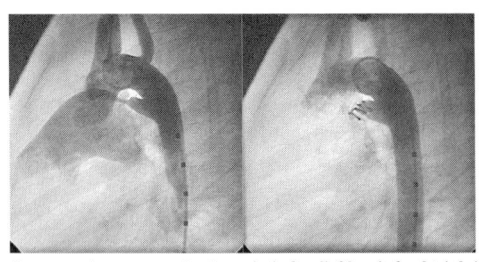

Ductus arteriosus apertus. Angiography before [left] and after [right] closure with a coil

patent ductus arteriosus → *ductus arteriosus apertus*
ductus venosus *Syn: canal of Arantius, canal of Cuvier, duct of Arantius*; anastomosis between the umbilical vein and inferior vena cava in the

fetal circulation; regresses after birth and forms the ligamentum teres

dysbetalipoproteinemia, familial → *type III familial hyperlipoproteinemia*

dysfibrinogen *Syn: nonclottable fibrinogen*; non-coagulable fibrinogen

dysfunction *Syn: abnormal function, parafunction*; functional disturbance, malfunction

dyskinesia *Syn: dyscinesia*; difficulty or abnormality in performing voluntary muscular movements

    intermittent dyskinesia → *Determann's syndrome*

dysplasia malformation or abnormal development of a tissue or organ

    atriodigital dysplasia *Syn: Holt-Oram syndrome, heart-hand syndrome*; autosomal dominant malformation of the thumb combined with an atrial septal defect

dyspnea *Syn: dyspnoea, shortness of breath, labored breathing, breathlessness, difficult respiration, labored respiration*; difficult breathing is a subjective symptom in increased work of breathing; both cardiac and pulmonary dyspnea can occur episodically, persist chronically, and increase with physical exertion; later these also occur at rest or when supine; cardiac and pulmonary dyspnea cannot be differentiated using the medical history

    cardiac dyspnea dyspnea in left ventricular failure; it develops in the sequence: exertional dyspnea – dyspnea at rest – orthopnea

    pulmonary dyspnea dyspnea caused by changes or diseases of the lungs

dysprothrombinemia autosomal recessive defect of prothrombin formation, which leads to a variably pronounced bleeding tendency

dysrhythmia defective rhythm

dystrophia → *dystrophy*

dystrophy *Syn: dystrophia*; disorder of the whole body, individual organs, or tissues caused by deficiency or malnourishment

E

ebullism → *aeroembolism*

echocardiogram image obtained by echocardiography

echocardiographic relating to echocardiography

echocardiography ultrasound examination; non-invasive technique in which electrical energy is converted into sound waves with a frequency of 2–10 MHz; absorption, reflection, and refraction of the sound waves in the tissues generate specific images that are displayed on a screen; three different processes are used in clinical practice: M-mode, 2-D echocardiography [B-mode imaging], and Doppler sonography; echocardiography is predominantly used to assess the pericardium, myocardium, endocardium, and heart valves

Doppler echocardiography procedure using the Doppler effect to measure the velocity of the bloodstream in the heart and in the pericardiac vessels; in **conventional Doppler echocardiography**, the Doppler signal is presented acoustically as well as graphically; in **color-coded Doppler echocardiography**, the direction and velocity of flow are coded using different colors and intensities and overlayed on a conventional B-mode or M-mode echocardiogram

epicardial echocardiography method used intra-operatively in which the transducer is applied directly to the epicardium

transesophageal echocardiography the probe is attached to the tip of an endoscope, which is introduced into the esophagus; the probe can usually point in any direction [**multiplanar transesophageal echocardiography**]; the proximity to the atria produces an extremely good visualization of intra-atrial structures

echography → *ultrasonography*

pulse echography Syn: *impulse echo technique*; *s.u. sonography*

echophonocardiography combined echocardiography and phonocardiography

ectasia → *ectasy*

arterial ectasia → *arteriectasis*

diffuse arterial ectasia *Syn: racemose aneurysm, cirsoid aneurysm; s.u. aneurysm*

ectasis → *ectasy*

ectasy *Syn: ectasia, ectasis*; permanent dilatation of hollow organs, vessels, and similar

ectocardia *Syn: cardiocele, exocardia*; congenital displacement of the heart out of the chest cavity, e.g., into the abdominal cavity [**ectocardia abdominalis/subthoracica**] or in front of the chest cavity [**ectocardia thoracica**] due to a cleft chest wall [thoracoschisis]; the displacement can be complete [**ectopia cordis completa**] or incomplete [**ectopia cordis incompleta**] and is mostly accompanied by other malformations [e.g., Fallot's tetralogy]

ectogenic → *exogenous*

ectogenous → *exogenous*

ectopic *Syn: atopic, heterotopic, aberrant*; relating to ectopia, arising from a different location than normal

edema *Syn: water thesaurismosis*; circumscribed or diffuse collection of water in tissues or cells; edema arises when the steady state between capillary filtration and capillary absorption and lymph drainage is disturbed; increase in the hydrostatic pressure [e.g., increased blood volume in renal or heart failure], reduction of oncotic pressure [protein deficiency in improper nutrition or malnutrition, nephrotic syndrome], increased capillary wall permeability [e.g., inflammation, allergic reactions, burns], and disturbances of lymphatic drainage [tumors, after surgery, parasites] lead to the development of edema; edema can also be subdivided into **primary edema** [in acute or chronic renal failure] and **secondary edema**; the first form is also called **overfill edema** and the second **underfill edema**; most edemas remain limited to interstitial tissue [**interstitial** or **extracellular edema**]; when the cell membrane is damaged or the extracellular volume cannot increase [e.g., in the cranial cavity], fluid can also flow into the cell [**cellular edema**]

angioneurotic edema subcutaneous swelling of the skin and mucous membranes caused by an allergic reaction; often combined with hives [urticaria]

cardiac edema secondary edema in heart failure; left ventricular failure leads to pulmonary edema and right ventricular failure primarily to ankle edema and pretibial edema

hereditary angioneurotic edema angioneurotic edema due to autosomal dominant deficiency of the C1-esterase inhibitor; the genesis of the swelling is not fully understood, but relates to increased vascular permeability; **clinical**: the recurrent attacks are impressive for their sudden [within a few hours], tense, swelling, which mostly affects the facial area and is associated with the risk of laryngeal edema and suffocation; the edema is painless, does not itch, and is not accompanied by urticaria; vomiting, colicky abdominal pain, and diarrhea are signs of angioedema of the intestinal mucosa; **therapy**: C1-INH replacement; antihistamines, and steroids are ineffective

intimal edema collection of fluid in the intima as a result of insudation; often a precursor to intimal fibrosis or sclerosis

edema of lung → *pulmonary edema*

lymphatic edema → *lymphedema*

primary edema *s.u. edema*

pulmonary edema *Syn: edema of lung, wet lung, pneumonedema*; accumulation of fluid in lung tissue [**interstitial pulmonary edema**] or air vesicles [**intra-alveolar pulmonary edema**]; the most frequent causes are left ventricular failure [**cardiac pulmonary edema**] or reduction of colloid osmotic pressure and increased vascular permeability [**non-cardiac pulmonary edema**]; the **clinical picture** includes restlessness, anxiety, sweating, tachypnea, hypoxemia, cyanosis, tachycardia, and foamy sputum; on auscultation, moist [and often in addition dry] rales are audible in intra-alveolar pulmonary edema, but these are not found in interstitial pulmonary edema; **diagnosis**: physical examination, ECG, chest X-ray, blood gas analysis, echocardiography; **therapy**: symptomatic treatment [upright body position, assisted ventilation with oxygen, nitroglycerin and furosemide to reduce preload, nifedipine or nitroprusside sodium to reduce afterload, sedation, CPAP ventilation if necessary] to improve the acute stage; treatment of the cause

secondary edema *s.u. edema*

edematigenous → *edematogenic*

edematogenic *Syn: edematigenous*; edema inducing, causing edema

edematous *Syn: tumid*; relating to or affected by edema

effect result of an action

Bohr effect dependence of the oxygen uptake and release in the blood on the pH and the carbon dioxide concentration; in the lung, the Bohr effect facilitates oxygen uptake, because the exhalation of carbon dioxide shifts the oxygen dissociation curve to the left; but in tissues, the high carbon dioxide concentrations causes a right shift in the dissociation curve and thereby a decline in the O_2 affinity, as well as increased oxygen diffusion into tissue

Doppler effect *Syn: Doppler phenomenon, Doppler principle*; changes in the wave frequency dependent upon the relative movements of transmitter and receiver; if these move toward each other, the frequency increases, and if they move apart, the frequency falls

effusion escape of fluid from the blood or lymph vessels into the tissue

pericardial effusion fluid collection in the pericardial sac as a facultative epiphenomenon of pericarditis; in idiopathic, viral, and autoimmune-reactive pericarditis, the effusion is serous or serofibrinous, in bacterial pericarditis cellular and purulent, and in tuberculosis and tumors mostly hemorrhagic; large effusions in acute pericarditis can lead to pericardial tamponade; in chronic pericarditis the pericardium stretches and in extreme cases up to 2 l of effusion can collect without any signs of pericardial tamponade; **diagnosis**: echocardiography can detect even small effusions of 5 ml [so-called **moist pericardium**]; in the X-ray, a large effusion is seen as a typical globular heart shadow; pericardiocentesis and microbiologic/serologic/biochemical laboratory tests/cytologic/immunologic examination of the aspirate helps in the search for the cause

pleural effusion *Syn: pleurorrhea, hydrothorax*; collection of fluid in the pleural cavity; it occurs primarily in pleurisy, heart failure, pericarditis, pulmonary infarction, pneumonia, pulmonary tuberculosis, hypoalbuminemia [nephrotic syndrome, malabsorption, cirrhosis of the liver], and primary and secondary pleural tumors; **diagnosis**: chest X-ray, CT, ultrasound, exploratory puncture; **therapy**: depends on the cause; in acute effusion [e.g., pulmonary infarction or inflammation], puncture and aspiration; in chronic effusions, permanent drainage and possibly pleurodesis

Eikenella corrodens facultatively pathogenic, Gram-negative bacterial rod; normally commensal in the oral and intestinal flora; occasionally found in wound infections, abscesses, meningitis or endocarditis; *s.a. HACEK group*

elasticin → *elastin*

elastin *Syn: elasticin*; skeletal protein of the elastic fibers with rubbery elasticity; consists of polypeptide chains, which are connected into a quaternary network by desmosine and isodesmosine; mainly occurs in elastic fibers and ligaments as well as the aortic wall

elastorrhexis fragmentation of elastic tissue

  systemic elastorrhexis generalized, degenerative disease of the elastic connective tissue with yellowish papules and skin blotches; inheritance is mostly autosomal recessive, partially also autosomal dominant; all organs, which contain elastic connective tissue, are affected, i.e., eye, skin, and cardiovascular system; the involvement of the eye can lead to blindness; the **clinical picture** is, however, dominated by the cardiovascular symptoms [hypertension, arteriosclerosis, myocarditis, internal bleeding]; the course is slowly progressive; there is no causal therapy available

elastosis angiopathy due to inclusion of altered elastic fibers in the vessel wall

electro- combining form denoting relation to electricity

electroatriogram recording of the spread of excitation in the atria

electrocardiogram as a result of the anatomic and electrophysiologic construction of the heart, there is a defined temporal and spatial progression of excitation of the individual heart muscle cells; simultaneous excitation of many muscle cells gives rise to sufficiently large potentials for these to be recorded from the body surface; **surface ECG**: a **standard ECG** usually comprises **12 recording sites**: 3 bipolar leads on the extremities after Einthoven, 3 unipolar leads on the extremities after Goldberger and 6 bipolar leads on the chest wall after Wilson; this allows the limb leads to acquire electric vectors in the coronal plane and the chest leads in the axial plane; in special cases, additional extended bipolar chest leads after Wilson as well as the 3 chest leads after Nehb can be recorded; the **bipolar leads after Einthoven** each record the potential difference between two limbs; the recording points make up the corners of an equilateral triangle in the coronal plane [**Einthoven's triangle**]; the positioning of the electrodes is proximal to the wrists or ankles with standardized electrode labeling: right arm – red, left arm – yellow, left leg – green, right leg – black [earth lead]; this is achieved by appropriate connection; **lead I**: right arm [–] → left arm [+], **lead II**: right arm [–] → left leg [+], **lead III**: left arm [–] → left leg [+]; the same electrode positions as used for the Einthoven recording are used for **unipolar limb lead recordings after Goldberger** by recording each individual limb as an active electrode with reference to an indifferent electrode; the electrode is formed by connection of the two uninvolved limbs, the active electrode is switched through resistors from the indifferent electrode; the unipolar recordings obtained are aligned from the mid-point of the **Einthoven triangle** to the respective corners of this triangle; Goldberger recordings are named "augmented" unipolar limb lead recordings as follows: **aVR** [right arm], **aVL** [left arm], and **aVF** [left foot]; the **unipolar chest wall recordings after Wilson** show the electric potential changes in the horizontal plane; each chest wall electrode is recorded relative to an indifferent electrode [connection of the three limb leads through resistors]; in addition to the standard leads V_1–V_6, there are extended precordial leads on the left side [V_7–V_9] and the right side [V_{3R}–V_{6R}]; for the **bipolar chest wall leads after Nehb**, the limb leads are placed on the chest wall in the following order: 1 = red electrode ["right arm"] over the right 2. rib parasternally, 2 = green electrode ["left leg"] over the cardiac apex beat and 3 = yellow electrode ["left arm"] at the level of the green electrode in the posterior axillary line on the left; corresponding to lead I, one records a dorsal lead [**Nehb D**], to lead II an anterior lead [**Nehb A**], and to lead III an inferior lead [**Nehb J**]; important **special ECG procedures** include the **esophageal ECG** [usually transnasal introduction of an electrode into the esophagus that permits recording of large atrial potentials; the probe is initially advanced into the stomach and then pulled back while recording the ECG until adequate atrial potentials are recorded approx. 40 cm from the teeth; used for differential diagnosis of supraventricular disturbances of rhythm], **late potential ECG** [late potentials are high frequency, low amplitude signals at the end of the QRS-complex, which arise in areas of damaged ventricular myocardium with slowed conduction; their amplitude in the surface ECG is very small, so they can only be recorded with high amplification and special noise-reduction techniques; this is achieved by **signal-averaged electrocardiography, SAECG** in temporal representations or by frequency analysis using the **fast Fourier transform (FFT)**], **stress-ECG** [ergometry; continuous ECG recording during physical exertion (bicycle ergometer, treadmill) can reveal disturbances of cardiac perfusion, stress-related disturbances of heart rhythm, as well as, using simultaneous recording of blood pressure, hyper- or hypotonic disturbances of circulatory control], **long-duration storage of ECG** [**Holter monitoring**; recording of the ECG with a portable magnetic tape recorder or solid state recording device; the gold standard is continuous recording, which permits detailed analysis of, e.g., ST-segment profiles, heart rate variability, and QT-variability] and **intracardiac ECG** [for this recording, several special electrodes are placed in the heart via a catheter introduced through the venous system]; in the **surface ECG**, the **atrial** component [electroatriogram], **atrioventricular conduction**, and the **ventricular component** [electroventriculogram] can be differentiated; following Einthoven, the waves recorded in this way are referred to by the letters **P** for the **atrial excitation**, **QRS** for the **ventricular excitation**, and T and U for the **ventricular relaxation**; **electroatriogram** [spread of excitation and repolarization in the atria]: the **P-wave** arises from the depolarization of the two atria with the beginning of the spread of excitation at the sinoatrial node: the early part of the P-wave is due to excitation of the right atrium, the second part is due to excitation of the left atrium; the normal duration of the P-wave is up to 0.10 s with an amplitude of 0.1–0.25 mV; the P-wave is generally positive in all leads except in III, V_1 and the right precordial leads; the repolarization of the atria is normally not recognizable in the surface ECG, since it is swamped by the higher amplitude QRS-complex; **atrioventricular conduction**: the **PQ-interval** is measured from the start of the P-wave to the start of the QRS-complex; the normal PQ-interval is rate-dependent 0.12–0.20 ms; **electroventriculogram** [spread of excitation and repolarization in the ventricles]: the **QRS-complex** characterizes the depolarization of the ventricles and can also be quite varied even in healthy individuals depending upon the recording; large amplitudes are labeled with capital letters [Q, R, S], small amplitudes with lower case letters [q, r, s]; a normal **Q-wave** in the limb leads is no more than ¼ the amplitude of the following R-wave and lasts no longer than 0.03 s [in aVL occasionally up to 0.04 s]; the **R-wave** reflects the primary electric vector; precordially, its amplitude increases through leads V_1–V_5, and declines again in V_6, with large inter-individual differences; the relationship between R-waves and S-waves is given as the **R/S-quotient** in the precordial leads; this increases from V_1 [< 1] to V_5, with the value 1 exceeded in V_2–V_4 [crossover or transition zone]; the **S-wave** arises as a result of the terminal depolarization of the ventricle with a mostly posterior and minimally cranial vector; one therefore finds deep S-waves [up to 2.0 mV] in V_1–V_3 as well as small S-waves in I, aVL, and V_6; occasional inflections or notches in the region of the crossover zone are generally not pathologic when the QRS-duration is normal; the **duration of a normal QRS-complex** without any disturbance of intraventricular conduction is 0.08 s; values above 0.10 s are pathologic and reflect a disturbance of intraventricular spread of excitation, whose **upper inflection point** can be used to characterize it; the **amplitude of the QRS-complex** in the limb leads varies depending upon the cardiac axis; the sums of the S in V_1 and R in V_5 or V_6 or the R in V_1 and S in V_5 are generally < 3.5 mV or < 1.05 mV respectively [**Sokolow-Lyon indices**]; the **ST-segment** represents the condition of complete ventricular depolarization and proceeds isoelectrically in the limb and left precordial leads, in contrast to the right precordial leads in which a slight convex upward curvature is usually found; horizontal or convexly curving ST-elevation leading from the R-wave as well as horizontal or descending ST-segments > 0.1 mV are considered to be pathologic; the **T-wave** arises from the repolarization of the ventricle, its duration is included in evaluation of the QT-interval; the vector of the T-wave is concordant with the vector of the QRS-complex except in lead III; the amplitude of the T-wave should be 1/8 to 2/3 that of the R-wave; the **QT-interval** characterizes the electric ventricular systole and is measured from the start of ventricular depolarization [start of the Q-wave] to the end of ventricular repolarization [end of the T-wave]; it is rate-dependent, so in addition to the **absolute QT-interval**, a **relative QT-interval** [determined using a nomogram, normal range: 80–120%] or a **corrected QT-interval** [QTc, calculated using **Bazett's formula**] is also given; **QT-dispersion** refers to the difference between the shortest and the longest QT-interval measurable from the surface ECG; occasionally, the T-wave can have a flat domed elevation – the **U-wave** – following it, whereby the border with the T-wave can be hard to define; the **determination of the cardiac axis** is achieved by assessing the main vector of ventricular depolarization in the limb leads; the types of axis are defined with reference to the angle α as follows: **over-rotated left type**: α > −30°, **left type**: α = +30° to −30° [using the Goldberger leads, this can be further subdivided into **semi horizontal type** and **horizontal type**], **indifferent type**: α = +30° to +60°, **steep type**: α = +60° to +90°, **right type**: α = +90° to +120°, **over-rotated right type**: α > +120°; if due to forward rotation of the heart, the main vector lies horizontally, that is, perpendicular to the coronal plane, this is described as a **sagittal type**; the QRS-amplitudes in the limb leads are only small; **ECG evaluation** [standard: 50 mm/s] is used to assess: **axis** [physiologic in adults are the right type, steep type, indifferent type, and left type; acute change of axis], **rhythm** [sinus rhythm, substitute rhythm, parasystole, cardiac pacemaker], **frequency** [normal rate 60–100/min,

electrocardiogram

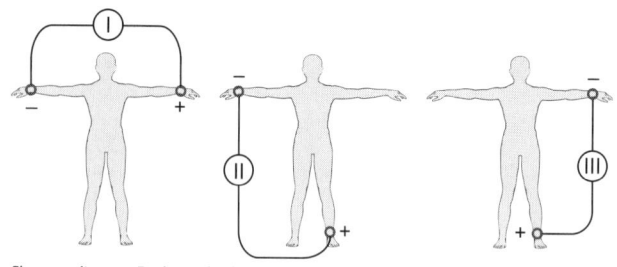

Electrocardiogram. Einthoven leads

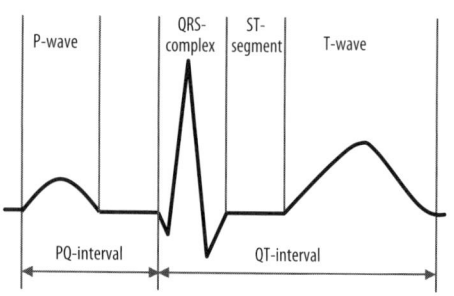

Electrocardiogram. Definitions

tachycardia, bradycardia], **time intervals** [P, PQ, QRS, QT], **atrial P-wave** [amplitude (≤ 0.25 mV), width (≤ 0.10 s), mono- or biphasic, positive or negative], **AV-conduction PQ-interval** [shortening (< 0.12 s), prolongation (> 0.20 s), AV-synchronicity, conduction ratio, pre-excitation (delta wave)] and **ventricular QRS-complex** [spread of excitation: QRS-morphology, QRS-amplitude, QRS-width (≤ 0.11 s), OUP, transition point; persistence of excitation: ST-segment isoelectric, elevation/depression; relaxation: T-wave dis-/concordant, peaked, flattened, terminal/preterminal negativity, U-wave; duration of ventricular excitation: QTc-time; disturbances of rhythm]; the ECG is a simple, uncomplicated investigation that is hardly any burden to the patient with a high predictive value; principal areas of use include diagnosis and therapeutic monitoring in coronary heart diseases [ST-segment analysis] with particular importance in the assessment of acute myocardial infarction, the assessment of disturbances of conduction, disturbances of heart rhythm, as well as of ventricular hypertrophy and the monitoring of cardiac pacemakers; in addition to the assessment of signs of ischemia [ST-segment analysis] and disturbances of heart rhythm, the state of the autonomic innervation of the heart can be assessed from heart rate variability using long-term ECG monitoring; for certain specific questions, the indications for additional investigations can be established using the ECG, e.g., cardiac catheterization for assessment of the coronary status, echocardiography for assessment of signs of hypertrophy, electrophysiologic tests for invasive clarification of disturbances of heart rhythm

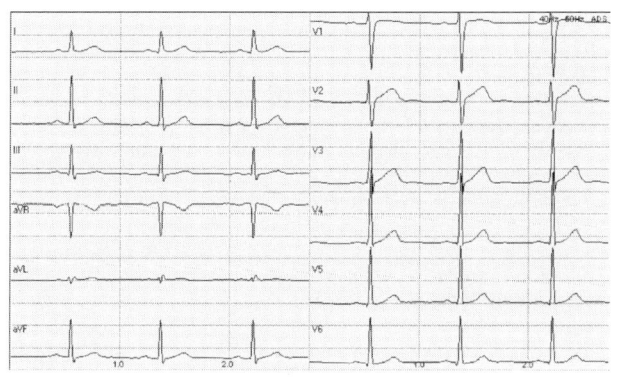

Electrocardiogram. Normal ECG with sinus rhythm

    late potential electrocardiogram *s.u. electrocardiogram*
    surface electrocardiogram *s.u. electrocardiogram*
electrocardiograph apparatus for electrocardiography
electrocardiographic relating to electrocardiography
electrocardiography recording of the action potential of the heart muscle
    exercise electrocardiography recording of an ECG during and after a defined exertion

His bundle electrocardiography intracardiac recording of the spread of excitation in the bundle of His

long term electrocardiography continuous ECG recording over 24–48 hours

signal-averaged electrocardiography *s.u. electrocardiogram*

electrocardiophonography combined electrocardiography and phonocardiography

electrocardioscope apparatus for the direct observation of the ECG trace

electrocardioscopy direct representation of the ECG trace on a display device; used, for example, on the Intensive Care Unit or as a miniature version in emergency doctors' cars

electrode that part of an electric conductor that serves as the entry or exit point for the electric current; electrodes come in all sizes [macroelectrodes for electrocardiography; microelectrodes for the measurement of cell membrane potentials] and shapes [button, disc, point, plate, needle, and ring electrodes]; for particular applications, electrodes can be mounted on endoscopes or catheters [**electrode catheter, catheter electrode**]

active electrode *Syn: exciting electrode, localizing electrode, therapeutic electrode*; the electrode from which the current exits during application of stimulating currents [**stimulating electrode**]; during conduction of an electric potential, the electrode which, with reference to a null electrode, has a potential difference [**recording electrode**]; in electrosurgery, the smaller electrode with higher current density, which cuts through the tissues, coagulates, etc. [**cutting electrode**]

catheter electrode *s.u. electrode*

coagulation electrode *s.u. coagulator*

exciting electrode → *active electrode*

localizing electrode → *active electrode*

therapeutic electrode → *active electrode*

electrodiagnostics recording and registration of bioelectric currents, e.g., electroencephalography, electrocardiography

electrokymography registration of the movement of the heart wall and great vessels using X-ray fluoroscopy; the pulsation of the heart causes variations in brightness on the screen, which is converted by photocells into fluctuating currents; rarely used today since ultrasound techniques [e.g., echocardiography] are simpler and do not involve exposure to ionizing radiation

electrostimulation the use of stimuli in diagnosis [electromyography, elec-

electroventriculogram section of the electrocardiogram, which relates to the spread of excitation in the ventricles

electroversion → *cardioversion*

elevation 1. the act of elevating **2.** the state of being elevated

ST segment elevation course of the ST-segment in the electrocardiogram above the (isoelectric) null line

embolectomy surgical removal of an embolus; it is performed either as a **direct** or **open embolectomy** after opening of the artery or as an **indirect embolectomy** using a balloon catheter [Fogarty balloon catheter], ring stripper, and the like

aspiration embolectomy *s.u. arterial embolism*

pulmonary embolectomy *Syn: Trendelenburg's operation*; a surgical removal of emboli in the pulmonary arteries is performed today only when there is a contraindication to thrombolysis

embolic relating to embolism or an embolus

emboliform like an embolus, stopper-like

embolism *Syn: embolic disease*; sudden blocking of a vessel by an embolus, air or gas bubbles, foreign bodies, fat droplets, etc.; the most frequent form is **thromboembolism** as a result of venous or arterial thrombosis; the clinical symptomatology depends on the type, localization, and extent of the embolism

air embolism *Syn: gas embolism, aeremia, aeroembolism, pneumatohemia, pneumathemia, pneumohemia*; embolism caused by air/gas bubbles in the arterial circulation [arterial air embolism] or in the venous system [venous air embolism]; it proceeds with sudden dyspnea, cyanosis, hypotension, and shock; the fatal amount of air is 0.5–1.5 ml/kg of body weight

arterial embolism embolic closure of an artery; mostly affects the pelvic and leg arteries [80%] and usually presents as an acute ischemic syndrome often with threat to life; the source of the embolus is mostly the heart [80–90%; cardiac aneurysm, heart valve prosthesis, mitral and aortic valve defects, bacterial endocarditis, atrial fibrillation] and proximal vessels [10–15%; aneurysms, atheromatous plaques]; air, fat, foreign body, tumor, and paradoxical embolism are all rarer; the **clinical** features depend upon the type, localization, and extent of the embolism; in extensive cases, the **6-Ps symptom complex of** Pain, Pallor, Pulselessness, Paresthesia, Paralysis develops in the affected limb, as well as the symptoms of shock [Prostration]; **therapy**: embolectomy is the method of choice; often performed as an **aspiration embolectomy**

capillary embolism embolization of capillaries by, e.g., dislodged cells, fat droplets, cholesterol crystals, or pathogens

cholesterol embolism embolization of the small arteries and capillaries by cholesterol crystals

crossed embolism → *paradoxical embolism*

fat embolism *Syn: oil embolism*; embolism caused by fat droplets in the bloodstream, e.g., after bone fracture and release of fat from the bone marrow; the emboli are found most frequently in the lungs, but can also occur in the systemic circulation [heart, brain, kidney, intestine, skin]; if a clinical symtomatology arises, the term **fat embolism syndrome** is used; if untreated, it leads to death in less than 24 hours; **clinical picture**: dyspnea, shortness of breath, restlessness, delirium, coma, petechial hemorrhages on the trunk and conjunctivas, cerebral symptoms [confusion, psychosis, apoplexy], signs of right ventricular failure; **therapy**: treatment of shock, volume replacement, improvement of microcirculation, treatment of respiratory failure, hypoxia, and acidosis

foreign-body embolism embolism caused by penetration of a foreign body into the circulation [cannula, catheter fragments]

gas embolism → *air embolism*

oil embolism → *fat embolism*

paradoxical embolism *Syn: crossed embolism*; arterial embolization of the systemic circulation by an embolus from the venous system, e.g., in ventricular or atrial septal defect

pulmonary embolism *Syn: pulmonary artery embolism*; blockage of a pulmonary artery by an embolus [thrombus, fat droplets, bone marrow particles, amniotic fluid, tumor cells, bacteria, parasites, foreign bodies]; the development of a pulmonary embolism is promoted especially by confinement to bed after surgery, accidents, childbirth, or internal diseases; overweight patients and patients with a history of deep leg vein thrombosis are especially at risk; the **clinical picture** depends on the narrowing of vessels and the localization of the blockage; the embolism can proceed as subclinical or clinically manifest diseases; the majority of the clinically manifest pulmonary embolisms proceeds with a clinical picture of acute cor pulmonale, but shock also occurs in some cases; patients complain of acute dyspnea, tachypnea, pleural pain, cough, palpitations, and angina symptoms; **diagnosis**: medical history, physical examination, auscultation [accentuated second heart sound], ECG, lung perfusion and lung ventilation scintigraphy; **differential diagnosis**: myocardial infarction, angina pectoris, pneumothorax, pulmonary edema, bronchial asthma, pneumonia, pleurisy, aortic dissection, and intercostal neuralgia; **therapy**: anticoagulation with heparin infusion [25,000–30,000 IU/24 hours as a continuous infusion], bed rest, sedation, analgesics, and oxygen; small and moderate pulmonary embolisms heal with the formation of an infarct scar; development of infarction pneumonia is rare; in massive pulmonary embolism with cardiogenic shock, the patient must be treated in an intensive care unit; a surgical pulmonary embolectomy in rare cases [blockage of central pulmonary arteries]; prophylaxis of recurrent pulmonary embolisms is important with treatment of the primary disease, long-term anticoagulant therapy, remedial exercises, surgical stockings, possibly treatment of varicose veins, vein ligation, or vena cava filters

pulmonary artery embolism →*pulmonary embolism*

venous embolism embolic blocking of a vein; the emboli generally stem from deep leg and pelvic veins or the right atrium and cause a pulmonary embolism

embolization Syn: *embolic therapy, therapeutic embolization*; therapeutic occlusion of a vessel by, e.g., coils, glues, etc.; usually performed as catheter embolization in order to stop bleeding or for palliative treatment of inoperable tumors [**tumor embolization**]

therapeutic embolization →*embolization*

embolomycosis embolization by a fungal plug in fungal sepsis or massive fungal invasion of the bloodstream

embolomycotic relating to embolomycosis

embolus non-soluble body in the circulation, which occludes a vessel and gives rise to an embolism; the most common are detached thrombi, fat droplets, air or gas bubbles, tumor cells, or foreign bodies [e.g., catheter tips]

cholesterol embolus →*atheroembolus*

pulmonary embolus an embolus causing pulmonary embolism

emergency a sudden unforeseen crisis that requires immediate action

hypertensive emergency exists when, as a result of a pathologically increased blood pressure a life-threatening situation has developed, and the clinical situation demands immediate reduction of the pressure in order to prevent further pressure-related organ damage; this is the case if, in addition to markedly elevated values for blood pressure, there are also signs of cardiovascular or cerebral end-organ damage [hypertensive encephalopathy, intracranial bleeding with neurologic deficits, dissecting aortic aneurysm, acute or threatened myocardial infarction, acute left heart failure with threatened pulmonary edema, eclampsia, malignant hypertension]; the immediate, but not abrupt, reduction in blood pressure, which is indicated in a hypertensive emergency, may require intravenous therapy with intensive care monitoring

empyema accumulation of pus in a body cavity

empyema of the pericardium → *pyopericardium*

enalapril ACE inhibitor; **usage**: arterial hypertension, cardiac insufficiency

encarditis → *endocarditis*

encephalomyocarditic relating to or marked by encephalomyocarditis

encephalomyocarditis → *EMC syndrome*

encephalorrhagia *Syn: cerebral hemorrhage*; bleeding into the brain is the cause of 10–15% of all strokes; men and women are equally affected; the frequency increases with increasing age; **etiology**: approx. 70% of patients have an elevated blood pressure; additional contributory factors include alcohol consumption, vessel malformations, anticoagulant therapy, and thrombolytic therapy [e.g., in pulmonary embolization]; the **diagnosis** is based upon history and clinical findings; computer tomography provides images with the best diagnostic yield; **therapy**: mostly conservative [treatment of the cause of bleeding, reduction of intracranial pressure]; cerebellar bleeds, lobar bleeds, and basal ganglia bleeds are sometimes operated upon, but the results are equivocal

endangeitis → *endangiitis*

endangiitic relating to or marked by endangiitis

endangiitis *Syn: endangeitis, endoangiitis, endovasculitis*; inflammation of the endangium

endangium → *intima*

endaortitis *Syn: endo-aortitis*; inflammation of the aortic intima; mostly in the setting of endarteritis obliterans or rheumatic diseases

endarterectomy *Syn: thromboendarterectomy*; operative removal of an arterial thrombus with cleaning of the inner wall of the vessel; for more superficial vessels, can be carried out as an **open** or **direct thromboendarterectomy**, but mostly carried out as a **half-closed** or **indirect**

thromboendarterectomy, in which a ring stripper or balloon catheter is passed into the opened artery

carotid endarterectomy opening of the carotid [external/internal/common] and removal of an old thrombus

endarterial in an artery

end-arteries → *end arteries*

endarteritic relating to or marked by endarteritis

endarteritis *Syn: endoarteritis*; inflammation of the intima of an artery

end-diastolic *Syn: telediastolic*; (occurring) at the end of diastole

end-expiratory *Syn: endexpiratory, end-tidal*; at the end of exhalation/expiration

endoaneurysmoplasty → *endoaneurysmorrhaphy*

endoaneurysmorrhaphy *Syn: endoaneurysmoplasty*; opening and cleaning out of an aneurysm with subsequent suturing

endo-aortitis → *endaortitis*

endoarteritis → *endarteritis*

endobronchial *Syn: intrabronchial*; occurring or proceeding in the bronchi

endocardiac → *endocardial*

endocardial *Syn: endocardiac*; relating to endocard

endocarditic relating to endocarditis

endocarditis *Syn: encarditis*; inflammation of the inner lining of the heart [endocardium], which generally also affects the heart valves [**endocarditis valvularis**]; causes include mechanical, ischemic, infective, immunologic, and toxic injury; nowadays, by far the most common in Central and Western Europe is **infective endocarditis**; the **rheumatic endocarditis** that previously dominated still plays a significant role in Eastern Europe, North Africa, Turkey, and in the Near and Far East; endocarditis of prosthetic heart valves is relatively common, whereas Löffler's endocarditis, endocardial fibroelastosis, endomyocardial fibrosis, and Libman-Sacks endocarditis are rare; patients with congenital or acquired heart valve defects have an increased risk of endocarditis, e.g., after dental treatment or tonsillectomy; they must be identified and treated with prophylactic antibiotics

parietal endocarditis *Syn: mural endocarditis*; endocarditis affecting mainly the lining of the chambers

atypical verrucous endocarditis → *nonbacterial thrombotic endocarditis*

constrictive endocarditis → *Löffler's endocarditis*

fungal endocarditis *Syn: mycotic endocarditis*; infective endocarditis caused by fungal attack [Candida species]

gonococcal endocarditis endocarditis caused by gonococci

infectious endocarditis → *infective endocarditis*

infective endocarditis *Syn: infectious endocarditis*; inflammation of the endocardium due to microorganisms [predominantly bacteria, fungi]; almost always affects the endocardium of the heart valves and parts of the adjacent mural endocardium; until the introduction of penicillin and other antibiotics approx. 50 years ago, the mortality was nearly 100%; nowadays it is around 10–15% in acute cases, although in fungal infections it is still up to 50%; the spectrum of pathogens has also changed [in part due to antibiotic treatment of other diseases]; streptococci are less frequent pathogens, but instead Gram-negative bacteria, fungi, and atypical pathogens are found more commonly; the average age of patients has increased from 30 to 50 years; i.v. drug abuse and indwelling venous catheters have led to the more frequent involvement of the right heart and tricuspid valve than previously; 55–75% of patients with infective endocarditis have predisposing factors, such as, e.g., anomalies of the valve apparatus, congenital heart defects, mitral valve prolapse, drug abuse; valve prostheses and other cardiac implants form an increasing problem [**prosthetic endocarditis**]; left-sided infective endocarditis mainly affects the aortic valve [50%], mitral valve [25%], and the suture ring of valve prostheses [20%]; in 90% of cases the course is that of a systemic infection or sepsis; right-sided infective endocarditis frequently manifests itself as septic thromboembolism with pneumonia; **acute infective endocarditis** arises in bacteremia with highly virulent pathogens; it mainly affects macroscopically unchanged heart valves; within two weeks, the patient develops fever, sweats, rigors, general malaise, ESR elevation, enlargement of the spleen; a new heart murmur is a cardinal symptom and can be an early sign of developing cardiac insufficiency; **subacute infective endocarditis** mainly develops based on a previously injured heart valve or congenital or acquired heart defects; in the form of subacute bacterial endocarditis due to Streptococcus viridans, it was formerly a classic rheumatic endocarditis; the course is insidious, with progression over weeks to months; metastatic spread is rare; anemia, hematuria, significant weight loss and anorexia, joint pains, and finger clubbing are all more common; the most common **complications** are embolism [up to 65% brain emboli], metastatic abscesses [lungs, brain, spleen] and cardiac insufficiency [mainly when the aortic or mitral valves are affected], with left-sided endocarditis, fungal endocarditis, and prosthetic endocarditis carrying the highest risks; **diagnosis**: history, physical findings, laboratory tests [ESR, blood picture, C-reactive protein], the most important is demonstration of the pathogen in blood cultures, generally positive identification occurs with 3 × 2 cultures within 24 h; in addition, so-called secondary criteria must be taken into consideration; **therapy**: specific antibiotic therapy, decontamination of the source of infection, symptomatic treatment of fever, anemia, cardiac insufficiency

Libman-Sacks endocarditis → *nonbacterial thrombotic endocarditis*

Löffler's endocarditis *Syn: constrictive endocarditis, eosinophilic endomyocardial disease, Löffler's disease, Löffler's fibroplastic endocarditis, Löffler's syndrome, Löffler's parietal fibroplastic endocarditis*; endocarditis following an acute course with predominant involvement of the right ventricle; histologically, there is eosinophilia and a fibrotic thickening of the apical and subvalvular endocardium, which frequently leads to thromboembolism; in addition to the heart, the lungs, bone marrow, brain, kidney, gastrointestinal tract, liver, and skin may all be affected [hypereosinophilic syndrome]; **therapy**: glucocorticoids, recombinant interferon-α, inhibitors of thrombocyte aggregation; possibly operative resection of endocardium and valve replacement

Löffler's fibroplastic endocarditis → *Löffler's endocarditis*

Löffler's parietal fibroplastic endocarditis → *Löffler's endocarditis*

marantic endocarditis → *nonbacterial thrombotic endocarditis*

mycotic endocarditis → *fungal endocarditis*

nonbacterial thrombotic endocarditis *Syn: atypical verrucous endocarditis, Libman-Sacks disease, Libman-Sacks endocarditis, Libman-Sacks syndrome, nonbacterial verrucous endocarditis, marantic endocarditis*; endocardial involvement in systemic lupus erythematosus; mainly affects the AV-valves; causes fibrinoid necrosis of the endocardium, particularly on the undersurfaces of the valves on which thrombi deposit, which become organized with granulation tissue; these nodules are mostly discovered for the first time after death, but in rare cases they can be dislodged and result in an embolism; valve damage plays hardly any role hemodynamically and only rarely causes insufficiency; mostly the illness remains uncertain or is concealed by the symptoms of the more common pericarditis or myocarditis

endocardium

nonbacterial verrucous endocarditis → *nonbacterial thrombotic endocarditis*

prosthetic endocarditis *Syn: prosthetic valve endocarditis; s.u. infective endocarditis*

prosthetic valve endocarditis *Syn: prosthetic endocarditis; s.u. infective endocarditis*

rheumatic endocarditis → *Bouillaud's disease*

rickettsial endocarditis relatively rare form of endocarditis caused by Coxiella burnetii

septic endocarditis acute bacterial endocarditis in the setting of septicemia

streptococcal endocarditis common form [up to 50%] of infective endocarditis; the subacute endocarditis caused by Streptococcus viridans plays an important role since it frequently damages heart valves

subacute bacterial endocarditis protracted course of endocarditis with minimal symptoms; afflicts mainly previously damaged heart valves; formerly mainly caused by Streptococcus viridans; today, enterococci, staphylococci, and Gram-negative cocci are also implicated; has become rarer as a result of the decline in acute rheumatic fever

thromboulcerative endocarditis hyperacute endocarditis with ulceration of the heart valves and thrombus formation

ulcerative endocarditis hyperacute endocarditis with ulceration of the heart valves

mural endocarditis parietal endocarditis

verrucous endocarditis endocarditis with formation of wart-like thrombi on the damaged heart valves; the thrombi can detach and cause pulmonary or cerebral embolization

viridans endocarditis subacute endocardial inflammation caused by Streptococcus viridans [endocarditis lenta]

endocardium innermost layer of the heart wall; single-layered endothelium of the heart chambers, which covers the ventricles, atria, heart valves, papillary muscles, tendons, and heart trabeculae; a basal membrane made of loose subendocardial connective tissue forms the connection to the heart wall muscles [myocardium]; the terminal branches of the excitation conduction system [subendocardial rami] run in the subendocardial connective tissue; the heart valves are often regarded as a differentiation of the endocardium

endocorpuscular situated within a corpuscle

endogenous 1. arising or lying within, not introduced from outside

2. from internal causes, arising within, constitutional
endoglobar situated within a blood corpuscle
endoglobular → *endoglobar*
endomyocardial relating to the endocardium and myocardium
endomyocarditic relating to or marked by endomyocarditis
endomyocarditis inflammation of endocardium and myocardium
endopericardiac → *intrapericardial*
endopericardial 1. *Syn:* endopericardiac; relating to endocardium and pericardium **2.** *Syn:* endopericardiac, intrapericardiac; within the pericardial cavity
endopericarditic relating to or marked by endopericarditis
endopericarditis inflammation of endocardium and pericardium
endoperimyocarditic relating to or marked by endoperimyocarditis
endoperimyocarditis → *pancarditis*
endophlebitic relating to or marked by endophlebitis
endophlebitis *Syn:* endovenitis; inflammation of the intima of a vein
    proliferative endophlebitis → *phlebosclerosis*
endosonography combination of endoscopy and sonography; endosonography is mainly performed rectally, vaginally, and trans-esophageal [transesophageal echocardiography]
endothelins vasoactive polypeptides made predominantly by the endothelium, as well as by neuronal, epithelial, and intestinal cells; since elevated plasma levels are found in patients with cardiogenic shock, pulmonary hypertension and acute renal failure, efforts are made to block its activation by **endothelin converting enzyme** with the so-called **ECE blockers**
endothoracic *Syn:* intrathoracic; (situated) within the ribcage/thorax
endovasculitis → *endangiitis*
end-systolic *Syn:* telesystolic; (occurring) at the end of systole
end-tidal → *end-expiratory*
enema the injection of a fluid into the rectum to cause a bowel movement; the fluid injected
    air-contrast barium enema → *double-contrast radiography*
enoximone phosphodiesterase inhibitor with positive inotropic and vasodilator action; coronary therapeutic; **usage**: arrhythmias, hypotension, gastrointestinal disorders
enterococcus class of Gram-positive, cocciform intestinal bacteria; **Enterococcus faecalis** and **Enterococcus faecium** play a role as nosocomial pathogens in immunosuppressed patients; the Vancomycin

resistance of many Enterococcus faecium strains is a particular problem; enterococci are sensitive to ampicillins, ureidopenicillins, and glycopeptides

Enterococcus. Species and infections

Species	Infections
Enterococcus faecalis, Enterococcus faecium	sepsis, endocarditis, urinary tract infections, peritonitis, cholecystitis, cholangitis, soft tissue infections, wound infections (burn wounds), catheter-associated infections

enzyme protein molecule that catalyzes chemical reactions without being changed or destroyed
  angiotensin converting enzyme *Syn: dipeptidyl carboxypeptidase, kininase II*; peptide that converts angiotensin I into angiotensin II
  endothelin converting enzyme *s.u. endothelins*
ephapse → *electrical synapse*
epi- combining form denoting relation to upon, above, or beside
epicardiac → *epicardial*
epicardial *Syn: epicardiac*; relating to the epicardium or epicardia
epicardiectomy partial removal of the epicardium
epicardium *Syn: cardiac pericardium, visceral layer of pericardium, visceral pericardium*; outermost layer of the heart wall; inside the pericardium, the epicardium forms the inner layer of the pericardium that covers the myocardium; the heart blood vessels run in the subepicardial fatty tissues
epicillin *Syn: dihydroampicillin*; penicillinase-resistant, semisynthetic penicillin; **indications**: same as for ampicillin
epinephrine *Syn: adrenaline, adrenine*; hormone synthesized in the adrenal cortex and sympathetic paraganglia; it is secreted primarily during stress, muscle activity, oxygen deficiency, and the premenstrual period; its secretion leads to tremors, weakness, cold sweat, tachycardia, and a feeling of anxiety; action: $alpha_1$- and $alpha_2$-sympathomimetic, increase in heart rate, cardiac output, and mean arterial pressure; reduction of intestinal peristalsis; relaxation of bronchial muscles and dilation of bronchi; pupillary dilation and piloerection; insulin-antagonistic activity [mobilization of glycogen reserves in the liver, breakdown of muscle glycogen]; epinephrine is used therapeutically

in circulatory arrest, anaphylactic shock, bronchospasm, bronchial asthma, and in addition to local anesthetics

epinephrinemia → *adrenalinemia*

epinephros → *adrenal gland*

episode → *attack*

eplerenone specific aldosterone receptor antagonist; in contrast to spironolactone, there is no increased menstrual disturbance [in women] or gynecomastia and impotence [in men] in comparison to placebo, but similar effects on the salt and water balance; not yet certified for clinical use

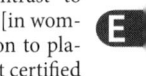

eptifibatide glycoprotein receptor IIb/IIIa antagonist; powerful, reversible inhibitor of thrombocyte aggregation, especially in the coronary arteries; **usage**: unstable angina pectoris, infarction without ST-segment elevation; **side effects**: bleeding complications, thrombocytopenia, hypotension, bradycardia

ergo- combining form denoting relation to work

ergocardiogram trace obtained by ergocardiography

ergocardiography recording of the work performed by the heart muscle

ergographic relating to ergography

ergometer an instrument for measuring the amount of work done by a muscle or group of muscles

    bicycle ergometer bicycle-like ergometer, mainly used to measure cardiac and circulatory parameters; the performance required by the subject can be kept constant or changed continuously

ergometry measurement of amount of work done and physiological changes occurring during the work; usually performance is measured, as well as exercise ECG [**stress ECG**], oxygen consumption [**exercise oxymetry**], or breathing time volume and oxygen uptake/carbon dioxide production [**ergospirometry**]

    oxymetric ergometry *Syn: exercise oxymetry; s.u. ergometry*

    treadmill ergometry ergometry in which the subject walks or runs on a treadmill; ECG, spirometry, respiratory gas analysis, etc., are usually performed during the exercise

ergospirometry *s.u. ergometry*

ergotropic impairing performance, energy sapping

erosion superficial destruction of a surface by friction, pressure, ulceration, or trauma

    plaque erosion *s.u. atherosclerosis*

erythema circumscribed, mostly inflammatory reddening of the skin, due

erythro-

to vessel dilatation as a result of physical, chemical, infectious, or psychic causes; it is a typical primary efflorescence [macula]; reddening of larger areas of skin or of the whole body are called erythroderma

erythro- combining form denoting relation to red or erythrocytes

erythroclasis *Syn: hemoclasia, hemoclasis*; erythrocyte fragmentation, e.g., due to mechanical damage by artificial heart valves

erythrocytes *Syn: red blood cells, red corpuscles*; disk-shaped, non-nucleated blood cells, which contain hemoglobin and transport oxygen from the lungs to tissues; **normal erythrocytes** [normocytes] are biconcave disks, which are about 2 µm thick at the edges and about 1 µm thick in the center; the diameter is 7–8 µm with an average of about 7.5 µm; the average lifespan of erythrocytes is 100–120 days

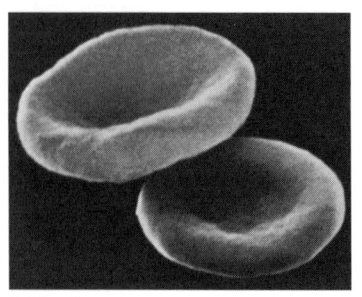

Erythrocytes

test erythrocytes washed and preserved erythrocytes for serologic and immunologic tests

erythrocythemia *Syn: erythrocytosis, hypercythemia, hypererythrocythemia*; rise in the erythrocyte count to values outside the normal range

erythrocythemic relating to or marked by erythrocythemia

erythrocytic relating to erythrocytes

erythrocytolysis → *hemolysis*

erythrocytopenia *Syn: erythropenia*; decrease in the number of erythrocytes in the peripheral blood

erythrocytopoiesis → *erythropoiesis*

erythrocytosis → *erythrocythemia*

erythrolysis → *hemolysis*

erythromycin macrolide antibiotic produced by **Streptomyces erythreus** with a limited action spectrum [gram-positive bacteria, Haemophilus influenzae, Bordetella pertussis, some rickettsias, chlamydias, and spirochaetes]; it can be given orally [erythromycin succinate] and intravenously [as the lactobionate or glucoheptonate]

erythropenia → *erythrocytopenia*

erythropoiesis *Syn: erythrocytopoiesis*; the formation of the red blood corpuscles initially occurs in the yolk sac, then in the liver and spleen [**hepatolienal blood formation**] after the 7. month of gestation, the bone marrow is the main site and following the 2.–4. week after birth the only site of blood formation; in adults, the blood forming bone marrow is concentrated in short flat bones [skull, spine, sternum, pelvis] and the distal and proximal ends of the long bones; when required [e.g., in tumors or severe blood loss], the entire bone marrow can reactivate hematopoiesis within a short time; the starting point of erythrocyte formation is a **lymphatic stem cell**, from which the **erythroid committed stem cell** for erythropoiesis arises; via various precursor cells [proerythroblasts, macroblasts, normoblasts] mature erythrocytes eventually form

escin glycoside mixture from the seed of the horse chestnut [Aesculus hippocastanum]; **usage**: treatment of edema or other conditions with swelling, predominantly of the legs; **side effects**: mucosal irritation

essential 1. critical to life **2.** *Syn: idiopathic, primary*; without recognizable cause, independent of other diseases

ester a compound produced by the reaction between an acid and an alcohol with the elimination of a molecule of water

ethacrynic acid loop diuretic; **usage**: edema

etilefrine α-sympatholytic, anti-hypotonic; **usage**: hypotension, circulatory collapse, shock-induced circulatory disturbances; **side effects**: dizziness, agitation, sweating, gastrointestinal symptoms, angina pectoris, disturbances of heart rhythm

etozolin loop diuretic; **usage**: edema

eutopic situated normally, arising from the normal location

evacuant → *diuretic*

evoked released by a stimulus

examination the act or process of inspecting or testing for evidence of disease or abnormality

   examination of blood → *hemanalysis*

exanimation → *unconsciousness*

exarteritis → *periarteritis*

excess an extreme or excessive amount or degree; superabundance
 base excess base concentration in the blood in mmol/l under standard conditions; in its narrowest sense, a deviation from the normal value of 48 mmol of buffer bases per l of blood

exchange the act, process, or an instance of exchanging
 diffusion limited exchange *s.u. microcirculation*
 perfusion limited exchange *s.u. microcirculation*

excitable sensitive, capable of being excited

excitative *Syn: excitatory*; exciting or arousing

excitatory → *excitative*

exhalation → *expiration*

exocardia → *ectocardia*

exocardial → *extracardial*

exogenetic → *exogenous*

exogenic → *exogenous*

exogenous *Syn: exogenetic, exogenic, exoteric, extrinsic, ectogenic, ectogenous*; introduced or arising or acting from outside, arising from external causes

exoteric → *exogenous*

expander any of several colloidal substances of high molecular weight used as a substitute for increasing the blood volume
 plasma expander *Syn: plasma volume expander*; plasma substitute, whose colloid osmotic pressure is higher than that of plasma; this leads to fluid shifts into the circulation
 plasma volume expander → *plasma expander*

expiration *Syn: exhalation, breathing out, exhaling*; under resting conditions or in normal respiration [eupnea], exhalation occurs passively by relaxation of the diaphragm and the inspiratory intercostal muscles; this state is often also called **postinspiration**; during **active** or **forced expiration**, the chest volume is reduced by contraction of the expiratory intercostal muscles; at the same time, contraction of the transverse muscle of the abdomen, internal and external oblique muscles of the abdomen, and the lumbar quadrate muscle leads to an increase in intra-abdominal pressure and a lifting of the dome of the diaphragm

expiratory relating to expiration

exsanguination death due to massive internal or external blood loss

exsanguinotransfusion → *exchange transfusion*

exterior on the outside, near the outside

external on the outside

extra- combining form denoting relation to outside of, beyond, or in addition

extracapillary outside a capillary

extracardial *Syn: exocardial*; outside the heart

extracellular outside a cell or cells

extracorporal *Syn: extracorporeal, extrasomatic*; outside the body

extracorporeal → *extracorporal*

extracorpuscular (occurring) outside the blood corpuscle

extraction the process of pulling or drawing out

   oxygen extraction → *oxygen utilization*

extrapericardial outside the pericardium

extrapulmonary (situated) outside the lung(s), not associated with the lung

extrasomatic → *extracorporal*

extrasystole *Syn: extra systole, premature beat, premature contraction, premature systole*; premature contraction of the heart muscle outside the normal rhythm; caused by a disturbance to the formation of the impulse [e.g., sinoatrial node syndrome] or conduction of the impulse [e.g., 3rd degree AV block]; **supraventricular extrasystoles** [arising in the atrium] and **ventricular extrasystoles** [arising in the ventricular muscles] are differentiated depending upon where the extrasystole arises; extrasystoles are the most common disturbances of rhythm of all and occur in people with healthy and diseased hearts; **extrasystoles are not an illness but a symptom** and need only be treated in the setting of acute myocardial infarction; otherwise, the main focus is on the diagnosis and treatment of any underlying illness

   atrial extrasystole *Syn: atrial premature contraction, auricular extrasystole, premature atrial beat, premature atrial contraction, premature atrial systole*; a supraventricular extrasystole arising from a focus in the atrium; occur frequently, with or without underlying cardiac disease; physical and emotional stress, coffee, nicotine, and alcohol can also provoke atrial extrasystoles in healthy individuals

   auricular extrasystole → *atrial extrasystole*

   idioventricular extrasystole *s.u. ventricular extrasystole*

   infranodal extrasystole → *ventricular extrasystole*

   junctional extrasystole *s.u. ventricular extrasystole*

   multiple extrasystoles runs of extrasystoles

   supraventricular extrasystole *s.u. extrasystole*

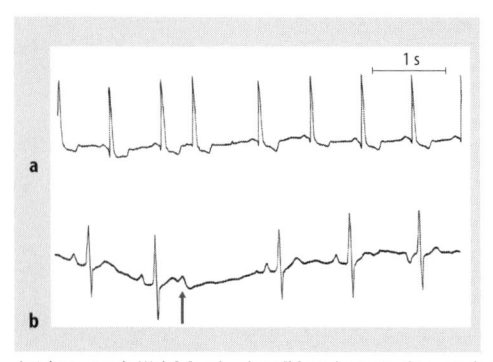

Atrial extrasystole. With [a] and without [b] conduction to the ventricle via the a-v bundle

ventricular extrasystole *Syn: infranodal extrasystole, premature ventricular beat, premature ventricular contraction, premature ventricular systole*; ventricular extrasystoles can be divided into monotopic and polytopic extrasystoles, ventricular bigeminy, pairs and triplets [salvos], as well as R-on-T-phenomenon; if there are **replacement systoles** due to failure of the sinoatrial node, these can be subdivided into **junctional extrasystoles** [narrow QRS-complex] and **idioventricular extrasystoles** [wide QRS-complex]; the **classification of Lown and Wolf** is used to assess the importance of these extrasystoles; however, it has significant disadvantages and is rejected by most cardiologists today

extravasate *Syn: extravasation*; fluid that has escaped from a vessel

extravasation → *extravasate*

extravascular outside a vessel or vessels

extraventricular outside a ventricle

extrinsic (arising or acting) from outside, external

exudate *Syn: exudation*; fluid exuding during inflammation, which, depending upon its constitution can be described as a **serous, hemorrhagic, fibrinous, purulent exudate**, etc.

cotton wool exudates → *cotton wool spots*

exudation formation of an exudate

exudative relating to or caused by exudation

ezetimibe cholesterol absorption inhibitor; taken orally ezetimibe local-

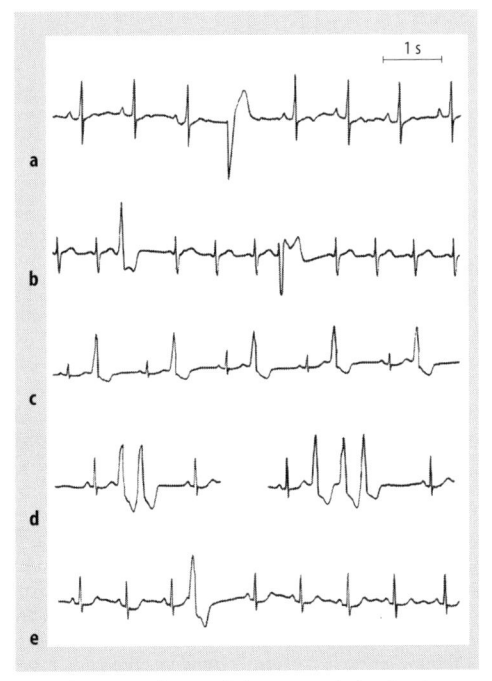

Ventricular extrasystole. **a** ventricular extrasystole; **b** polytopic extrasystoles; **c** ventricular bigeminy; **d** pairs and triplets; **e** R-on-T-phenomenon

izes in the brush border of the small intestine inhibiting cholesterol absorption from the diet; **usage**: in combination with a statin [simvastatin] for treatment of hypercholesterolemia

facies 1. face **2.** outer surface, anterior surface

facies anterior cordis *Syn: sternocostal surface of heart*; the anterior surface of the heart that faces the breastbone [sternum]

facies diaphragmatica cordis diaphragmatic surface of the heart

mitral facies *Syn: mitrotricuspid facies*; pale face with reddish-blue cheeks and cyanosed lips due to severe mitral stenosis or other diseases associated with markedly reduced cardiac minute volume

mitrotricuspid facies → *mitral facies*

facies pulmonalis cordis the side of the heart turned toward the right [**facies pulmonalis cordis dextra**] or left [**facies pulmonalis cordis sinistra**] lung

factitious → *artificial*

factor (decisive) factor, determining feature

factor I → *fibrinogenous*

factor II *Syn: plasmozyme, prothrombin, serozyme, thrombogen*; vitamin K-dependent blood clotting factor made in the liver; inactive precursor of thrombin [factor IIa]; also belongs to the acute phase proteins; deficiency leads to hypoprothrombinemia

factor IIa *Syn: fibrinogenase, thrombase, thrombin, thrombosin*; proteolytic factor in blood clotting, which converts fibrinogen to fibrin; formed from prothrombin [factor II]

factor III *Syn: tissue factor, tissue thromboplastin*; lipoprotein complex consisting of several factors [among others activated factor V, factor X], which converts prothrombin [factor II] into thrombin; develops both in intravascular and extravascular activation of the clotting system and thereby represents the final common pathway in both systems

factor V → *accelerator globulin*

factor VI → *accelerin*

factor VII *Syn: autoprothrombin I, cofactor V, convertin, cothromboplastin, prothrombin conversion factor, proconvertin, prothrombin* *converting factor, prothrombokinase, serum prothrombin conversion accelerator, stable factor*; factor made in the liver; deficiency causes hypoproconvertinemia

factor VIII *Syn: antihemophilic factor, antihemophilic factor A, antihemophilic globulin, plasma thromboplastin factor, platelet cofactor, plasmokinin, thromboplastic plasma component, thromboplastinogen*; factor made in the liver; deficiency or absence causes hemophilia A

factor IX *Syn: antihemophilic factor B, autoprothrombin II, Christmas factor, plasma thromboplastin component, platelet cofactor, plasma thromboplastin factor B, PTC factor*; vitamin K-dependent factor in the intrinsic pathway of blood clotting that is synthesized in the liver; deficiency leads to hemophilia B

factor X *Syn: autoprothrombin C, Prower factor, Stuart factor, Stuart-Prower factor*; blood clotting factor made in the liver, which forms the final common pathway in both the intravascular and extravascular systems; together with factor V, calcium, and phospholipids, it forms an enzyme complex [**prothrombinase**], which catalyzes the conversion of prothrombin [factor II] to thrombin; deficiency leads to an increased bleeding tendency

factor XI *Syn: antihemophilic factor C, plasma thromboplastin antecedent, PTA factor*; factor in the intrinsic pathway of the blood clotting cascade; congenital deficiency leads to hemophilia C

factor XII *Syn: activation factor, contact factor, glass factor, Hageman factor*; blood clotting factor made in the reticulohistiocyte system

factor XIII *Syn: fibrin stabilizing factor, fibrinase, Laki-Lorand factor*; blood clotting factor formed in the liver and thrombocytes, which is activated by thrombin [factor IIa]; cross-links fibrin monomers by forming peptide bonds and thereby forms insoluble [stable] fibrin; a deficiency can lead to disturbances of wound healing and secondary bleeding

accelerator factor → *accelerator globulin*
activation factor → *Hageman factor*
angiogenic factors description of substances that promote the development or new formation of blood vessels
antihemophilic factor → *factor VIII*
antihemophilic factor A → *factor VIII*
antihemophilic factor B → *factor IX*
antihemophilic factor C → *factor XI*
atrial natriuretic factor → *atrial natriuretic peptide*

Christmas factor →*factor IX*

coagulation factors the blood clotting cascade has 12 factors in total, which are all required for it to run smoothly

colony-stimulating factor *s.u. blood formation*

contact factor →*factor XII*

Day's factor →*folic acid*

fibrin stabilizing factor →*factor XIII*

glass factor →*factor XII*

growth factors of hemopoiesis *s.u. blood formation*

Hageman factor *Syn: activation factor, contact factor, factor XII, glass factor*; factor made in the reticuloendothelial system

labile factor →*accelerator globulin*

Lactobacillus casei factor →*folic acid*

Laki-Lorand factor *Syn: factor XIII, fibrin stabilizing factor, fibrinase*; blood clotting factor made in thrombocytes and the liver, which is activated by thrombin [factor IIa]; cross-links the fibrin monomers by forming peptide bonds and thereby forms insoluble [stable] fibrin; a deficiency can lead to disturbances of wound healing and secondary bleeding

liver Lactobacillus casei factor →*folic acid*

plasma labile factor →*accelerator globulin*

plasma thromboplastin factor →*factor VIII*

plasma thromboplastin factor B →*factor IX*

plasmin prothrombin conversion factor →*accelerator globulin*

platelet factors factors released during thrombocyte aggregation, which promote clotting

platelet factor 3 phospholipoprotein complex of the outer thrombocyte membrane; in the intrinsic pathway of blood clotting it forms an enzyme complex together with factor IXa, factor VIIIa, and calcium ions that activates factor X

platelet factor 4 →*antiheparin*

prothrombin conversion factor →*factor VII*

prothrombin converting factor →*factor VII*

Prower factor →*Stuart-Prower factor*

PTA factor →*factor XI*

PTC factor →*factor IX*

stable factor →*factor VII*

Stuart factor →*Stuart-Prower factor*

Stuart-Prower factor *Syn: autoprothrombin C, factor X, Prower fac-*

tor, Stuart factor; blood clotting factor made in the liver, which forms the final common pathway in both the intravascular and extravascular systems; together with factor V, calcium, and phospholipids, it forms an enzyme complex [**prothrombinase**], which catalyzes the conversion of prothrombin [factor II] to thrombin; deficiency leads to an increased bleeding tendency

tissue factor → *factor III*

factor VIII:vWF → *von Willebrand factor*

von Willebrand factor *Syn: factor VIII-associated antigen, factor VIII:vWF*; oligomeric glycoprotein, which occurs subendothelially and in thrombocytes; facilitates the adhesion of thrombocytes to the damaged vessel wall and protects blood clotting factor VIII from premature proteolysis; severe deficiency therefore leads to factor VIII deficiency and disturbances of secondary hemostasis

Wills' factor → *folic acid*

failure inability to perform; state of insufficient function or performance

acute heart failure often arises following extensive myocardial infarctions, in disturbances of rhythm or in acute decompensation of chronic cardiac insufficiency; the main causes of acute worsening of a pre-existing insufficiency are insufficient medication of hypertension, cessation of antihypertensives, pulmonary embolization, inflammation of the heart muscle [myocarditis] or lungs [pneumonia], disturbances of rhythm and ischemia; **therapy**: treatment of the underlying cause or the cardiogenic shock which it gives rise to; a central point is to reduce the afterload and blood pressure using nitrates, diuretics, and vasodilators

cardiac failure → *heart failure*

chronic heart failure most common cardiac disease of all; the classification of chronic cardiac insufficiency according to the New York Heart Association rests upon restriction of the body's physical capacity due to restrictions in the physical capacity of the heart; the most important causes of chronic cardiac insufficiency are pressure overload [hypertension, coronary heart disease, aortic stenosis, cor pulmonale], volume overload [aortic or mitral insufficiency, heart defects with shunt formation], impaired filling [mitral stenosis, constrictive pericarditis, restrictive cardiomyopathy], reduction in the heart muscle mass [post-infarct state, coronary heart disease], and primary and secondary diseases of the myocardium [cardiomyopathy, myocarditis, toxic injury]; **clinical**: in addition to the reduction in physical capacity, there are **symptoms of backward failure** [orthopnea, exertional dyspnea, cardiac asthma, pulmonary edema, venous engorgement, liver enlargement, generalized edema] and **symptoms of forward failure** [hypotension, dizziness, symptoms of cerebral ischemia, intermittent abdominal pains, concentrated urine]; **therapy**: the medical treatment consists of a combination of diuretics, ACE inhibitors, and digitalis; additional targeted treatment of the underlying disease and general measures [physical conditioning, weight reduction, fluid restriction, salt-poor diet, avoidance of alcohol] are also used; the goal is to improve the hemodynamics, exertional capacity, quality of life, and prognosis; in therapy-resistant cardiac insufficiency, a heart transplant may be considered for certain patients [under 60 years of age, no generalized arteriosclerosis, liver, or kidney damage]

decompensated heart failure *s.u. heart failure*

global heart failure *Syn: total heart failure, global insufficiency, total heart insufficiency; s.u. heart failure*

heart failure *Syn: cardiac failure, myocardial insufficiency, cardiac insufficiency, Beau's disease, heart insufficiency*; inability of the heart to perform sufficient pumping; the insufficiency can be limited to certain parts of the heart [left ventricular failure, right ventricular failure] or affect the entire heart [global insufficiency, global heart failure]; a distinction is made between failure during exercise and insufficiency at rest depending on the severity of the failure; the clinical picture of congestive heart failure develops when the body's compensation mechanisms are exhausted

heart failure at rest *s.u. heart failure*

left-sided heart failure → *left-ventricular failure*

left-ventricular failure *Syn: left-sided heart failure, left-ventricular heart failure; s.u. heart failure*

left-ventricular heart failure → *left-ventricular failure*

multiorgan failure *Syn: multiple organ failure*; simultaneous failure of two or more vital organ functions [liver, lung, kidney, respiratory, or cardiovascular function, acid-base balance, metabolism and energy metabolism, water and electrolyte metabolism, coagulation system, thermoregulation]; it occurs particularly after trauma, due to poisoning, sepsis, and shock

multiple organ failure → *multiorgan failure*

respiratory failure *Syn: pulmonary insufficiency, respiratory insuf-*

ficiency; disturbance of the gas exchange, which leads to a deficient oxygen supply and inadequate CO_2 release; it can be due to a disturbance in internal or external respiration; a distinction is made clinically between acute and chronic respiratory insufficiency; **acute respiratory insufficiency** is due to a rapidly progressing loss of respiratory pump function or gas exchange function; the most frequent underlying diseases are pneumonia, asthma attack, pulmonary embolism, pneumothorax, and cardiogenic pulmonary edema; a life-threatening condition [shock lung] develops clinically within a very short time; **chronic respiratory insufficiency** is much more frequent than the acute form, because about 20% of adults suffer from chronic-obstructive pulmonary disease and about 1/3 of these develop chronic respiratory insufficiency; a compensated or latent form usually exists for years; it is not noticeable under resting conditions and is manifested only upon exertion; this is often followed by acute progression and terminal decompensation; the priority **therapy** is to treat the specific primary disease [e.g., pneumoconiosis, bronchial asthma, pleural thickening, or obesity] or to eliminate exposure factors; symptomatic treatment of chronic respiratory insufficiency consists primarily of long-term O_2 therapy, intermittent self-ventilation [usually at night as mask ventilation], and individually tailored stimulation or dampening of the respiratory center; breathing exercises and physical therapy for draining mucus in mucus-producing diseases

right-sided heart failure → *right-ventricular failure*

right-ventricular failure *Syn: right-sided heart failure, right-ventricular heart failure*; inability of the right ventricle to pump a sufficient amount of blood in the pulmonary circulation; it leads to congestion in the venous circulation; the most frequent causes are acute or chronic recurrent pulmonary embolisms, decompensated cor pulmonale, and acute [posterior/inferior] myocardial infarction; cyanosis, dyspnea, venous congestion, and edema are seen **clinically**; examination reveals hepatic congestion, ascites, pleural and pericardial effusion, and increased central venous pressure; **therapy**: afterload reduction, improvement of myocardial contractility, and optimization of heart rate and fluid balance

right-ventricular heart failure → *right-ventricular failure*

total heart failure *Syn: global insufficiency, global heart failure, total heart insufficiency*; s.u. heart failure

faint *Syn: swoon, unconsciousness*; sudden, brief loss of consciousness

fainting → *syncope*

fascicle a small bundle of nerve or muscle fibers

fat ester of glycerol and saturated and unsaturated fatty acids; often equated with lipid; subdivided, depending upon the esterified OH-groups, into **monoacylglycerides**, **diacylglycerides**, and **triacylglycerides**, which are also known as **neutral fats**; the number and type of fatty acids determine the physical characteristics of the fats; fats made from medium or short chain fatty acids are liquid at room temperature [oils], fats with long chain fatty acids are solids; triacylglycerides are hydrophobic and can therefore not take part in the formation of structures forming interfaces, whereas the mono- and diacylglycerides also contain hydrophilic groups and therefore play an important role in the formation of micelles, membranes, and the emulsification of lipids during their reabsorption from the intestine; the main function of fats in the body is as an energy source [1 g of fat delivers 39.1 kJ or 9.3 kcal] or store [depot fat] source of carbohydrate for the biosynthesis of glucose, building blocks for membranes, and as the precursor of important molecules such as, e.g., prostaglandins and leukotrienes; the body contains approx. 10% triacylglycerides [approx. 8 kg], which can provide the body's energy requirements for around 37 days; in severe obesity, these amounts can increase to more than 50 kg; it is clear why weight reduction in the obese is such a protracted process that often exceeds their staying power

febris → *fever*

fendiline calcium antagonist, coronary therapeutic; **usage**: aftercare following myocardial infarction

ferroprotoporphyrin → *heme*

fever Syn: *febris*; **1.** elevation of body temperature above normal **2.** febrile disease; disease with fever as the cardinal symptom

atropine fever temperature elevation occurring in atropine poisoning

rheumatic fever Syn: *acute articular rheumatism, acute rheumatic arthritis, acute rheumatic polyarthritis, inflammatory rheumatism, rheumatopyra, rheumapyra*; acute inflammation of the large joints [polyarthritis] belonging to the post-streptococcal diseases; characterized by, among others, fever, involvement of the heart [endocarditis, myocarditis, pericarditis], Sydenham's chorea, erythema marginatum, and soft tissue swelling; **diagnosis**: rheumatic fever is a rare condition in Central Europe nowadays and is often misdiagnosed; this can be avoided by strict adherence to the Jones criteria; **therapy**: in the acute

septic fever → *septicemia*

fiber a slender, threadlike element or cell, as of nerve, muscle, or connective tissue

impulse-conducting fibers → *Purkinje's fibers*

James fibers accessory conduction bundle in the atrial myocardium; possible cause of disturbances to the conduction of excitation [Lown-Ganong-Levine syndrome]

Mahaim fibers accessory conducting pathway in the excitation conduction system between the bundle of His and the ventricular septum; can lead to pre-excitation

Purkinje's fibers *Syn: impulse-conducting fibers*; terminal fibers of the excitation conduction system of the heart within the myocardium; individual Purkinje fibers can run through the ventricular cavity as so-called false tendon fibers

fibremia → *fibrinemia*

fibrillation disorganized muscle contractions following rapidly one after the other; mostly applied to disorganized contraction of parts of the heart musculature [ventricular fibrillation, atrial fibrillation]

atrial fibrillation *Syn: auricular fibrillation*; disturbance of heart rhythm, in which the atria fibrillate in uncoordinated fashion; frequently found in cardiac insufficiency, mitral valve defects, arterial hypertension, coronary heart disease, and hyperthyroidism; increasingly frequent with increasing age, 3–5% of all over-65-year olds have atrial fibrillation; the atrial fibrillation destroys the pumping action of the atrium and leads to irregular conduction to the ventricles and to absolute arrhythmia; **clinically** apparent features are palpitations and signs of cardiac insufficiency; depending upon the ventricular rate, there may be either bradycardia or tachycardia; the **therapy** depends upon the nature of the atrial fibrillation; **paroxysmal atrial fibrillation** [stops spontaneously within hours or days] usually responds well to β-blockers, propafenone, flecainide, or amiodarone; in **persistent atrial fibrillation** [shows no sign of spontaneous arrest], medical or electric cardioversion is tried; the most difficult is the treatment of **permanent atrial fibrillation**, which cannot be converted back to sinus rhythm; this often requires pacemaker implantation or catheter

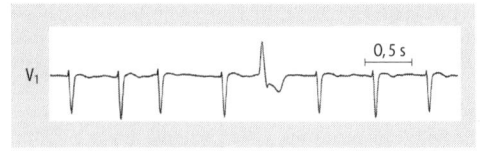

Atrial fibrillation. Atrial fibrillation in V_1

ablation of the AV-node

auricular fibrillation → *atrial fibrillation*

ventricular fibrillation asynchronous, extremely rapid [300–500/min] beats of the atria and ventricles; leads to functional circulatory standstill; **acute therapy**: external DC cardioversion [200–400 Ws] is the only lifesaving measure in ventricular fibrillation; **long-term therapy**: sotalol and amiodarone are the agents of choice for medical management

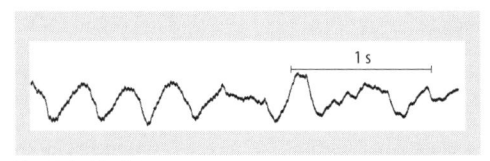

Ventricular fibrillation

fibrin *Syn: antithrombin I*; high molecular weight, water insoluble protein; develops from fibrinogen [factor I] during blood clotting; the soluble fibrin monomers form layers under the influence of electrostatic forces; in the presence of factor XIIIa and calcium ions, the monomers are connected by covalent bonds, and insoluble fibrin polymers result

fibrinase 1. → *factor XIII* **2.** → *fibrinolysin*

fibrinemia *Syn: fibremia, inosemia*; occurrence of fibrin in the blood

fibrinogen → *fibrinogenous*

   nonclottable fibrinogen → *dysfibrinogen*

fibrinogenase → *factor IIa*

fibrinogenemia *Syn: hyperfibrinogenemia*; increased fibrinogen content of the blood, e.g., due to infections, rheumatic diseases, or tumors

fibrinogenesis formation of fibrin from fibrinogen in the context of blood

fibrinogenolysis dissolution of fibrin, e.g., by plasmin; leads in certain circumstances to a disturbance of blood clotting

fibrinogenopenia → *hypofibrinogenemia*

fibrinogenous *Syn: factor I, fibrinogen*; factor made in the liver; precursor of fibrin, fibrin

fibrinolysin *Syn: fibrinase, plasmin*; seropeptidase, which cleaves soluble peptides [fibrin degradation products] from fibrin and also cleaves fibrinogen, prothrombin, and the clotting factors V, VIII, IX, XI and XII; plasmin therefore acts not only as a fibrinolytic, but also as an inhibitor of blood clotting

streptococcal fibrinolysin → *streptokinase*

fibrinolysis enzymatic cleavage of fibrin or fibrin clots; formation and dissolution of fibrin are in equilibrium, which is pushed toward fibrin formation by injury; the most important limb of the fibrinolytic system is plasmin, which, in a similar way to thrombin, is activated from its precursor [plasminogen] via an **extrinsic** or **intrinsic pathway**; plasmin is a seropeptidase, which cleaves soluble peptides from fibrin [fibrin degradation products] and also cleaves fibrinogen, prothrombin, and factors V, VIII, IX, XI and XII; plasmin thus acts not only as a fibrinolytic, but also inhibits blood clotting; the extrinsic pathway is activated by tissue activators, which are called **tissue-type plasminogen activator** [t PA]; they are found in, e.g., uterus or urine [urokinase]; the blood activators of the intrinsic pathway require proactivators [e.g., prekallikrein], which are released from blood cells in response to inflammatory or traumatic injury

fibrinolytic → *fibrinolysis inhibitor*

fibrinopenia → *hypofibrinogenemia*

fibroelastosis excessive proliferation of collagenous and elastic fibrous tissue

endocardial fibroelastosis *Syn: African endomyocardial fibrosis, endocardial sclerosis, endomyocardial fibrosis*; disease of uncertain etiology, with massive thickening of the endocardium, particularly of the left ventricle; frequent involvement of mitral and aortic valves; it may possibly be some form of post-infective or immunologic reaction; mostly starts within the first two years of life; if the disease affects a normally developed heart, then it is called **primary endocardial fibroelastosis**; it leads primarily to marked left heart dilatation with accompanying valve insufficiency; in **secondary endocardial fibroelastosis**, there are also congenital heart defects [aortic stenosis, restriction of the outflow tract]; in this case, marked hypertrophy of the myocardium usually develops; the **therapy** is symptomatic; often a heart transplant is the only therapeutic option

fibrosis *Syn: fibrous degeneration, fibroid degeneration*; abnormal formation of connective tissue by increased fiber production and reduced breakdown; examples of causes are chronic edema, organized inflammation, necrosis, thrombosis or hematoma, mechanical stress [e.g., in chronic blood stasis] and proliferative inflammation [e.g., chronic hepatitis]; it is often equated with sclerosis

African endomyocardial fibrosis → *endomyocardial fibrosis*

congestive fibrosis *Syn: congestive induration*; consolidation of organ tissue, caused by chronic blood stasis, with an increase in collagen fibers

endocardial fibrosis disease leading to fibrotic thickening of the endocardium

endomyocardial fibrosis *Syn: African endomyocardial fibrosis, endocardial fibroelastosis, endocardial sclerosis*; disease of uncertain etiology, with massive thickening of the endocardium particularly of the left ventricle; frequent involvement of mitral and aortic valves; very rare in Europe, but common in central Africa [Uganda, Nigeria]; the only therapy is resection of the affected region of endocardium, though the mortality is high [15–25%]; most patients die within 2–5 years

intimal fibrosis proliferation of the connective tissue in the intima; often a transition into intimal sclerosis

myocardial fibrosis fibrosis and hardening of the heart muscle tissue leading to cardiac insufficiency

filling *s.u. intracranial aneurysm*

filter device that removes something from whatever passes through

vena caval umbrella filter *Syn: vena cava filter; s.u. vena caval block*

finger any of the digits of the hand

clubbed fingers *Syn: drumstick fingers, clubbed digits, hippocratic fingers, digiti hippocratici*; roundish distension of the distal phalanges of the fingers occurring in various diseases; it often occurs together with hippocratic nails; it is a frequent concomitant symptom of chronic arterial hypoxemia of pulmonary [bronchial asthma] or cardiac [cyanotic heart defect] origin

drumstick fingers → *clubbed fingers*

hippocratic fingers → *clubbed fingers*

fistula 1. spontaneously formed, duct-like connection between an organ and the body surface [**external fistula**] or another organ [**internal fistula**]; most fistulas arise due to chronic inflammations [Crohn's disease] or proceed from an abscess; apart from these, there are also traumatically acquired and congenital fistulas [e.g., median cervical fistula] **2.** *Syn: anastomosis, fistulation, fistulization*; surgically created connection between an organ and the body surface or another organ

arteriovenous fistula congenital or acquired connection of an artery to a vein

carotid-cavernous fistula fistula that develops following trauma [usually basal skull fracture] between the internal carotid artery and the cavernous sinus; often presents like an aneurysm with exophthalmus, double vision, pressure atrophy of the optic nerve, and trigeminal neuralgia

cavernous sinus fistula traumatic fistula between the cavernous sinus and the internal carotid artery; can lead to unilateral, pulsatile exophthalmos

fistulation *Syn: fistulization*; surgically created connection between an organ and the body surface or another organ

fistulization → *fistulation*

fit a sudden, acute attack or manifestation of a disease

apoplectic fit → *cerebrovascular accident*

flaccid → *atonic*

flecainide class IC antiarrhythmic; acts as a negative dromotrope and inotrope **usage**: tachycardia, ventricular, and supraventricular heart rhythm disturbances

flow an act of flowing; blood flow

decreased blood flow → *hypoperfusion*

impaired cerebral blood flow underperfusion of the brain is mostly caused by arteriosclerosis of the cerebral vessels, which can lead to an ischemic infarct [stroke]

flucloxacillin semisynthetic, penicillinase-resistant penicillin, which is highly effective against penicillinase-forming staphylococci and enterococci; **indications**: meningitis, infections of the skin, mucosa, and soft tissues

fluctuation 1. variation, undulation **2.** deviation of the null line in the electrocardiogram

fludrocortisone fluorocorticoid with powerful mineralocorticoid action; **usage**: essential hypotension, Addison's disease, adrenogenital syndrome, disturbances of peripheral perfusion

fluorescein *Syn: dihydroxyfluorane, resorcinolphthalein*; fluorescent xanthine dye; used among other things to determine the circulation time, to diagnose corneal defects, as an indicator and pigment

flutter a rapid pulsation

atrial flutter *Syn: auricular flutter*; disturbance of heart rhythm, in which the atria beat at a rate of 220–350 beats per minute; a potentially life-threatening disturbance of rhythm due to the danger of 1:1 conduction; the **clinical** features are determined by the ventricular rate; at 3:1 or 4:1 conduction ratios, patients are asymptomatic; however, higher ventricular rates can lead to hypotension, angina pectoris, left heart insufficiency, or cardiogenic shock; **therapy**: cardiac glycosides or verapamil i.v. for acute management; long-term treatment with β-blockers or calcium antagonists

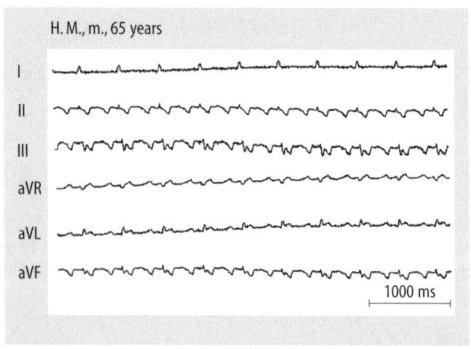

Atrial flutter

auricular flutter → *atrial flutter*

mediastinal flutter respiration-synchronous pendulum-like movement of the mediastinum in open pneumothorax or flail chest; during inspiration the mediastinum shifts toward the affected side and returns to the starting position during expiration; it results in impairment of the breathing mechanics and of the venous reflux to the heart

ventricular flutter disturbance of heart rhythm with rapid [220–350/min] and regular contractions; conversion to ventricular fibrillation possible; **acute therapy**: lidocaine or ajmaline are the agents of choice for acute medical therapy; if this is unsuccessful, anti-tachycardic stimulation or cardioversion

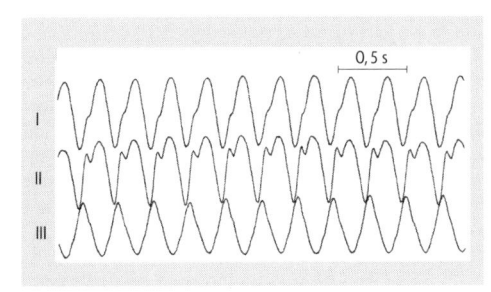

Ventricular flutter

focal relating to a focus
folacin → *folic acid*
fold wrinkle, crease
  fold of left vena cava *Syn: Marshall's fold, Marshall's vestigial fold, vestigial fold of Marshall*; pericardial fold over the left atrium
  Marshall's fold → *fold of left vena cava*
  Marshall's vestigial fold → *fold of left vena cava*
  vestigial fold of Marshall → *fold of left vena cava*
folic acid *Syn: Day's factor, folacin, Lactobacillus casei factor, liver Lactobacillus casei factor, pteroylglutamic acid, pteropterin, Wills' factor*; essential nutrient that belongs to the vitamin B complex; converted in the body to its biologically active form **tetrahydrofolic acid**; deficiency leads to neurologic disorders and anemia
foramen natural opening or passage, aperture
  Botallo's foramen → *oval foramen of heart*
  oval foramen → *oval foramen of heart*
  foramen ovale → *oval foramen of heart*
  foramen ovale cordis → *oval foramen of heart*
  oval foramen of fetus → *oval foramen of heart*
  oval foramen of heart *Syn: Botallo's foramen, foramen ovale, oval foramen, oval foramen of fetus*; physiologically normal connection between the right and left atria in the fetus

foramina of smallest veins of heart openings of the small cardiac veins [venae cordis minimae] in the right atrium

foramina venarum minimarum → *foramina of smallest veins of heart*

formation the process of giving form and shape; a structure

blood formation *Syn: hemapoiesis, hematogenesis, hematopoiesis, hematosis, hemogenesis, hemocytopoiesis, hemopoiesis, sanguification*; formation of cellular blood elements; the **embryonal blood formation** initially occurs in the yolk sac, then in the liver and spleen [**hepatolienal blood formation**]; after the 7. month of pregnancy, the bone marrow is the main site, and following the 2.–4. week after birth, the only site of blood formation; in adults, the blood forming bone marrow is concentrated in short flat bones [skull, spine, sternum, pelvis] and the distal and proximal ends of the long bones; when required [e.g., in tumors or severe blood loss], the entire bone marrow can reactivate hematopoiesis within a short time; the starting point of blood cell formation is a **pluripotent stem cell** in the bone marrow, from which the **precursor cells** for the lymphatic series [**lymphatic stem cell**] and the myeloid series [**myeloid stem cell**] arise; these give rise to the **committed stem cells** of lymphopoiesis [B- and T-lymphocyte formation], erythropoiesis [erythrocyte formation], myelopoiesis [granulocyte formation], monocytopoiesis [monocyte formation], and megakaryocytopoiesis [thrombocyte formation]; proliferation and differentiation of the stem cells and various intermediate stages are controlled by **growth factors** made by, e.g., endothelial cells, T-helper cells, or the kidney [erythropoietin]; since they often lead to the formation of colonies of identical cells, most are called **colony-stimulating factors** [CSF], while the precursor cells are called **colony-forming units** [CFU]

microthrombus formation → *microthrombosis*

thrombus formation → *thrombosis*

N-formimidoyl thienamycin → *imipenem*

formula a rule or principle, frequently expressed in algebraic symbols

Bazett's formula *s.u. electrocardiogram*

Read's formula formula for approximate calculation of the basal metabolic rate variation [BMRV] as a % of normal: BMRV = $0.75 \times$ [pulse rate + ($0.74 \times$ blood pressure amplitude)] − 72

foromacidin → *spiramycin*

fosfomycin *Syn: phosphonomycin*; bactericidal broad-spectrum antibiotic; inhibitor of bacterial pyruvyl transferase; it is active against staphylococci, streptococci, gonococci, Haemophilus influenzae, salmonellas,

fossa → *fovea*

Gerdy's hyoid fossa → *carotid triangle*

Malgaigne's fossa → *carotid triangle*

oval fossa of heart indentation of the atrial septum in the right atrium as a relic of the foramen ovale

fossa ovalis → *oval fossa of heart*

foudroyant sudden or abrupt (onset)

fovea *Syn: depression, pit, fossa*; small pit or depression

foxglove → *digitalis*

fraction a small part or segment of something

ejection fraction pumping performance of the heart, i.e., the proportion of the blood in the left ventricle ejected during systole; the normal value is approx. 65%; in cardiac insufficiency, the ejection fraction is reduced in spite of an increased filling volume; it is measured by means of contrast agent delineation of the ventricle

residual fraction relationship between end-systolic residual volume and end-diastolic filling volume of the heart

fragile *Syn: brittle, frail*; easily broken or damaged; vulnerable

fragility *Syn: fragileness, fragilitas*; quality or state of being easily broken or destroyed

fragility of blood → *erythrocyte resistance*

capillary fragility *s.u. capillary resistance*

erythrocyte fragility → *erythrocyte resistance*

osmotic fragility → *osmotic erythrocyte fragility*

osmotic erythrocyte fragility *Syn: osmotic fragility*; resistance of the erythrocytes to osmosis; determined in hypotonic salt solutions; reduced in various hematologic diseases [spherocytosis, pernicious anemia]

frail → *fragile*

fremitus palpable or audible vibration, thrill

pericardial fremitus → *pericardial friction sound*

frusemide → *furosemide*

α-L-fucosidase *s.u. fucosidosis*

fucosidosis lysosomal storage disease caused by an autosomal recessive deficiency of α-L-fucosidase [oligosaccharidosis]; the main clinical features are hepatosplenomegaly, cardiomegaly, short stature, and mental retardation

fulminant sudden or abrupt (onset)

fulminating → *fulminant*
function a factor related to or dependent upon other factors
   abnormal function → *dysfunction*
   pressure reservoir function *Syn: windkessel function*; description of the conversion of the discontinuous blood flow from the heart into a continuous bloodstream; relies upon the elasticity of the walls of the large arteries, which stretch during systole and thus store blood, which they then push forwards during diastole
   vasomotor function → *vasomotoricity*
   windkessel function → *pressure reservoir function*
fundus base, bottom
   fundus arteriosclerticus change in the optic fundus in arteriosclerosis
   fundus hypertonicus change in the optic fundus in benign hypertension
fungal *Syn: fungous*; relating to a fungus
fungemia *Syn: mycethemia*; occurrence of fungi in the blood
fungicidal lethal to fungi
fungiform *Syn: fungilliform, fungus-shaped, mushroom-shaped*; fungal, like a fungus
fungilliform → *fungiform*
fungistatic *Syn: mycostatic*; inhibiting fungal growth
fungoid *Syn: fungous*; fungal, like a fungus
fungous → *fungoid*
fungus-shaped → *fungiform*
furosemide *Syn: frusemide*; potent loop diuretic; **indications**: [cereberal, pulmonary] edema, forced diuresis in poisonings, arterial hypertension, hyperkalemia, hypercalcemia; **side effects**: hypokalemia, hypocalcemia, hyponatremia, reduced bicarbonate excretion, hyperglycemia, hyperuricema, nausea, vomiting, tachycardia, increased risk of thrombosis
fusiform spindle-shaped
futile pointless, without purpose, useless, ineffective

G

gallop *Syn: cantering rhythm, gallop rhythm, Traube's bruit, Traube's murmur*; auscultation of a triple rhythm due to an additional sound [e.g., 3. heart sound]

  atrial gallop → *presystolic gallop*

  presystolic gallop *Syn: atrial gallop*; gallop rhythm with a muffled atrial sound [4. heart sound], e.g., in left-sided hypertrophy and in the acute phase of myocardial infarction

  protodiastolic gallop gallop rhythm with a loud 3. heart sound at the start of diastole, mainly found in myocarditis, mitral stenosis or insufficiency, and atrial septal defect

  summation gallop *s.u. fourth heart sound*

gallopamil calcium antagonist, coronary vasodilator; **usage**: prophylaxis and intermittent treatment of angina pectoris

gamma-hemolysis → *γ-hemolysis*

gamma-hemolytic → *γ-hemolytic*

ganglion *Syn: nerve ganglion*; collection of nerve cells in the peripheral nervous system; ganglia have a capsule [**capsula ganglii**], which surrounds the stroma [**stroma ganglii**], consisting of nerve cells and the connective tissue lying between them

  Bidder's ganglia *Syn: Remak's ganglia, sinoatrial ganglia*; ganglion cells of the vagus nerve in the atrial septum

  cardiac ganglia *Syn: Wrisberg's ganglia*; ganglia of the cardiac plexus, in which fibers of the vagus nerve relay

  ganglia cardiaca → *cardiac ganglia*

  caudal vagal ganglion → *lower ganglion of vagus nerve*

  caudal ganglion of vagus nerve → *lower ganglion of vagus nerve*

  inferior vagal ganglion → *lower ganglion of vagus nerve*

  inferior ganglion of vagus nerve → *lower ganglion of vagus nerve*

  ganglion inferius nervi vagi → *lower ganglion of vagus nerve*

  jugular vagal ganglion → *superior ganglion of vagus nerve*

  jugular ganglion of vagus nerve → *superior ganglion of vagus nerve*

lower vagal ganglion → *lower ganglion of vagus nerve*
lower ganglion of vagus nerve Syn: *caudal ganglion of vagus nerve, caudal vagal ganglion, inferior ganglion of vagus nerve, inferior vagal ganglion, nodose ganglion, lower vagal ganglion*; ganglion lying immediately beneath the jugular foramen
nodose ganglion → *lower ganglion of vagus nerve*
Remak's ganglia → *Bidder's ganglia*
rostral vagal ganglion → *superior ganglion of vagus nerve*
rostral ganglion of vagus nerve → *superior ganglion of vagus nerve*
sinoatrial ganglia → *Bidder's ganglia*
superior vagal ganglion → *superior ganglion of vagus nerve*
superior ganglion of vagus nerve Syn: *jugular ganglion of vagus nerve, jugular vagal ganglion, rostral ganglion of vagus nerve, rostral vagal ganglion, superior vagal ganglion*; superior ganglion of the vagus nerve lying in the jugular foramen
ganglion superius nervi vagi → *superior ganglion of vagus nerve*
Wrisberg's ganglia → *cardiac ganglia*

gap opening, cleft, hiatus
  synaptic gap Syn: *synaptic cleft; s.u. chemical synapse*

gas a fluid substance or a mixture of fluid substances with the ability to expand
  blood gases gases present in bound or dissolved form in the blood
  sweet gas → *carbon monoxide*

gastrocardiac relating to stomach and heart

gemmangioma → *hemangioendothelioma*

generation the act or process of generating
  impulse generation the heart rhythm is controlled by the excitation that arises spontaneously in the heart [autorhythm]; the origin of the excitation usually lies in the sinoatrial node in the right atrium, which at rest maintains a heart rate of 60–90/min; the conduction of the impulse proceeds via the excitation conduction system of the heart

gepefrine sympathomimetic, anti-hypotonic

germ a microorganism, especially a pathogen
  nosocomial germs generally antibiotic-resistant germs, which cause nosocomial infections

gitoxin digitalis glycoside derived from Digitalis purpurea and Digitalis lanata

gland organized aggregation of cells that secretes or excretes materials
  adrenal gland Syn: *adrenal body, adrenal capsule, epinephros, reni-*

capsule, paranephros, suprarenal, suprarenal capsule, suprarenal gland, suprarene; an endocrine gland sitting on the upper pole of the kidney, which is divided into two different portions [adrenal cortex, adrenal medulla]; each adrenal gland is approx. 4–6 cm long, 1–2 cm wide, and 4–6 cm thick; they are surrounded by a very cellular connective tissue capsule, which also contains vessels; under the capsule lies the **adrenal cortex**], which looks yellowish due to its lipid content; three layers can be identified: **zona glomerulosa**: outermost layer, which contains acidophil cells; synthesizes aldosterone and other mineralocorticoids; **zona fasciculata**: consists of parallel pillars of lipid-containing cells, which synthesize the glucocorticoids [cortisone, cortisol] and to a small extent also estrogens and androgens; **zona reticularis**: contains small, pigmented, acidophil epithelial cells, which synthesize the glucocorticoids [cortisone, cortisol]; the activity of the adrenal cortex is influenced by adrenocorticotrophic hormones and sympathetic nerves; the **adrenal medulla** contains specific medullary cells [chromaffin or pheochrome cells] and sympathetic nerve cells; the majority of the medullary cells [80%] synthesize adrenaline [**A-cells**], the remainder noradrenaline [**N-cells**]

carotid gland → *carotid glomus*
glomiform gland → *glomiform body*
lymph gland → *lymph node*
lymphatic gland → *lymph node*
suprarenal gland → *adrenal gland*

globulin generic term for globular proteins, which are water soluble thanks to their shape; this includes most enzymes, plasma proteins, hemoglobin, myoglobin, and peptide hormones [e.g., insulin]; they are often also described as **functional proteins**

accelerator globulin *Syn: accelerator factor, cofactor of thromboplastin, component A of prothrombin, factor V, plasma labile factor, labile factor, plasmin prothrombin conversion factor, proaccelerin, thrombogene*; heat-labile blood clotting factor; involved in the conversion of prothrombin to thrombin

antihemophilic globulin → *factor VIII*
plasma globulins *s.u. plasma protein*

glomangioma → *angiomyoneuroma*
glome → *glomus*
glomus *Syn: glome*; tuft of blood vessels, tuft of nerves
  glomus caroticum → *carotid glomus*

carotid glomus *Syn: carotid body, carotid gland, intercarotid body, glomus caroticum*; paraganglion of the carotid bifurcation; reacts to changes in oxygen partial pressure and pH value

jugular glomus *Syn: glomus jugulare*; paraganglion in the wall of the superior bulb of the jugular vein

glomus jugulare → *jugular glomus*

glucemia → *glycemia*

glucohemia → *glycemia*

glutamic-oxaloacetic transaminase → *aspartate aminotransferase*

glycemia *Syn: glucemia, glucohemia, glycohemia, glycosemia, glykemia*; sugar content of the blood

glyceride ester of glycerol and saturated or unsaturated fatty acids; subdivided, depending upon the number of esterified alcohol groups, into **monoglycerides**, **diglycerides**, and **triglycerides**

glyceryl trinitrate → *nitroglycerin*

glycohemia → *glycemia*

glycosemia → *glycemia*

glycoside any compund containing a carbohydrate molecule

digitalis glycosides glycoside obtained from digitalis species and other plants [Adonis vernalis, Convallaria majalis], which increase the contractile strength of the heart; includes, among others, digitoxigenin, digitoxin, lanatoside A, B, and C, digoxigenin, digoxin, gitoxigenin, k-strophanthin-α, -β and -γ; **action**: 1. positive inotrope [increase in the contraction strength and increase in the stroke volume] 2. negative chronotrope [reduction in the heart rate] 3. negative dromotropy [slowing of the conduction of excitation] 4. positive bathmotrope [increase in the excitability, mainly of the ventricular myocardium]; **usage**: cardiac insufficiency, tachycardic arrhythmias, atrial extrasystoles; **side effects**: gastrointestinal pains, vomiting, lightheadedness, sleepiness, color vision, visual field disturbances; disturbances of heart rhythm with extrasystoles

triterpene glycosides glycoside belonging to the tri-terpenes, digitalis glycoside

glycyl betaine → *betaine*

glykemia → *glycemia*

graft → *transplant*

composite graft *Syn: combination transplant, multi-organ transplant*; transplant consisting of two or more organs, e.g., heart-lung transplant

heterogenous graft →*heterotransplant*
heterologous graft →*heterotransplant*
heteroplastic graft →*heterotransplant*
heterospecific graft →*heterotransplant*
vascular graft transplantation of autogenous [e.g., long saphenous vein], allogeneic [umbilical cord vessels, cadaveric donation], or xenogeneic [bovine, porcine] blood vessel segments as vessel substitutes or for plastic procedures on vessels
xenogeneic graft →*heterotransplant*

granule grain
alpha granules *Syn:* α-*granules*; *s.u. thrombocyte granules*
electron-dense granules *s.u. thrombocyte granules*
thrombocyte granules in activated thrombocytes one can differentiate, based on morphologic and chemical aspects, electron-dense granules, α-granules, and lysosomes; the substances contained in the electron dense granules and α-granules are released during thrombocyte aggregation and play an important role in hemostasis and blood clotting; the importance of the lysosomes remains unclear

granulocyte *Syn: granular leukocyte, polynuclear leukocyte*; polymorphonuclear white blood cell with stainable granules; 60% of all leukocytes in the blood are granulocytes, i.e., approx. 3000–6000/ml blood; of these approx. 95% are neutrophil granulocytes, approx. 4% eosinophil granulocytes, and approx. 1% basophil granulocytes; they are capable of ameboid movement like the other leukocytes and can actively penetrate through the wall of blood vessels [leukodiapedesis]; more than half of the granulocytes are therefore found in the extravascular space, where they act as phagocytes, ingesting organisms and destroying them

granulocytic relating to or characterized by granulocytes

granulocytopenia →*neutropenia*

granuloma *Syn: granulation tumor*; nodular lesion consisting of granulation tissue with histiocytic cells [often epithelioid cells] and possibly central exudative necrosis and giant cells; it occurs, for example, in tuberculosis or poorly degradable foreign bodies [foreign body granuloma, asbestosis, silicone]

granulomatosis occurrence of multiple granulomas
allergic granulomatosis →*allergic granulomatous angiitis*
Wegener's granulomatosis *Syn: Wegener's syndrome*; systemic disease of uncertain etiology, with necrosis of the blood vessels and forma-

tion of granulomas in the nasal, oral, and pharyngeal cavities; **therapy**: prednisone in combination with cyclophosphamide; operative removal of granulomas and plastic reconstruction of the damaged structures

granulopenia → *neutropenia*

groove shallow linear depression

anterior interventricular groove → *anterior interventricular sulcus*
atrioventricular groove → *coronary sulcus of heart*
auriculoventricular groove → *coronary sulcus of heart*
inferior interventricular groove → *posterior interventricular sulcus*

group a number of similar or related objects

blood group *Syn: blood type*; properties caused by specific antigens on the erythrocyte membrane [blood group antigens], which can be demonstrated with the help of specific antibodies; the most important blood groups are the **AB0 blood group** [blood groups A, AB, B, 0], **Rhesus blood groups**, and **MNSs blood groups**; the different blood groups play a particular role as triggers of hemolytic transfusion reactions and erythroblastosis of the newborn and in forensic medicine in the determination of paternity and identification of perpetrators or victims of violent crime

Bombay blood group rare variant of the AB0 blood group system; the blood group antigens A, B, and H are suppressed and the serum contains both Anti-A and also Anti-B and Anti-H; this renders transfusion practically impossible

Diego blood group blood group that only occurs in Indians, Chinese, and Japanese; the antigens Di^a and Di^b are inherited in autosomal codominant fashion; a rare cause of transfusion reactions or hemolytic disease of the newborn

Duffy blood group blood group system, whose antigens [Anti-Fy^a, Anti-Fy^b] can provoke a severe hemolytic disease of the newborn or cause a transfusion reaction; named after the first patients

HACEK group generic term for Haemophilus aphrophilus, Actinobacillus actinomycetemcomitans, Cardiobacterium hominis, Eikenella corrodens, and Kingella kingae, which can all cause endocarditis, are difficult to culture, and can therefore easily evade diagnosis; Haemophilus paraphrophilus is also included nowadays

Kell blood groups blood group system, which can lead to incompatibility reactions in transfusions and in pregnancy; was named after the first two patients [Kellacher and Cellano]

Kidd blood groups *Syn: Kidd blood group system*; blood group system, which can lead to incompatibility reactions in transfusions and in pregnancy; was named after the first two patients

Le blood groups → *Lewis blood groups*

Lewis blood groups *Syn: Le blood groups*; blood group system, whose antigens also occur in saliva and blood plasma; can lead to transfusion reactions

Lu blood groups → *Lutheran blood groups*

Lutheran blood groups *Syn: Lu blood groups*; blood group system, whose antigens [Lu^a, Lu^b] can cause a mild transfusion reaction

MN blood groups → *MNSs blood group system*

MNSs blood groups → *MNSs blood group system*

P blood groups *Syn: P blood group system*; blood group system of the erythrocytes and thrombocytes; can in rare cases cause transfusion reactions and miscarriages

Rhesus blood groups *Syn: Rh blood group system, Rh system, rhesus system*; blood group system, which was discovered because of antibodies against the erythrocytes of rhesus monkeys; most common cause of transfusion reactions and the development of hemolytic disease of the newborn; the rhesus antigens sit on various surface regions of the erythrocytes; the most important are C-antigen, D-antigen, E-antigen, c-antigen, and e-antigen, of which the D-antigen has the strongest antigenic action; blood containing erythrocytes bearing the D-antigen is called **Rh-positive**; if the antigen is absent, then this is called **Rh-negative**; in Europe and North America 85% of the population is Rh-positive and 15% Rh-negative; since D is dominant over d, the phenotype D can have the genotype DD or Dd, whereas the phenotype d always has the genotype dd; in contrast to the AB0-blood group system, antibodies against rhesus-antigens are only formed after a first exposure [sensitization]; for this reason, the first transfusion of Rh-positive blood into a Rh-negative recipient does not provoke a transfusion reaction; it is also important that the antibodies of the Rh-system, which are incomplete IgG-antibodies, can cross the placental barrier and cause hemolytic disease of the newborn

Wright blood groups rare blood group system described in 1953, whose antigens Wr^a and Wr^b are inherited in autosomal dominant fashion; may rarely cause transfusion reactions or hemolytic disease of the newborn

Xg blood group blood group, with X-linked inheritance; of no clinical importance; used in determination of paternity and genetic research

G-strophantin cardiac glycoside from **Strophanthus gratus**

H

haem → *heme*

Haemophilus gram-negative, facultatively anaerobic, rod-shaped bacteria that do not form spores; they grow only on blood-containing media; they require growth factors X [hemin] and V [NAD]

Haemophilus. Species and infections

Species	Infection(s)
H. influenzae B [HiB]	meningitis, sepsis, epiglottitis, arthritis, pneumonia
H. influenzae [without capsule]	otitis media, sinusitis, conjunctivitis, tracheobronchitis, pneumonia
H. aegypticus [Koch-Week's bacillus]	conjunctivitis
H. parainfluenzae	respiratory tract infections, endocarditis
H. ducreyi	soft chancre
H. acrophilus	endocarditis
H. paraphrophilus	endocarditis

Haemophilus acrophilus *s.u. HACEK group*

Haemophilus influenzae *Syn: Pfeiffer's bacillus, influenza bacillus*; causative agent of purulent laryngitis, conjunctivitis, endocarditis, meningitis, and atypical pneumonia [primarily as a secondary infection in influenza]; some strains have polysaccharide capsules and can be divided into serotypes A-F; of these, Haemophilus influenzae B [HiB] is a dangerous causative agent of meningitis or sepsis; before the introduction of protective vaccinations against HiB, meningitis caused by HiB was the most frequent purulent meningitis; Haemophilus influenzae is susceptible to aminopenicillins, ureidopenicillins, cephalosporins, and chloramphenicol

Haemophilus parainfluenzae part of the normal flora of the upper respiratory tract; in rare cases, it is the causative agent of respiratory tract infections, sepsis, meningitis, or endocarditis

Haemophilus paraphrophilus *s.u. HACEK group*

haemorrhagia → *bleeding*

heart *Syn: cor*; the heart is the central organ of the circulation; like a suction-pressure pump, it sucks in blood during diastole and pumps it back into the circulation during systole; functionally and anatomically, a right and left half can be differentiated, which are each subdivided into an atrium and a ventricle; the **right heart** receives the oxygen-poor [venous] blood returning from the body periphery and head into the **right atrium** and pumps it through the **right ventricle** into the pulmonary circulation; the oxygen-rich [arterial] blood flows out of the lungs into the **left atrium** and is then pumped out of the **left ventricle** into the systemic circulation; the excitation conduction system of the heart initiates and coordinates the formation and spread of excitation in the heart muscle of the various segments; externally, three surfaces can be discerned [sternocostal, diaphragmatic, and pulmonary surfaces of the heart], a right border [margo dexter cordis], although this is only obvious on the cadaveric heart, the superior **heart base** [basis cordis] with exiting and entering great vessels and the **heart apex** formed from the left ventricle [apex cordis]; the **anterior interventricular sulcus** is a groove on the front of the heart, which marks the border between the right and left ventricles; in it, the anterior interventricular branch of the left coronary artery runs to the cardiac apex; correspondingly, there is a **posterior interventricular sulcus** on the back of the heart; in it, the posterior interventricular branch of the right coronary artery runs to the cardiac apex; the **coronary fissure of the heart** [coronary sulcus] runs on the atrioventricular border; in it lie the coronary vessels [right and left coronary arteries]; both atria possess blind sacs called the **left/right auricle**; the two ventricles are separated by the **ventricular septum**; its inferior portion is muscular [**pars muscularis**], the superior membranous [**pars membranacea**]; the **atrial septum** is purely membranous; the **heart wall** consists of a connective tissue **cardiac skeleton**, which makes the fibrous ring around the cardiac ostia [annulus fibrosus dexter/sinister cordis], endocardium, myocardium, and epicardium; the **endocardium** forms the innermost layer of the heart wall; it consists of a one cell thick

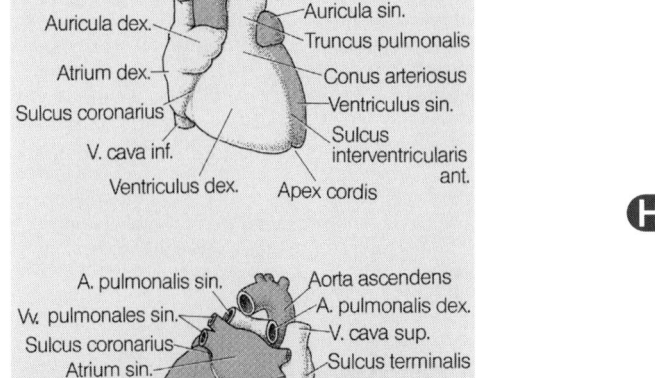

Heart. View onto the sternocostal surface

endothelium, which covers the ventricle, atria, heart valves, papillary muscles, tendons, and cardiac trabeculae; the terminal branches of the excitation conduction system [rami subendocardiales] run in the subendocardial connective tissue; a basal membrane made from loose connective tissue forms the connection to the heart wall musculature [**myocardium**]; it is the working muscle, from which the papillary muscles [musculi papillares] and the trabeculae carneae arise; in the atria, the myocardium is mostly smooth, in the ventricles it forms macroscopically visible ridges, which surround the left ventricle in three layers [**outer oblique, middle circular, and inner longitudinal layers**]; the outermost layer of the heart wall is called the **epicardium**; within the heart sac, the epicardium forms the inner layer of the pericardium, which covers the myocardium; the heart vessels run in the

heart

subepicardial fatty tissue; ventricles and atria are separated by valve systems, which prevent backward flow of blood into the atria while allowing blood out of the atria into the ventricles during diastole; the right valve has three cusps and is therefore called the **tricuspid valve**; the left only has two cusps and is called the **mitral valve** because of its shape; the **pulmonary valve** closes the exit from the right ventricle in the pulmonary trunk; the **aortic valve** sits in the aortic orifice of the left ventricle

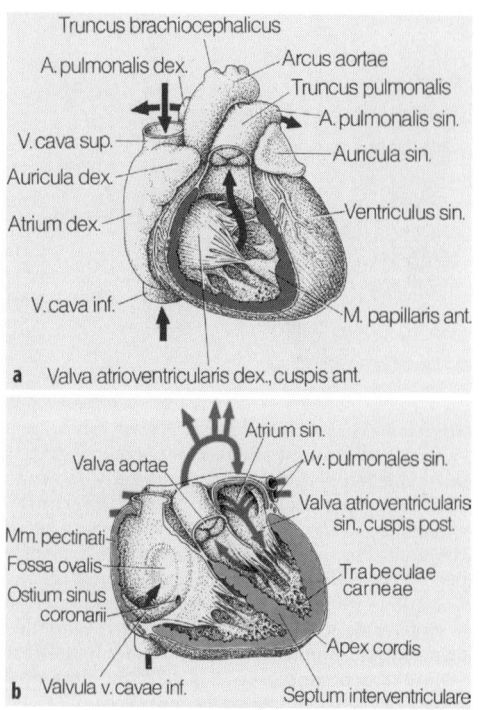

Heart. **a** view into the right ventricle; **b** view into both ventricles and atria

armored heart *Syn: armour heart, panzerherz*; constrictive pericardial inflammation with calcification of the pericardium

armour heart →*armored heart*

athletic heart enlarged heart in performance athletes who perform endurance sports [long-distance runners, cyclists]; the heart muscle hypertrophies and the weight can increase to up to 500 g [normal 300–350 g]; because of the increased stroke volume, the pulse rate falls at rest

beer heart dilated cardiomyopathy caused by excessive beer consumption

boat-shaped heart typical appearance of the heart on an X-ray with enlargement of the left ventricle in aortic insufficiency

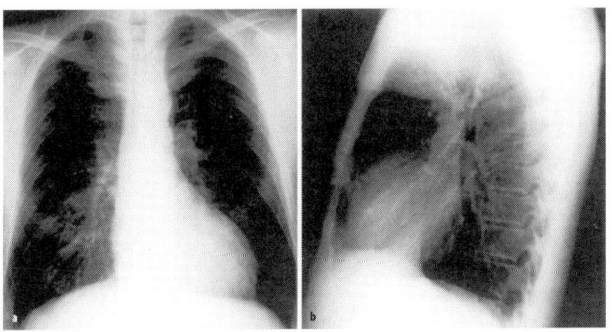

Boat shaped heart. Typical X-ray in aortic insufficiency

bovine heart *Syn: bucardia, ox heart*; extreme enlargement of the heart, e.g., in dilated cardiomyopathy due to chronic alcohol abuse

drop heart →*bathycardia*

fat heart *Syn: fatty heart*; subepicardial fat deposition, e.g., in diphtheric myocardial injury

fatty heart →*fat heart*

hairy heart *Syn: cor villosum, trichocardia*; gritty cardiac surface that develops following fibrin deposition in the pericardium

irritable heart →*neurocirculatory asthenia*

ox heart →*bovine heart*

pendulous heart teardrop-shaped heart due to a low-lying dia-

phragm
pulmonary heart → *right heart*
right heart *Syn: pulmonary heart*; right heart chamber, right ventricle
sabot heart → *wooden-shoe heart*
soldier's heart → *neurocirculatory asthenia*
tiger heart striation of the heart muscle due to fat deposition
wooden-shoe heart *Syn: coeur en sabot, sabot heart*; typical heart shape of tetralogy of Fallot seen on the chest X-ray

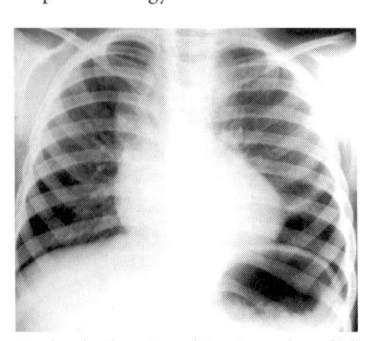

Wooden-shoe heart. Typical X-ray in tetralogy of Fallot with right aortic arch

heartbeat a complete cardiac cycle
heart-lung machine *Syn: pump-oxygenator*; apparatus for maintaining extracorporeal circulation in, e.g., open heart surgery; it consists in principle of a pump, which pumps the blood out of the body to an oxygenator/heat exchanger and then through a blood filter back into the body
hem- combining form denoting relation to blood
hema- combining form denoting relation to blood
hemacytes → *hemocytes*
hemadostenosis → *arteriostenosis*
hemadsorption adhesion of red blood corpuscles, e.g., onto a surface
hemafacient → *hemopoietic*
hemagglutination *Syn: hemoagglutination*; blood clumping caused by hemagglutinins; in **direct** or **active hemagglutination** the clumping is caused by antibodies against the surface antigens of the erythrocytes;

if the agglutination only occurs after loading the erythrocyte surface with an antigen, then this is called **indirect** or **passive hemagglutination**

hemagglutinative relating to or causing hemagglutination

hemagglutinins substances [e.g., agglutinating antibodies, phytoagglutinins], which lead to clumping of erythrocytes

hemanalysis *Syn: analysis of blood, examination of blood*; examination of blood, blood analysis

hemangioblast vessel-forming cell

hemangioblastoma *Syn: angioblastic meningioma, angioblastoma, Lindau's tumor*; benign tumor arising from the vessel wall

hemangioendothelioma *Syn: angioendothelioma, gemmangioma, hemendothelioma, hypertrophic angioma*; semi-malignant tumor arising in the endothelium of blood vessels; grows slowly locally with only minimal tendency to metastasize; **kaposiform hemangioendothelioma** [mainly occurs in children in the deep soft tissues of the upper extremity], **retiform hemangioendothelioma** [tumor occurring mainly in middle age with net-like branching], **epitheloid hemangioendothelioma** [solitary, painful tumor, mostly attached to a large vessel in the deep soft tissues], and **spindle-cell hemangioendothelioma** [red-blue, solitary or multiple lumps in the dermis or subcutaneous tissues, mainly in the distal extremities] are differentiated histologically; all forms progress over a protracted period of years; there is a general tendency to recur, but almost none to metastasize; **therapy**: excision

fusiform hemangioendothelioma *Syn: spindle-cell hemangioendothelioma; s.u. hemangioendothelioma*

malignant hemangioendothelioma → *hemangiosarcoma*

spindle-cell hemangioendothelioma *Syn: fusiform hemangioendothelioma; s.u. hemangioendothelioma*

hemangioendotheliosarcoma → *hemangiosarcoma*

hemangioma *Syn: hemartoma*; benign tumor of vessels, which is mostly present at birth or develops in the first months of life [**infantile hemangioma**]; there are, however, also forms that first arise in later life [**senile angioma, pyogenic granuloma**]; hemangiomas also occur in the setting of malformation syndromes [blue rubber bleb nevus syndrome, Maffucci syndrome]

sinusoidal hemangioma large sinusoidal cavities, predominantly on the trunk of young women

target hemangioma solitary angioma with target-like shape; mostly on the trunk of middle-aged males; histology shows marked iron deposition

hemangiomatosis occurrence of multiple hemangiomas; in infants as **benign neonatal hemangiomatosis** with up to several hundred small [1–10 mm] hemangiomas; if there is an association with malformation of the liver or intestinal tract, then this is a case of **diffuse neonatal hemangiomatosis**

hemangiosarcoma *Syn: hemangioendotheliosarcoma, malignant hemangioendothelioma*; degenerate hemangioendothelioma with metastasis; found, e.g., in the thyroid gland and bones

hemapoiesis → *blood formation*

hemapoietic → *hemopoietic*

hemartoma → *hemangioma*

hemat- combining form denoting relation to blood

hematherapy → *hemotherapy*

hematin *Syn: hematosin, hydroxyhemin, oxyheme, oxyhemochromogen, metheme, phenodin*; blue to blackish-brown compound formed in the oxidation of hemoglobin

reduced hematin → *heme*

hemato- combining form denoting relation to blood

hematoblast → *hemopoietic stem cell*

hematocrit proportion of the red blood cells [erythrocytes] in the total blood volume; in adult males, it is 0.44–0.46, in women 0.41–0.43; in the newborn, it is approx. 20% higher and in toddlers approx. 10% lower; it is measured either by the **Wintrobe** method [centrifugation of blood prevented from clotting in standardized hematocrit tubes] or in the setting of automated blood analysis by calculation [$Hct = MCV \times Z_E$]

hematocrystallin → *hemoglobin*

hematocytes → *hemocytes*

hematocytoblast → *hemopoietic stem cell*

hematocytoblasts → *stem cells*

hematocytolysis → *hemolysis*

hematogenesis → *blood formation*

hematogenic → *hematogenous*

hematogenous *Syn: hematogenic, hemogenic*; **1.** originating in the blood, arising from the blood **2.** transmitted through blood, via the circulation, blood-borne

hematoglobin → *hemoglobin*

hematoglobulin → *hemoglobin*
hematolysis → *hemolysis*
hematolytic → *hemolytic*
hematoma a localized swelling filled with blood
  aneurysmal hematoma *Syn: spurious aneurysm, false aneurysm; s.u. aneurysm*
hematopenia reduction in the blood volume
hematopericardium → *hemopericardium*
hematophilia → *hemophilia*
hematopiesis → *blood pressure*
hematopoiesis → *blood formation*
hematopoietic → *hemopoietic*
hematorrhea *Syn: hemorrhea*; severe/massive bleeding
hematosepsis → *septicemia*
hematoseptic relating to or caused by hematosepsis
hematosis → *blood formation*
hematostatic → *hemostatic*
hematotherapy → *hemotherapy*
hematotoxic *Syn: hematoxic, hemotoxic*; injuring blood cells
hematotropic *Syn: hemotropic*; with particular affinity for blood or blood cells
hematoxic → *hematotoxic*
heme *Syn: ferroprotoporphyrin, haem, protoheme, reduced hematin*; iron-containing porphyrin; pigment portion of hemoglobin and myoglobin, which transports oxygen and carbon dioxide; made in almost all cells, but particularly in the erythroblasts of the bone marrow, erythrocytes in the flowing blood, and in the liver
hemendothelioma → *hemangioendothelioma*
hemi- combining form denoting relation to one half
hemiblock interruption of a fascicle of the Tawara crus of the conducting system of the heart
  left anterior hemiblock *s.u. intraventricular block*
  left posterior hemiblock *s.u. intraventricular block*
hemisystole unilateral contraction of the heart muscle, i.e., only the right ventricle contracts; this leads to a prominent venous pulse in the absence of a radial pulse
hemo- combining form denoting relation to blood
hemoagglutination → *hemagglutination*
hemoblast → *hemopoietic stem cell*

hemoblasts → *stem cells*
hemoclasia → *erythroclasis*
hemoclasis → *erythroclasis*
hemocoagulin enzyme [protease] made by the poisonous snake Bothrops atrox; formerly used as a hemostyptic; nowadays only used to determine the reptilase time
hemoconcentration water deficiency in the blood
hemoculture → *blood culture*
hemocytes *Syn*: hemacytes, hematocytes, blood cells; generic term for the cells contained in the blood, i.e., **red blood corpuscles** [erythrocytes], **white blood corpuscles** [leukocytes], and **blood platelets** [thrombocytes] as well as their precursors
hemocytoblast pluripotent stem cells in the bone marrow
hemocytolysis → *hemolysis*
hemocytometer an instrument for counting blood cells
  Thoma-Zeiss hemocytometer → *Thoma-Zeiss counting cell*
hemocytopoiesis → *blood formation*
hemodilution thinning of the blood caused by an increase in the proportion of fluid or a reduction in the red blood corpuscles; used therapeutically in thromboprophylaxis or to improve cerebral perfusion or the microcirculation; treatment with coumarin derivatives is often incorrectly described as blood thinning, but actually works by inhibiting the vitamin K-dependent blood clotting factors
hemodynamic relating to hemodynamics
hemodynamics study of the movement of blood in the circulation
hemogenesis → *blood formation*
hemogenic → *hematogenous*
hemoglobin *Syn*: blood pigment, hematocrystallin, hematoglobin, hematoglobulin; blood pigment contained in the red blood corpuscles, which consists of a globin portion and an iron-containing prosthetic group [heme]; hemoglobin transports oxygen from the lungs to the tissues and carbon dioxide from the tissues to the lungs; in addition, it is part of the protein buffering system that maintains a constant pH value in the blood; an adult weighing 70 kg has approx. 800 g hemoglobin; of this approx. 6–6.5 g per day is broken down or synthesized; hemoglobin is a globular molecule, which is made up of four polypeptide chains and one prosthetic group [heme]; the various hemoglobins differ in the structure of the polypeptide chains; **embryonal hemoglobin** [also called **hemoglobin Gower 1 and 2**] consists of two ε and ζ chains;

after the third month, **fetal hemoglobin** [two α and two γ chains] dominates, but by birth this has already been partially replaced by adult hemoglobin [hemoglobin A]; the hemoglobin of children and adults consists of two α and two β chains [hemoglobin A_1]; approx. 2.5% contains δ chains instead of β chains [hemoglobin A_2] and as a result has a higher oxygen affinity; the combination of four chains to make a functioning unit [quaternary structure] is achieved thanks to complementary regions on the surfaces of the chains; the subunits are held together by oxygen bridging as well as by hydrophobic and electrostatic forces; this allows them to be packed tightly without using large amounts of energy, which is very important for the function of hemoglobin; the binding of oxygen to the heme moiety of the hemoglobin is called **oxygenation**, the release of oxygen **deoxygenation**; correspondingly, oxygen-loaded hemoglobin is called **oxyhemoglobin**, hemoglobin without oxygen is called **deoxyhemoglobin**; since the two forms have different spectra of light absorption in the red and infrared wavelengths, the oxygen saturation of the blood can be measured non-invasively by photo detectors [**pulse oximetry**]

mean cell hemoglobin → *mean corpuscular hemoglobin*

mean corpuscular hemoglobin *Syn: erythrocyte color coefficient, mean cell hemoglobin*; hemoglobin content of individual erythrocytes; calculated as the quotient of hemoglobin content of the blood [g/l] and the erythrocyte count [10^{12}/l]; the normal range is around 26.4–34 pg or 1.7–2 mmol; decreased in hypochromic anemias and increased in hyperchromic anemias

muscle hemoglobin → *myoglobin*

hemoglobinopathy *Syn: hemoglobin disease*; hereditary disease with formation of anomalous hemoglobin types, e.g., thalassemia, sickle cell anemia

hemoglobinuric relating to hemoglobinuria

hemogram → *differential count*

hemokinesis blood flow, blood circulation

hemolysin 1. toxin causing hemolysis, hemolytic poison **2.** antibody causing hemolysis

hemolysis *Syn: cythemolysis, erythrocytolysis, erythrolysis, hematocytolysis, hemocytolysis, hematolysis*; disruption/destruction of the red blood corpuscles, erythrocyte disruption, erythrocyte destruction; also a description of erythrocyte breakdown in the setting of physiologic blood turnover; increased hemolysis is found in, e.g., hemolytic anemia, chronic inflammation, hemoglobinopathies, artificial heart valves, etc.; jaundice may develop [icterus] as a result of the increased production of hemoglobin breakdown products [bilirubin]

α-hemolysis *Syn: alpha-hemolysis*; bacterial growth with hemolysis on blood agar, which is characterized by the formation of a green zone around the colony

β-hemolysis *Syn: beta-hemolysis*; bacterial growth with total hemolysis of the erythrocytes in blood agar

colloid osmotic hemolysis *Syn: osmotic hemolysis*; destruction of the red blood corpuscles provoked by a change in the colloid osmotic pressure

conditioned hemolysis → *immunohemolysis*

γ-hemolysis *Syn: gamma-hemolysis*; bacterial growth without hemolysis, non-hemolytic/non-hemolyzing growth

immune hemolysis → *immunohemolysis*

osmotic hemolysis → *colloid osmotic hemolysis*

hemolytic *Syn: hematolytic*; relating to or causing hemolysis

α-hemolytic *Syn: alpha-hemolytic*; relating to, characterized by, or producing α-hemolysis

β-hemolytic *Syn: beta-hemolytic*; relating to, characterized by, or producing β-hemolysis

γ-hemolytic *Syn: gamma-hemolytic*; relating to γ-hemolysis, non-hemolytic

hemopericardium *Syn: hematopericardium*; blood collection in the pericardial sac; bloody pericardial effusion

hemophilia *Syn: hematophilia*; hereditary blood clotting disorder with reduced activity of blood clotting factors VIII [hemophilia A], IX [hemophilia B], or XI [hemophilia C]; clinical differentiation is based upon the residual levels and the clinical symptoms

hemophilia A *Syn: classical hemophilia*; classical blood clotting disorder caused by deficiency of blood clotting factor VIII; occurs with an incidence of 1:5000 in males and is therefore the most common severe blood clotting disorder; inherited as an X-linked recessive trait and therefore practically only affects men; heterozygous women are asymptomatic carriers; due to the deficiency of factor VIII, the activation of factor X in the intrinsic system is disturbed and the activation of prothrombin is slowed or does not occur; hemophilia A does not have a unique clinical picture, rather there are both the most severe forms that cause bleeding in neonates and also subclinical forms that only become apparent in adulthood or may even be discovered completely by chance; four grades of severity are therefore defined, distinguished by the residual factor VIII activity: severe: < 1%, intermediate: 1–5%, mild: 5–15%, and sub-hemophilic: 15–35%; **clinical**: generally, the first symptoms develop when children start to stand or walk; the bleeds affect mainly the large joints [ankle, knee, elbow joints] and untreated lead to joint deformities [bleeder's joint]; in addition, there may be soft tissue and muscle bleeds, more rarely hematuria or intracerebral bleeds; **diagnosis**: determination of the factor VIII level; **therapy**: lifelong replacement therapy, which usually means i.v. infusion that can be performed by the patient, or in children by their parents; the factor concentrates used contain highly purified factor VIII and traces of von Willebrand factor; to some extent, genetically engineered factor concentrates are now being used; DDAVP [1-desamino-8-D-arginine-vasopressin] is a derivative of the antidiuretic hormone, which leads to an increase in the concentration of factor VIII and von Willebrand factor in the blood; before operative interventions, the blood level must be increased to a value appropriate to the procedure; the most feared complication is the formation of antibodies to the infused factor, which leads to inhibitory body hemophilia

hemophilia B *Syn: Christmas disease, factor IX deficiency*; disturbance of blood clotting caused by congenital deficiency of the Christmas factor; **therapy**: lifelong replacement therapy, which generally consists of i.v. administration performed by the patient, or in children by their parents; the factor concentrates used contain highly purified factor IX

hemophilia C *Syn: factor XI deficiency, PTA deficiency*; autosomal recessive deficiency of factor XI with an inherited bleeding tendency

classical hemophilia → *hemophilia A*

mild form of hemophilia rarely used term for clinically silent hemophilia with only mildly reduced factor levels and without a bleeding tendency

vascular hemophilia → *angiohemophilia*

hemophilic relating to hemophilia

hemopneumopericardium *Syn: pneumohemopericardium*; collection of air and blood in the pericardial sac

hemopoiesic → *hemopoietic*

hemopoiesis → *blood formation*

antenatal hemopoiesis the **embryonic blood formation** initially occurs in the yolk sac, then in the liver and spleen [**hepatolienal blood formation**]; after the 7. month of gestation, the bone marrow is the main site and following the 2.–4. week after birth the only site of blood formation

extramedullary hemopoiesis the formation of blood outside the bone marrow

hepatolienal hemopoiesis the formation of blood in the liver and spleen; physiologic during the embryonic period

medullary hemopoiesis *Syn: myelopoietic hemopoiesis*; the formation of blood in the bone marrow

myelopoietic hemopoiesis → *medullary hemopoiesis*

postnatal hemopoiesis after the 2.-4. post-partum weeks, blood formation occurs exclusively in the bone marrow

hemopoietic *Syn: hematogenic, hemogenic, hemafacient, hemapoietic, hematopoietic, hemopoiesic, sanguinopoietic, sanguifacient*; relating to blood formation/hemopoiesis

hemorrhage *Syn: bleeding*; escape of blood from a vessel

arterial hemorrhage → *arterial bleeding*

cerebral hemorrhage → *encephalorrhagia*

concealed hemorrhage bleeding inside a body cavity or an organ [internal bleeding]

decompression hemorrhage description of hemorrhage by diapedesis in the setting of reactive hyperemia

external hemorrhage bleeding on the body surface

fibrinogen deficiency hemorrhage bleeding caused by deficiency of fibrinogen

parenchymatous hemorrhage internal bleeding into an organ

hemorrhage per rhexin bleeding following a tear in the vessel wall

petechial hemorrhage → *petechia*

venous hemorrhage → *venous bleeding*

hemorrhagic relating to or characterized by hemorrhage

hemorrhea → *hematorrhea*

hemostasia → *hemostasis*

hemostasis *Syn: hemostasia*; mechanisms initiated by the body to protect itself from blood loss; in the first step [**primary hemostasis**], smaller bleeds are quelled by vasoconstriction and sealing of the vessel defect by a platelet plug [white thrombus]; even during this process, blood clotting is activated [**secondary hemostasis**], which closes the vessel with a red thrombus, which contracts and hardens following clotting;

disturbances of hemostasis lead to a bleeding tendency or to thromboses; defects in primary hemostasis can be caused by the vessels [vascular] or the thrombocytes [thrombocytic]; disturbances of secondary hemostasis are due to inborn or acquired deficiencies of one or more clotting factors

hemostatic Syn: *hematostatic, hemostyptic, antihemorrhagic, anthemorrhagic*; **1.** an agent with hemostatic properties **2.** arresting hemorrhage

hemostyptic → *hemostatic*

hemotherapeutics → *hemotherapy*

hemotherapy Syn: *hematherapy, hematotherapy, hemotherapeutics*; therapeutic transfusion of blood or blood components

hemotoxic → *hematotoxic*

hemotropic → *hematotropic*

heparin Syn: *heparinic acid*; glycosaminoglycan inhibitor of clotting, which occurs, among other sites, in the mast cell granules and which is used therapeutically as an anticoagulant; heparin acts indirectly by activating antithrombin III as well as by inhibiting thrombokinase, factor V, IX, and XII; in high doses, it inhibits thrombocyte aggregation; because of its activating effect on lipoprotein lipase, it has positive actions in arteriosclerosis; endogenous or parenterally given heparin is catabolized in the liver through hepariniases; **usage**: temporary systemic anticoagulation [mostly intravenous **total heparinization**] and thrombo-prophylaxis [**low-dose heparin** subcutaneously]

heparinic acid → *heparin*

heparinization transient systemic anticoagulation [mostly intravenous **complete heparinization**] or thrombo-prophylaxis [**low-dose heparin** subcutaneously] produced by parenteral treatment with heparin **total heparinization** s.u. *heparin*

hereditary inherited, heritable, related to heredity; inborn

hetero- combining form denoting relation to other, different, or abnormal, denoting relationship to another

heterochronic → *heterochronous*

heterochronous Syn: *heterochronic*; shifted in time or delayed

heterodromous (running) in the opposite direction

heterogeneic → *heterogenetic*

heterogenetic Syn: *heterogeneic, heterogenic, heterogenous*; of mixed origin, (derived) from another species

heterogenic 1. inconsistent, disparate, diverse **2.** of different provenance,

heterogenous

(derived) from another species

heterogenous → *heterogenetic*

heterograft → *heterotransplant*

heterologous 1. aberrant, non-autologous **2.** *Syn:* xenotypic; derived from another species

heterophile *Syn:* heterophil, heterophilic; having an affinity for foreign antigens

heterophilic → *heterophile*

heteroplastid → *heterotransplant*

heteroplasty *Syn:* heterologous transplantation, heteroplastic transplantation, heterotransplantation, xenogeneic transplantation, xenotransplantation; plastic procedure with implantation of tissues from a different species

heterotopic → *ectopic*

heterotransplant *Syn:* heterogenous graft, heterograft, heterologous graft, heteroplastic graft, heterospecific graft, heteroplastid, xenogeneic graft, xenograft, xenograft; tissue derived from another species [e.g., porcine heart valves]

heterotransplantation → *heteroplasty*

hexamethylenamine → *hexamethylentetramine*

hexamethylentetramine *Syn:* aminoform, hexamethylenamine, hexamine, methenamine; decomposes in an acidic solution of ammonia and formaldehyde; **usage:** antiseptic predominantly in urinary infections, diuretic

hexamine → *hexamethylentetramine*

hiatus gap, cleft, opening

    aortic hiatus *Syn:* hiatus aorticus; opening in the diaphragm for passage of the aorta and the thoracic duct at the level of the first lumbar vertebra

    hiatus aorticus → *aortic hiatus*

hilum *Syn:* hilus; site of entry and exit of nerves and vessels

    hilum of lung *Syn:* pulmonary hilum, hilus of lung; the opening on the side of both lungs, which faces the mediastinum, where the pulmonary arteries and veins, primary bronchi [bronchus principalis dexter and sinister], and nerves of the hilum of the lung enter and exit

    pulmonary hilum → *hilum of lung*

hilus → *hilum*

hirudin inhibitor of blood clotting found in the saliva of the leech [Hirudo medicinalis]; **usage:** externally for the treatment of hematomas, ve-

nous inflammation, and inflamed varices
Hirudo medicinalis leech used both in traditional medicine and in alternative medicine
histo- combining form denoting relation to tissue
histocompatibility *Syn: tissue tolerance*; tolerability/compatibility of foreign substances with the body tissues
histocompatible relating to histocompatibility
holodiastolic throughout diastole
holosystolic *Syn: pansystolic*; throughout systole
homochronous →*synchronous*
homodromous (running) in the same direction
homogeneous of uniform composition, of identical structure, of similar type, uniform, analogous
homogenous →*homologous 2.*
homological →*homologous 2.*
homologous 1. *Syn: analogous, autologous, akin, autologous*; corresponding in structure, position, etc. **2.** *Syn: homogenous, homological, isologous, allogeneic, allogenic*; derived from the same species
hormone a substance produced by one tissue and conveyed by the bloodstream to another to effect physiological activity
  antidiuretic hormone *Syn: vasopressin*; hormone formed in the hypothalamus, which regulates renal reabsorption of water; used in the treatment of diabetes insipidus
  atrial natriuretic hormone →*atrial natriuretic peptide*
hum humming noise
  venous hum →*bruit de diable*
hump a rounded mass or protuberance
  heart hump swelling of the chest wall in cardiac hypertrophy
hyalin light microscopic description of transparent, homogenous, eosinophilic deposits in cells or tissues, which mainly consist of collagen and proteins; **intracellular hyalin** includes, e.g., Councilman bodies, Mallory bodies, and Russell bodies; **vascular hyalin** is part of the changes in the wall caused by atherosclerosis
hyalinosis hyaline degeneration
  arteriolar hyalinosis hyaline degeneration of arterioles
hydr- combining form denoting relation to water or hydrogen
hydralazine antihypertensive; vasodilator; works primarily by its action on the smooth muscle of smaller arteries and arterioles; **usage**: intermediate and severe arterial hypertension, cardiac insufficiency,

impaired renal function, retinopathy as well as hypertensive emergencies; in pregnancy, for hypertension of pregnancy, eclampsia, and pre-eclampsia; the combination of **hydralazine and isosorbide mononitrate** is used for the treatment of cardiac insufficiency in African Americans or those who cannot tolerate ACE inhibitors/ARB

hydremia increase in the volume of blood/blood plasma due to increased water intake or reduced water excretion, e.g., in renal insufficiency

hydro- combining form denoting relation to water or hydrogen

hydrocardia → *hydropericardium*

hydrochlorothiazide oral diuretic [saluretic] with a half-life of 6–14 hours

hydrodiuresis → *water diuresis*

hydropericarditic relating to or marked by hydropericarditis

hydropericarditis formation of an effusion [hydropericardium] accompanying pericardial inflammation [pericarditis]

hydropericardium *Syn: cardiac dropsy, hydrocardia*; collection of water in the pericardial sac, e.g., in cardiac insufficiency, renal insufficiency

hydroperitoneum → *ascites*

hydroperitonia → *ascites*

hydropneumatosis combined emphysema and edema

hydropneumopericardium *Syn: pneumohydropericardium*; air and fluid collections in the pericardial sac

hydrops *Syn: dropsy*; collection of fluid in a body cavity or in the interstitial space; collection of fluid in the tissues is called edema

hydrothorax → *pleural effusion*

3-hydroxytyramine → *dopamine*

hyoscyamine → *d/l-hyoscyamine*

hyper- combining form denoting relation to above, beyond, more than normal, or excessive

hyperacute *Syn: fulminant, fulminating, peracute, superacute*; (course, reaction) extreme, acute

hyperbetalipoproteinemia elevated β-lipoprotein content of the blood familial hyperbetalipoproteinemia → *LDL-receptor disorder*

hyperbicarbonatemia → *bicarbonatemia*

hypercalcemia *Syn: calcemia, hypercalcinemia*; increased calcium content of the blood [> 2.6 mmol/l]; the main causes are increased intestinal absorption, decreased renal excretion, and increased mobilization from bone in, e.g., primary hyperparathyroidism or tumors [**malignant hypercalcemia, tumor hypercalcemia**]; occasionally hypercalcemia occurs due to increased vitamin D intake

hypercalcemic relating to or marked by hypercalcemia
hypercalcinemia → *hypercalcemia*
hypercardia → *cardiac hypertrophy*
hypercholesteremia → *hypercholesterolemia*
hypercholesterinemia → *hypercholesterolemia*
hypercholesterolemia *Syn: cholesteremia, cholesterinemia, cholesterolemia, hypercholesteremia, hypercholesterinemia*; increased cholesterol content of the blood; in addition to familial hypercholesterolemia, **secondary hypercholesterolemia** in diabetes mellitus, hypothyroidism, alcoholism, liver diseases, etc., play a role; however, the most common is the so-called **polygenic hypercholesterolemia**, which is probably caused by a minor aberration in several enzymes, transfer factors, and binding proteins involved in cholesterol metabolism; however, hypercholesterolemia only develops following an increased intake of saturated fatty acids and cholesterol in the diet; the long-term damage that develops [arteriosclerosis, coronary heart disease, arterial occlusive disease] make this dietary hypercholesterolemia one of the most important clinical entities requiring treatment with dietary modification and/or medication [lipid-lowering drugs], particularly in patients in middle age or older
    familial hypercholesterolemia → *LDL-receptor disorder*
    polygenic hypercholesterolemia *s.u. hypercholesterolemia*
    secondary hypercholesterolemia *s.u. hypercholesterolemia*
hypercholesterolemic relating to or marked by hypercholesterolemia
hyperchylomicronemia *Syn: Bürger-Grütz disease, Bürger-Grütz syndrome, chylomicronemia, familial apolipoprotein C-II deficiency, familial hyperchylomicronemia, familial fat-induced hyperlipemia, familial hypertriglyceridemia, familial lipoprotein lipase deficiency, familial LPL deficiency, idiopathic hyperlipemia, type I familial hyperlipoproteinemia*; increased chylomicrons in the blood
    familial hyperchylomicronemia → *hyperchylomicronemia*
hyperchylomicronemic relating to or marked by hyperchylomicronemia
hypercoagulability increased tendency for the blood to clot
hypercythemia → *erythrocythemia*
hypercytosis increased numbers of cells in the blood; also equated with polycythemia and leukocytosis
hyperelectrolytemia elevated concentrations of electrolytes in the blood
hyperemia *Syn: congestion*; increased blood volume in an organ or body segment

active hyperemia → *active congestion*
arterial hyperemia → *active congestion*
compensatory hyperemia hyperemia due to compensatory increase in perfusion
reactive hyperemia hyperemia due to local reaction and dilatation of the vessels
venous hyperemia → *venous congestion*

hyperemic relating to or marked by hyperemia
hypererythrocythemia → *erythrocythemia*
hyperfibrinogenemia → *fibrinogenemia*
hyperfibrinolysis increased fibrinolysis due to release of plasminogen
hypergammaglobulinemia elevated gammaglobulin content of the blood
hyperglobulia *Syn:* hyperglobulism; increased numbers of red blood corpuscles in the peripheral blood
hyperglobulinemic relating to or marked by hyperglobulinemia
hyperglobulism → *hyperglobulia*
hyperglyceridemia elevated triglyceride content of the blood
hyperhydration *Syn:* overhydration; excessive water content of the body
hypertonic hyperhydration hyperhydration predominantly due to salt excess; mostly a result of excessive salt intake [e.g., drinking of sea water]
hypotonic hyperhydration hyperhydration predominantly due to excessive water; mostly caused by excessive water intake [infusions!] or increased water retention in ADH excess

hyperkalemia increased potassium content of the blood [> 6.5 mmol/l]; the most common causes are renal failure, adrenal insufficiency, massive potassium administration, heavy hemolysis, or muscle trauma; in acidosis, potassium is displaced from the cells into the extracellular space [**extracellular hyperkalemia**], in alkalosis, it is displaced into the cells, which therefore leads to **intracellular hyperkalemia**
hyperkalemic relating to or marked by hyperkalemia
hyperlipemia → *lipemia*
carbohydrate-induced hyperlipemia → *type IV familial hyperlipoproteinemia*
combined fat-induced and carbohydrate-induced hyperlipemia → *type V familial hyperlipoproteinemia*
familial fat-induced hyperlipemia → *hyperchylomicronemia*
idiopathic hyperlipemia → *hyperchylomicronemia*
mixed hyperlipemia 1. → *type IIb familial hyperlipoproteinemia*

2. →*type V familial hyperlipoproteinemia*

hyperlipemic relating to or marked by hyperlipemia

hyperlipidemia *Syn: hyperlipoidemia, lipidemia*; increased total lipid content in the blood, elevation of the serum lipids

familial combined hyperlipidemia 1. →*type II familial hyperlipoproteinemia* **2.** →*type IIb familial hyperlipoproteinemia* **3.** →*type IV familial hyperlipoproteinemia*

mixed hyperlipidemia →*type IIb familial hyperlipoproteinemia*

multiple lipoprotein-type hyperlipidemia 1. →*type II familial hyperlipoproteinemia* **2.** →*type IV familial hyperlipoproteinemia*

hyperlipoidemia →*hyperlipidemia*

hyperlipoproteinemia increased lipoprotein content of the blood; both primary and secondary forms potentially carry increased cardiovascular risk; in order to determine the individual risk, however, other risk factors must also be taken into account, including smoking, lack of exercise, stress, diabetes mellitus, hypertension, etc.; since the cardiovascular risk increases exponentially with the LDL-cholesterol level, all hyperlipoproteinemias with elevated LDL [types IIa, IIb, III; IV] have a high risk, whereas the forms in which VLDL and chylomicrons are elevated [types I, V] have no arteriosclerosis risk; the goal of **therapy** for the hyperlipoproteinemias is to keep the LDL-cholesterol values in the region of < 160 mg/dl [< 4 mmol/l]; if there are other risk factors too, then this value has to be adjusted downwards; in high-risk patients [e.g., diabetics with hypertension], the levels should be less than 100 mg/dl

acquired hyperlipoproteinemia *Syn: nonfamilial hyperlipoproteinemia*; hyperlipoproteinemia caused by nutrition or other diseases [diabetes mellitus]

familial hyperlipoproteinemia autosomally inherited disease, which is divided into 5 types according to Frederickson

familial combined hyperlipoproteinemia 1. →*type II familial hyperlipoproteinemia* **2.** →*type IIb familial hyperlipoproteinemia*

mixed hyperlipoproteinemia 1. →*type IIb familial hyperlipoproteinemia* **2.** →*type V familial hyperlipoproteinemia*

nonfamilial hyperlipoproteinemia →*acquired hyperlipoproteinemia*

type I familial hyperlipoproteinemia →*hyperchylomicronemia*

type IIa familial hyperlipoproteinemia →*LDL-receptor disorder*

type IIb familial hyperlipoproteinemia *Syn: familial combined hyperlipidemia, familial combined hyperlipoproteinemia, mixed hyper-*

lipemia, mixed hyperlipidemia, mixed hyperlipoproteinemia; hyperlipoproteinemia with elevated cholesterol, LDL and VLDL; leads to premature development of severe arteriosclerosis

type II familial hyperlipoproteinemia *Syn: familial combined hyperlipidemia, familial combined hyperlipoproteinemia, multiple lipoprotein-type hyperlipidemia*; form characterized by elevation of the cholesterol and β-lipoprotein

type III familial hyperlipoproteinemia *Syn: broad-beta disease, broad-beta proteinemia, familial dysbetalipoproteinemia, floating-beta disease, floating-beta proteinemia*; hyperlipoproteinemia with elevated triglycerides and VLDL and a typical widened β-lipoprotein band; the risk of arteriosclerosis is high

type IV familial hyperlipoproteinemia *Syn: carbohydrate-induced hyperlipemia, familial combined hyperlipidemia, familial hypertriglyceridemia, multiple lipoprotein-type hyperlipidemia*; hyperlipoproteinemia marked by elevated triglycerides, VLDL and prebetalipoproteinemia with a high risk of arteriosclerosis

type V familial hyperlipoproteinemia *Syn: apolipoprotein C-II deficiency, combined fat-induced and carbohydrate-induced hyperlipemia, familial hyperchylomicronemia and hyperprebetalipoproteinemia, familial lipoprotein lipase deficiency, mixed hyperlipemia, familial LPL deficiency, mixed hyperlipoproteinemia*; hyperlipoproteinemia due to endogenous factors, as well as by intake of carbohydrates and fat, which carries a low risk of arteriosclerosis

hypermagnesemia increased magnesium content of the blood [> 1.1 mmol/l], e.g., in renal insufficiency or uremia

hypernatremia *Syn: hypernatronemia, natremia, natriemia*; increased sodium content of the blood [< 145 mmol/l]; the most common causes are hyperaldosteronism, Cushing's syndrome, disturbances of water balance [hypertonic hyperhydration]

hypernatremic relating to or marked by hypernatremia

hypernatronemia → *hypernatremia*

hyperoxemia *Syn: hyperoxia*; increased oxygen content of the blood, e.g., in hyperbaric oxygenation

hyperoxia *Syn: hyperoxemia*; increased oxygen tension in the blood [hyperoxemia] or tissue [hyperoxidosis] during oxygen therapy

hyperoxic relating to or marked by hyperoxia

hyperpiesia → *essential hypertension*

hyperpiesis → *essential hypertension*

hyperplasia *Syn: quantitative hypertrophy, numerical hypertrophy*; enlargement of a tissue or organ by multiplication of its cells, i.e., there is an increased cell count

angiolymphoid hyperplasia with eosinophilia rare, chronic-persistent capillary proliferation with epitheloid endothelial cells invading the lumen; forms multiple, skin-colored to reddish nodules in the scalp and in the region of the ear and neck; predominantly affects middle-aged women; a condition that occurs in Japan with similar symptoms is called the **Kimura syndrome**, which is a pseudolymphoma or lymphoma of low malignant potential; **therapy**: excision

hypertension 1. *Syn: hypertonicity, hypertonia*; increased tension, increased tone **2.** →*arterial hypertension*

arterial hypertension *Syn: high-blood pressure, hypertonus, hypertension, vascular hypertension*; in the past hypertension was defined as persistent elevation of the blood pressure in the arterial system to values of > 140 mmHg systolic pressure before age 65 or > 160 mmHg after age 65 and > 90 mmHg diastolic pressure; based on multinational studies **manifest hypertension** is now defined as a blood pressure of greater than 140/90; the vast majority of patients [95%] has **essential** or **idiopathic hypertension**; however, this diagnosis can only be made after secondary hypertension has been ruled out; the most common causes for **secondary hypertension** are renal and renovascular hypertension, pheochromocytoma, diabetes mellitus, oral contraceptives, and non-steroidal antiphlogistics; arterial hypertension is directly or indirectly responsible for a variety of organ and vascular damages, such as coronary heart disease, left ventricular hypertrophy, heart failure, aortic stenosis, benign and malignant nephrosclerosis, atherosclerosis, aneurysm, ocular damage, and intracerebral hemorrhage; such damage is further increased by additional risk factors [diabetes mellitus, nicotine and alcohol abuse, hyperlipidemia]; the main goals of therapy are reduction of the blood pressure, elimination or at least reduction of risk factors, improvement of existing damage as well as avoidance of further damage; it is apparent that these goals can only be achieved by a combination of medical and non-medical measures, and that the patients need to be fully informed and have to comply with the therapy strategy; non-medical measures include a permanent life-style change encompassing restrictions on the intake of salt and fat, weight loss, no smoking and only moderate drinking, stress avoidance and regular physical activity; the drug therapy depends upon the severity of the hypertension, concomitant disorders, existing organ damage, risk factors, age, quality of life considerations, cost of treatment as well as side effects of the different drugs; whenever possible an individualized sequential monotherapy should be attempted to find the right antihypertensive; still, some 25% of patients need a combination therapy; substances suitable for long-term medication are beta-blockers, diuretics, calcium antagonists, ACE inhibitors, alpha$_1$-blockers, vasodilators, and central antihypertensives [clonidine, indoramin, α-methyldopa, urapidil]

borderline hypertension *Syn: labile hypertension*; clinical description of an only moderately increased blood pressure, i.e., the diastolic pressure lies between 90 and 94 mmHg at rest

cardiac-output hypertension hypertension due to increased cardiac minute volume, e.g., in hyperthyroidism

continued arterial hypertension → *Huchard's disease*

endocrine hypertension hypertension due to various diseases of the endocrine system [Cushing's syndrome, hyperthyroidism]

essential hypertension *Syn: hyperpiesia, hyperpiesis, idiopathic hypertension, primary hypertension*; hypertension without obvious cause; diagnosis of exclusion, which can only be made after excluding all secondary causes of hypertension; there is a familial predisposition, which is augmented by risk factors [mainly adiposity, alcohol and nicotine consumption, stress, lack of exercise]; makes up approx. 95% of all cases

Goldblatt hypertension high blood pressure due to restriction of the renal perfusion resulting from intrinsic or extrinsic reduction in the diameter of the renal arteries

Goldblatt's hypertension → *Goldblatt's mechanism*

idiopathic hypertension → *essential hypertension*

labile hypertension → *borderline hypertension*

latent pulmonary hypertension *s.u. pulmonary hypertension*

malignant hypertension *Syn: pale hypertension*; hypertension with persistent diastolic values of > 120 mmHg; untreated leads to death within 2 years; particularly frequent in renal hypertension and pheochromocytoma; **therapy**: ACE inhibitors, calcium antagonists

manifest pulmonary hypertension *s.u. pulmonary hypertension*

neurogenic hypertension high blood pressure and tachycardia due to loss of neural regulatory mechanisms, e.g., in polyneuritis, injury to pressure receptors, skull base fracture

pale hypertension → *malignant hypertension*

portal hypertension elevation of the portal venous pressure to values 10 mmHg higher than those in the right atrium; caused by increased outflow resistance due to post-hepatic [hepatic vein thrombosis], intra-hepatic [liver cirrhosis], or pre-hepatic [portal vein thrombosis] obstruction; leads to esophageal varices, intestinal bleeding, ascites, or encephalopathy; **diagnosis**: endoscopy, sonography, angiography, Duplex sonography; the goal of **therapy** is long-term reduction of the pressure and the formation of a shunt circulation by placement of a portacaval shunt or **transjugular intrahepatic portosystemic shunt** [TIPS]

primary hypertension → *essential hypertension*

pulmonary hypertension *Syn: pulmonary artery hypertension*; chronic elevation of mean pulmonary pressure above 20 mmHg at rest and above 30 mmHg during exercise [**manifest pulmonary hypertension**]; the condition in which the resting value is below 20 mmHg, but increases with exercise to > 30 mmHg is called **latent pulmonary hypertension**; in **severe pulmonary hypertension**, the pressure is often > 55 mmHg and cardiac output is reduced; for **causes**, **clinical picture**, and **therapy** *s.u. chronic cor pulmonale*

pulmonary artery hypertension → *pulmonary hypertension*

renal hypertension hypertension secondary to kidney disease; may also be due to disorders of the renal artery [**renovascular hypertension**] or the parenchyma [**renoparenchymal hypertension**]

resistance hypertension arterial hypertension caused by increased peripheral resistance

secondary hypertension *Syn: symptomatic hypertension*; hypertension as a consequence of other diseases; approx. 5% of all forms of arterial hypertension; the most common causes are renovascular and renoparenchymal hypertension, pheochromocytoma, diabetes mellitus, hormonal contraceptives, and non-steroidal anti-inflammatories

severe pulmonary hypertension *s.u. pulmonary hypertension*

symptomatic hypertension → *secondary hypertension*

systolic hypertension permanent systolic pressure of more than 140 mmHg with normal diastolic pressure

vascular hypertension → *arterial hypertension*

hypertensive relating to or marked by high blood pressure/hypertension

hyperthrombinemia increased thrombin content of the blood

hypertonia increased tension, increased tone

hypertonic 1. with increased tension/increased tone **2.** *Syn: hyperisotonic*; with increased osmotic pressure

hypertonus → *arterial hypertension*

hypertriglyceridemia increased triglyceride content of the blood; **secondary hypertriglyceridemia** relates like polygenic hypolipoproteinemia to a combination of disposition plus overnutrition and malnutrition; it is significantly more common than primary hypertriglyceridemia

essential hypertriglyceridemia congenital hypertriglyceridemia; generic term for exogenous and familial hypertriglyceridemia

familial hypertriglyceridemia hyperlipoproteinemia characterized by increased triglycerides, VLDL and prebetalipoproteins with a high risk of arteriosclerosis

secondary hypertriglyceridemia *s.u. hypertriglyceridemia*

hypertrophia → *hypertrophy*

hypertrophy *Syn: hypertrophia*; enlargement of an organ or tissue due to an increase in the volume of its cells

biventricular hypertrophy hypertrophy of both ventricles of the heart

cardiac hypertrophy *Syn: heart hypertrophy, hypercardia*; increased thickness of the heart muscle due to pressure overload of the ventricle in stenosis of the outflow tract or in chronic valve insufficiency; leads to **left heart hypertrophy** in aortic or aortic valve stenosis and aortic or mitral valve insufficiency, or to **right heart hypertrophy** in pulmonary stenosis and pulmonary or tricuspid insufficiency

heart hypertrophy → *cardiac hypertrophy*

left heart hypertrophy → *left-ventricular hypertrophy*

left-ventricular hypertrophy *Syn: left heart hypertrophy*; exertional hypertrophy of the left ventricle, e.g., in aortic stenosis or aortic valve stenosis

numerical hypertrophy → *hyperplasia*

quantitative hypertrophy → *hyperplasia*

right-ventricular hypertrophy *Syn: right heart hypertrophy*; exertional hypertrophy of the right ventricle, e.g., in pulmonary valve stenosis or tricuspid valve insufficiency

right heart hypertrophy → *right-ventricular hypertrophy*

ventricular hypertrophy hypertrophy of a cardiac ventricle

hypervolemia *Syn: plethora*; increased plasma volume, increased circulating blood volume in hyperhydration

hypervolemic relating to or marked by hypervolemia

hypisotonic → *hypotonic*

hypoadrenalism → *adrenocortical insufficiency*

hypoadrenocorticism → *adrenocortical insufficiency*

hypoaldosteronism *Syn: aldosteronopenia*; diminished aldosterone production is found in primary or secondary adrenal insufficiency, adrenogenital syndrome with salt loss, disturbances of aldosterone synthesis, reduced renin or angiotensin-II levels or in therapy with β-blockers, ACE inhibitors, and non-steroidal anti-inflammatories; as a result of the aldosterone deficiency, hyperkalemia with bradycardic disturbances of heart rhythm develop; **therapy**: potassium restriction, kaliuretic diuretics [furosemide, thiazide]

hypocalcemia reduced calcium content in the blood [< 2.0 mmol/l]; the most important causes are reduced intake and/or reabsorption, vitamin D deficiency, hypoparathyroidism, renal insufficiency, and renal tubular acidosis; **clinical**: increased neuromuscular hyperexcitability [Chvostek's sign, carpopedal spasm, tetany], shortening of the ST interval in the ECG, trophic changes in the skin, tooth damage, cataracts; **therapy**: oral or parenteral calcium replacement; on occasion cholecalciferol

hypocalcemic relating to or marked by hypocalcemia

hypocapnia *Syn: hypocarbia*; reduced carbon dioxide tension in the blood, e.g., in hyperventilation, respiratory alkalosis

hypocapnic relating to or marked by hypocapnia

hypocarbia → *hypocapnia*

hypocholesteremia → *hypocholesterolemia*

hypocholesteremic → *hypocholesterolemic*

hypocholesterinemia → *hypocholesterolemia*

hypocholesterolemia *Syn: hypocholesteremia, hypocholesterinemia*; reduced content of cholesterol in the blood, e.g., in damage to the liver parenchyma or hyperthyroidism

hypocholesterolemic *Syn: hypocholesteremic*; relating to or marked by hypocholesterolemia

hypochromemia → *hypochromic anemia*

hypocoagulability reduced clotting potential of the blood; can be due to an increase in substances that inhibit clotting or a reduction in factors that promote clotting [e.g., hemophilia]; treated with anticoagulants to prevent thromboses and emboli

hypocoagulable with lower clotting potential

hypocorticalism → *adrenocortical insufficiency*

hypocorticism → *adrenocortical insufficiency*

hypocythemia reduction in the cell count of the blood or more particularly the erythrocyte count

hypocytosis reduction in the number of blood cells; also equated with hypocythemia or leukocytopenia

hypoelectrolytemia reduced electrolyte content of the blood

hypoemia → *ischemia*

hypofibrinogenemia *Syn: factor I deficiency, fibrinogen deficiency, fibrinogenopenia, fibrinopenia*; reduced fibrinogen content in the blood; may be [rarely] an autosomal recessive **congenital hypofibrinogenemia** or acquired as **acquired hypofibrinogenemia** if utilization is increased [consumptive coagulopathy] or production reduced [liver parenchymal damage]

hypogammaglobinemia → *hypogammaglobulinemia*

hypogammaglobulinemia *Syn: hypogammaglobinemia, panhypogammaglobulinemia*; reduced gammaglobulin content of the blood may be congenital or acquired; infants go through a period of physiologic hypogammaglobulinemia between the 2. and 6. months

hypoglobulia reduced erythrocyte count in the peripheral blood

hypohydration insufficient hydration of the body

   hypotonic hypohydration → *hypotonic dehydration*

hypoisotonic → *hypotonic*

hypokalemia reduced potassium content in the blood [< 3.5 mmol/l]; the most common **causes** are: reduced intake, increased renal excretion [renal tubular acidosis, aldosteronism] or gastrointestinal losses [vomiting, diarrhea, malabsorption], medications [diuretics, laxative abuse], hyperinsulinemia, alkalosis, sweating; **symptoms**: sleepiness, muscle weakness, paralysis, heart rhythm disturbances [among others, ST depression, U waves in the ECG], hypodynamic ileus, reduced glucose tolerance, reduction in the insulin level; **therapy**: oral or parenteral potassium replacement

hypokalemic *Syn: hypopotassemic*; relating to or marked by hypokalemia

hypokinesia reduced motility of the myocardium following an infarct

hypolipemia reduced lipid content of the blood

hypolipidemic relating to or marked by hypolipidemia

hypolipoproteinemia reduced lipoprotein content of the blood

hypolymphemia → *lymphopenia*

hypomagnesemia reduced magnesium content in the blood [< 0.65 mmol/l]; most commonly **caused by** renal [aldosteronism, alcoholism, osmotic diuresis] or intestinal electrolyte losses [diarrhea], extreme sweating, loop diuretics; **clinical**: muscle weakness, agitation, neuromuscular excitability, atrial tachycardia or fibrillation, ventricular and supraventricular rhythm disturbances, ventricular fibrillation, calf cramps; **therapy**: oral or parenteral magnesium replacement

hyponatremia reduced sodium content in the blood [< 135 mmol/l]; the **cause** is either an excess of body water [hyperhydration] or a lack of sodium [**absolute hyponatremia**]; **clinical**: reduction in blood pressure [predominantly orthostatic], reduction of the cardiac minute volume and renal perfusion, dryness of the skin and mucous membranes, reduced skin turgor, weakness, lethargy and, on occasion, confusion; **therapy**: in mild cases increased dietary salt intake, otherwise infusion therapy with hypertonic NaCl solutions [3%] in sodium deficiency or isotonic NaCl solutions [0.9%] in hypovolemic hypohydration

depletional hyponatremia hyponatremia caused by increased excretion of sodium

dilutional hyponatremia hyponatremia caused by an increase in the plasma or blood fluid

hypo-osmolar with reduced osmolality

hypoperfused underperfused

hypoperfusion *Syn: decreased blood flow*; less perfusion

peripheral hypoperfusion restriction of perfusion of the periphery of the body in various shock states

hypophosphatemia *Syn: hypophosphoremia*; reduced phosphate content of the blood [< 0.8 mmol/l]; **clinical**: weakness [asthenia], muscle weakness or myopathy, cardiac muscle weakness, impaired function of erythrocytes, leukocytes, and thrombocytes, neurologic problems; **therapy**: removal of the cause; oral or intravenous phosphate replacement

hypophosphoremia → *hypophosphatemia*

hypoplasia incomplete development, underdevelopment

thymic hypoplasia → *DiGeorge syndrome*

hypopotassemic → *hypokalemic*

hypoproaccelerinemia → *factor V deficiency*

hypoproconvertinemia → *factor VII deficiency*

hypoproteinemia reduced protein content in the blood [< 60 g/l]; in **relative hypoproteinemia** the cause is an increase in the extracellular water [hyperhydration], while in **absolute hypoproteinemia**, there is protein deficiency

hypoprothrombinemia → *factor II deficiency*

hyposalemia reduced salt content of the blood

hypostasis *Syn: hypostatic congestion*; passive blood filling in the lower regions of the body when it sinks due to cardiovascular insufficiency

hypostatic relating to or caused by hypostasis

hyposystole incomplete or diminished systole

hypotension → *low blood pressure*

  acute hypotension a sudden fall in the systolic blood pressure to values below 90 mmHg

  asympathicotonic hypotension *Syn: autonomic-neurogenic hypotension*; *s.u. low blood pressure*

  autonomic-neurogenic hypotension *Syn: asympathicotonic hypotension*; *s.u. low blood pressure*

  chronic arterial hypotension → *low blood pressure*

  chronic idiopathic hypotension → *idiopathic orthostatic hypotension*

  chronic orthostatic hypotension → *idiopathic orthostatic hypotension*

  essential hypotension *Syn: primary hypotension*; hypotension without demonstrable cause

  idiopathic orthostatic hypotension *Syn: chronic idiopathic hypotension, chronic orthostatic hypotension, Shy-Drager syndrome*; multi-system disease of uncertain etiology with loss of neurones in the substantia nigra, spinal cord, and nucleus dorsalis of the vagus nerve; usually starts between 35 and 70 years of age and affects men more frequently than women; dangerous hypotension can develop during standing on reaching 45° and there is no compensatory increase in heart rate or stroke volume; later, disturbances of sweating, potency, bowel, and bladder function also develop; in the late stages, there is an akinetic Parkinsonian state; the average survival is 7–8 years

  non-autonomic-neurogenic hypotension *Syn: sympathicotonic hypotension*; *s.u. low blood pressure*

  non-orthostatic hypotension *Syn: non-postural hypotension*; *s.u. low blood pressure*

  non-postural hypotension *Syn: non-orthostatic hypotension*; *s.u. low blood pressure*

  orthostatic hypotension *Syn: postural hypotension*; fall in blood pressure on standing up or after prolonged standing

  postural hypotension → *orthostatic hypotension*

  primary hypotension → *essential hypotension*

  secondary hypotension *Syn: symptomatic hypotension*; hypotension caused by a different disease [myocardial infarct, cardiac insufficiency]

sympathicotonic hypotension *Syn: non-autonomic-neurogenic hypotension*; *s.u. low blood pressure*

symptomatic hypotension → *secondary hypotension*

hypotensive relating to or marked by or causing hypotension

hypothrombinemia reduced thrombin content of the blood

hypotonia reduction of pressure, reduction of tone, reduction of tension

hypotonic *Syn: hypisotonic, hypoisotonic*; with or due to low tone or pressure; with lower osmotic pressure

hypotriglyceridemia reduced triglyceride in the blood

hypovolemia *Syn: oligemia, oligohemia*; reduction in the circulating blood volume, after heavy bleeding or fluid losses; if the cell:plasma ratio is unchanged, this is referred to as **simple hypovolemia**, if the cell count is elevated, as **polycythemic hypovolemia** and, if reduced, as **oligocythemic hypovolemia**

hypovolemic *Syn: oligemic*; relating to or marked by hypovolemia

hypoxemia *Syn: arterial hypoxia*; reduced oxygen content in arterial blood

hypoxemic relating to, affected with, or characterized by hypoxemia

hypoxia *Syn: hypoxemia, oxygen deficiency*; local or generalized oxygen deficiency; it occurs most often as **ischemic** or **anemic hypoxia**; **respiratory hypoxia** caused by alveolar hypoventilation and **hypoxic hypoxia** caused by a reduction in the oxygen partial pressure during exposure to high altitudes are also frequent; hypoxia begins as **arterial hypoxia** and can lead to a decline in venous oxygen partial pressure and development of **venous hypoxia**; both **acute hypoxia** and **chronic hypoxia** can lead to reversible or irreversible tissue damage

anemic hypoxia → *anemic anoxia*

arterial hypoxia *Syn: hypoxemia*; reduced oxygen content in arterial blood

circulatory hypoxia → *ischemic hypoxia*

ischemic hypoxia *Syn: stagnant hypoxia, circulatory hypoxia*; hypoxia caused by an insufficient blood supply

stagnant hypoxia → *ischemic hypoxia*

hypoxic relating to, affected with, or characterized or caused by hypoxia

hysteresis prolongation of the QT interval in the ECG due to a sudden change in the heart rhythm

ictus 1. sudden attack, bout, syncope, symptoms developing suddenly **2.** blow, jolt
  ictus cordis heartbeat; apex beat
idiopathetic → *idiopathic*
idiopathic *Syn: agnogenic, autopathic, essential, idiopathic, protopathic, primary*; (arising) without recognizable cause, independent of other diseases, independent
idioventricular relating to or affecting one ventricle only
illness → *disease*
iloprost oral prostaglandin; inhibitor of thrombocyte aggregation; **usage**: thromboangiitis obliterans with severe disturbances of perfusion, arterial occlusive disease, Raynaud's phenomenon
imipenem *Syn: N-formimidoyl thienamycin*; carbapenem antibiotic with a broad action spectrum; **indications**: severe infections of the respiratory tract, kidneys, urinary tract, bones, joints, genital organs, skin, and soft tissues, sepsis
immedicable → *incurable*
immunocoagulopathy coagulopathy caused by antibodies against coagulation factors [immune inhibitors]
immunodiagnosis → *serodiagnosis*
immunogenic → *antigenic*
immunohemolysis *Syn: conditioned hemolysis, immune hemolysis*; disintegration of red blood corpuscles due to complement-mediated immune reactions
impermeable *Syn: impervious*; impenetrable
impervious → *impermeable*
impulse a progressive wave of excitation over a nerve or muscle fiber
  apex impulse → *apex beat*
  apical impulse → *apex beat*
inapparent *Syn: latent*; symptomless, with few symptoms, not clinically apparent, not visible, imperceptible

incisure notch, incision, sulcus, cleft
  incisure of apex of heart incision into the apex of the heart at the meeting point of the anterior and posterior interventricular septum
incompatibility *Syn: incompatibleness*; the state or quality of being incompatible
  blood group incompatibility incompatibility of blood groups; mixing of incompatible blood leads to agglutination or destruction of the erythrocytes by specific antibodies
  Rh incompatibility blood group incompatibility in the rhesus system; mainly the rhesus incompatibility between a Rh-negative mother and a Rh-positive fetus; if Rh-positive erythrocytes from the fetus enter the maternal circulation, formation of Anti-D-antibodies will follow; as incomplete IgG-antibodies, these can cross the placental barrier and cause hemolytic disease of the newborn
incompetence → *insufficiency*
  incompetence of the cardiac valves → *valvular regurgitation*
  mitral incompetence → *mitral insufficiency*
  tricuspid incompetence → *tricuspid regurgitation*
  valvular incompetence → *valvular regurgitation*
incompetency → *insufficiency*
incurable *Syn: immedicable*; (*illness*) not curable
indapamide saluretic, antihypertensive
index a numerical scale used to compare variables with one another or with some reference number
  cardiac index cardiac minute volume per square meter of body surface area; normal value 3–4 l/min/m^2; in manifest left heart insufficiency, less than 2.2 l/min/m^2
  color index → *blood quotient*
  left ventricular mass index left ventricular mass as measured by echocardiography or cardiac MRI indexed to body surface area and expressed as g/m^2; complex index often calculated by means of a formula described by Devereux; increased LVMI indicates hypertrophy of the left ventricle usually as a consequence of hypertension and has been shown to be associated with higher mortality
  shock index quotient of pulse rate and systolic blood pressure; has proved useful as a crude tool in emergency medicine
  Sokolow-Lyon index ECG criteria for left and right ventricular hypertrophy
indicated (*therapy*) appropriate

indolent *Syn: painless*; indifferent, inert; insensitive to (pain); painless
indoramin peripheral α-sympatholytic, antihypertensive
indurated *Syn: indurate*; hardened
induration hardening and consolidation of a tissue
   brown induration →*cyanotic induration*
   congestive induration →*congestive fibrosis*
   cyanotic induration *Syn: red/brown induration*; reddish-brown discoloration [hemosiderin] and hardening of lung tissue, generally caused by a mitral valve defect or left ventricular failure
   red induration →*cyanotic induration*
indurative relating to induration, affected by induration, characterized by induration
infarct *Syn: infarction*; death of a tissue [necrosis] due to acute interruption of its blood supply; the most common causes are thrombosis, embolism, arteriosclerosis, and internal bleeding; vessel constriction or spasm are rare causes
   anemic infarct *Syn: ischemic infarct, pale infarct, white infarct*; infarct with pale, dry, infarcted area
   bland infarct non-infected infarct
   hemorrhagic infarct *Syn: red infarct*; brown-red infarct due to hemorrhage into the tissue
   ischemic infarct →*anemic infarct*
   pale infarct →*anemic infarct*
   red infarct →*hemorrhagic infarct*
   septic infarct infarct caused by an infected embolus; also a description of secondary infection of a simple infarct
   thrombotic infarct anemic infarct due to a thrombus
   white infarct →*anemic infarct*
infarction →*infarct*
   anterior myocardial infarction myocardial infarction affecting the anterior wall of the heart
   anteroinferior myocardial infarction myocardial infarction affecting the anterior wall of the heart and the cardiac apex
   anterolateral myocardial infarction myocardial infarct of the front and side wall
   cardiac infarction →*myocardial infarction*
   lateral myocardial infarction myocardial infarction at the border between the anterior and posterior walls of the heart
   myocardial infarction *Syn: cardiac infarction*; necrosis of a circum-

scribed region of the heart muscle caused by an acute shortage of oxygen; **myocardial necrosis** develops if coronary ischemia persists for longer than 20 minutes; the time required for ischemia to develop depends upon the available collaterals, which can preserve perfusion, whether the occlusion is persistent or intermittent and upon the vulnerability of the myocytes; **epidemiology**: diseases of the cardiovascular system are the most common cause of death in the industrialized nations; myocardial infarcts lie in second position; the incidence of infarction increases with increasing age, however, in recent years more and more infarcts are occurring in younger people [< 40 years old]; in the population under 65 years of age, men are mainly affected, with women in this age band suffering an infarct more rarely; the reason for this is the formation of female sex hormones, which continues until the menopause and which are thought to exert an anti-arteriosclerotic effect; the concentration of the sex hormones falls after the menopause and the arteriosclerotic processes proceed; in the age range > 65 years old, women are at least as frequently affected by myocardial infarcts as men; the important **risk factors** include advanced age, male gender, arterial hypertension, hyperlipoproteinemia, nicotine usage, diabetes mellitus, lack of exercise, and familial predisposition; the most common **cause** of a transmural infarct is the formation of an occluding intravascular thrombus; in about 10–20% of cases, there is no coronary thrombosis; additional causes include vasospasm, vasculitis, coronary embolism, aortic dissection or dissection of the coronary arteries, coronary anomalies [e.g., aneurysms], intracoronary thrombosis [e.g., polycythemia rubra vera, thrombocytosis], conditions with increased oxygen demand in the myocardium [e.g., aortic malformations, thyrotoxicosis]; depending upon the amount of necrotic tissue, infarcts are subdivided into: **microscopic** [focal necrosis], **small** [< 10% of the left ventricular mass], **medium** [10–30% of the left ventricular mass], or **large** [> 30% of the left ventricular mass]; biochemical tests can detect even small infarcts [at least 1g of necrotic myocardium] by demonstrating a positive troponin test; with increasing infarct size, the troponin value increases; the CK-MB is first positive following medium-sized infarcts, where there is a correlation between the total amount released and the size of the infarct; the healing process of an infarct lasts at least 5 weeks, in which time a myocardial scar forms; **clinically**, an infarct is defined by the criteria of typical angina pectoris, increase in the cardiac biomarkers, and corresponding ECG changes; one of the following **criteria** is sufficient for the **diagnosis** of infarction: **1. typical time course of the cardiac biomarkers** [troponins or CK-MB] with at least one of: infarct symptoms, development of Q-waves in the ECG [also in the absence of prior development of ST-segment changes], ST-segment changes [elevation or depression], or T-wave inversion **2. pathologic anatomic findings**; in addition, account should be taken of other features such as infarct size, stage [ongoing, healing, healed infarct], and the circumstances in which the infarct arose [spontaneous or after coronary intervention]; clinically, **transmural** [through the entire wall] and **non-transmural myocardial infarction** are differentiated, with the distinction being made based on ECG changes; in transmural infarcts, all the typical ECG changes can be seen, in the non-transmural infarcts these are missing; particularly characteristic is the absence of Q-waves in the later stages, for which reason the term **non-Q-wave infarct** [NQWI] is often used synonymously; **clinical**: angina pectoris which lasts at least 20 minutes is typical; the pain begins in the chest and can be felt both in the retrosternal and left thoracic regions; generally the pain radiates into the left arm, into the jaw, neck, nape, back, or into the epigastrium; the character of the pain varies widely and can be perceived as burning, stabbing, gouging, pressure, or dragging; the pain is intense [**overwhelming pain**]; some patients feel dyspnea in addition to pain; in some patients, this is the only symptom, while about 15–20% of people affected have no symptoms at all [so-called **silent infarct**]; women and diabetic patients are particularly prone to this; **atypical symptoms** can include: dyspnea associated with pulmonary edema, weakness, fatigue, vomiting, nausea, attacks of sweating, dizziness, syncope, arrhythmias, peripheral embolism; the atypical symptoms can develop separately or together with the typical symptoms; the **most common triggers** for an infarct are physical exertion, psychologic stress, and severe illness; infarcts are more common in the early morning; in about 30% of cases, unstable angina pectoris precedes an infarct, in another 30%, the infarct is the first manifestation of coronary heart disease; **the laboratory test parameters and the ECG are indispensable for diagnosis**; echocardiography can provide valuable information regarding the left ventricular function, while coronary angiography is crucial for decisions about further therapy [invasive vs. operative]; **ECG**: 4 stages can be differentiated, which represent the time course of evolution of the infarct, and allow determination of the age of an infarct: **1. stage 0** [acute stage, asphyxia-T]: changes usually only visible in the first minutes, with the T-wave recorded in the infarct leads being much higher than its R-wave; the so-called **asphyxia-T** mirrors transmural ischemia, which advances from the subendocardial to the subepicardial layers **2. stage 1** [acute stage]: the asphyxia-T is regressing, and the ST-segment becomes elevated, often to the point of fusion of the ST-segment and the T-wave; this stage lasts several days; in the leads that lie opposite the infarct area, there is depression of the ST-segment **3. stage 2** [intermediate stage]: possibly while the ST-elevation is still present, the next development is inversion of the T-wave; after some time, the ST-elevation disappears completely and the inverted T-waves persist; gradually Q-waves form; this stage can last several weeks **4. stage 3** [chronic stage]: is characterized by the development of Q-waves; they are pathologic if they last at least 0.04s and their amplitude is at least ¼ that of the R-wave [**Pardee-Q**]; in addition, the R-wave is flatter; the terminal negative T-waves may still be present or they may have returned to normal; this stage is observed after about 2 weeks and is characterized as the chronic stage; ST-segment elevation can persist, and if they have a convex shape, they may indicate a cardiac aneurysm; a further sign of infarction is the development of a left bundle branch block [LBB] in a previously normal ECG; the LBB in such cases indicates a large anterior wall infarct with involvement of the ventricular septum and is a sign of an unfavorable prognosis; the named changes occur in transmural infarcts, but no stages are defined for the non-transmural infarcts; there is no asphyxia-T and no Q-waves in the subsequent course; also, the ST-segment elevations and the loss of R-waves are absent, instead of which ST-segment depression and T-wave inversion are seen [negative T-waves]; the following **laboratory test parameters** change pathologically following an infarct: **creatine kinase** [CK] and its isoenzyme **CK-MB**, **troponin I** and **T**, **myoglobin**, **GOT** [ASAT], **GPT** [ALAT], and **LDH**; because of their specificity, CK-MB and the troponins are important in the diagnosis of infarction; they are released at different rates and therefore permit temporal analysis of the infarct; in addition, the total amount of marker released can allow estimation of the size of the infarct, although the peak value is of lesser importance; the **creatine kinase** rises within 8–24 h of the infarct; it reaches its peak, dependent upon reperfusion measures, within the first 48 h after the infarct and returns to normal values after 72 h; the CK-MB shows a similar time course; its myocardial specificity has also been increased in recent years using enzyme immunoassay, using monoclonal antibodies; the **cardiac troponins** rise within 3–12 h after the start of ischemia; troponin T reaches its peak after 12–48 h and troponin I after 24 h; the values can still be elevated after 14 days; the biochemical laboratory differentiation between cardiac and musculoskeletal isoforms is achieved by means of enzyme immunoassay using antibodies; proof of the smallest myocardial necrosis is achieved by the troponins, since their sensitivity is higher; if a normal CK-MB and an elevated troponin are measured in unstable angina pectoris or in a non-transmural infarct, then the latter is a predictor of increased mortality; **complications** can be subdivided into mechanical complications [heart wall aneurysm, septal defect, pericardial tamponade, papillary muscle rupture, pericarditis] and bradycardic [e.g., SA-block, AV-block] and tachycardic [atrial fibrillation, ventricular extrasystoles, ventricular tachycardia up to ventricular fibrillation] disturbances of heart rhythm; both can favor cardiac insufficiency; in about 5–10% of all infarct patients, a **true aneurysm of the heart wall** can form; the most common locations are the anterior wall and the cardiac apex; in the ECG, one typically finds persistent ST-elevation over several years; false aneurysms, i.e., perforations of the heart wall covered by an organized hematoma and the pericardium, can also form; false aneurysms carry a risk of rupture, whereas true aneurysms rarely rupture, but instead can lead to calcification of the heart wall after a number of years; about 10% of patients, who die in hospital from an acute myocardial infarct, are affected by **rupture** of the free wall of the left ventricle; early thrombolytic therapy appears to reduce the risk of rupture, the simultaneous administration of corticosteroids or non-steroidal anti-inflammatories favors its development; free rupture leads to **pericardial tamponade**, which may be lethal within a few minutes or may run a subacute course with circulatory disturbances as the main symptomatology; a covered perforation by contrast leads to a **pseudoaneurysm**; covered perforations are observed more frequently in patients who receive systemic thrombolysis; a **septal rupture** leads, depending upon its size, to a variably large left-to-right shunt; in addition to these hemodynamic effects, AV-block, bundle branch block, or atrial fibrillation are also often seen, which further reduce the likelihood of survival; smaller infarcts may be enough to cause a **papillary muscle rupture**; generally the posteromedial muscle is affected during an inferobasal infarct, and anterolateral infarcts can lead to rupture of the anterolateral papillary muscle; the rupture can be partial or complete; it results in mild to severe mitral insufficiency, which can have fatal consequences; most **pericardial effusions** cause no or only mild hemodynamic disturbances; their occurrence can be correlated with the infarct size and it is more common in anterior wall infarcts; **pericarditis** is a consequence of a local inflammatory reaction and almost exclusively seen in transmural infarcts; it causes thoracic pain, which radiates to the trapezius muscles [pathognomonic], is made worse by breathing in and improved by standing up or bending over; triphasic rub sounds on auscultation of the heart are the diagnostic clue and echocardiography confirms the diagnosis by showing a fluid collection in the pericardium; **Dressler's syndrome** is a form of pericarditis, which can develop 1–8 weeks after an infarct; it is characterized by malaise, fever, leukocytosis, high ESR, and pericardial effusion; an autoimmune pathologic process is presumed to be the cause; the manifestation of **arrhythmias** depends upon the extent of the infarct, the presence of collaterals and the level of autonomic activity; they are divided into **early** [< 30 min after the start of ischemia] and **late arrhythmias**, with the early ones being responsible for the high mortality of infarcts [30%] before reaching a hospital; there are three pillars of **therapy**: 1. optimal analgesia, calming, sedation, administration of O_2 and β-blockers to reduce the oxygen consumption of the heart 2. acetylsalicylic acid and heparin i.v. to prevent the growth of thrombus, organic nitrates i.v. to improve coronary perfusion 3. reperfusion as soon as possible; a coronary intervention [**coronary angioplasty**, PTCA] should, if possible, be performed as the first measure [**primary PTCA**]; if an emergency intervention is not possible, then lytic therapy should be used; it is widely available and has a success rate of approx. 60% [vessel recanalization], with the number being dependent upon the time of lysis; the earlier lytic drugs are given after the onset of symptoms, the higher the success rate; if more than 12 h have passed since the start of symptoms, the success rate of lysis falls relative to the complication rate; lysis during transport to the hospital has been able to produce a 17% reduction in mortality, if the treatment is performed in the first 90 minutes after the start of symptoms; the recanalization rates for PTCA are over 90%; at the same time, the risk of hemorrhagic complications from this procedure is far less than that of lytic therapy; the patency rate of the coronary arteries is favorably influenced by using **inhibitors of thrombocyte aggregation**; a newly developed class of substances is the **GP-IIb/IIIa antagonists**, which are administered intravenously before the intervention; patients with non-transmural infarcts also benefit from the administration of a GP-IIb/IIIa receptor antagonist; the relative risk for transmural infarcts and the mortality are reduced by up to 20% in these patients, and in combination with PTCA the relative risk is reduced by up to 40%; the use of **stents** in the treatment of acute myocardial infarction has improved both the acute result and also the long-term patency rate of the coronary arteries; the ADP-antagonist **clopidogrel** can produce a significant reduction in the short and long-term prognosis of patients with acute coronary syndrome; after PTCA, all patients with non-Q-wave infarcts should receive combination therapy with acetylsalicylic acid 100 mg and clopidogrel for at least 1–9 months; patients with a transmural infarct should receive the same therapy following stent insertion for 4 weeks; indications for **aortocoronary bypass** [ACB] include severe arteriosclerosis of all three coronary arteries, involvement of the main stem, or a proximal high grade stenosis of the LAD; furthermore, it appears that the patients who benefit most from the operation are those with restricted LV pump function; **prevention**: use of **acetylsalicylic acid** in all patients with confirmed coronary heart disease leads to a reduction in frequency of infarcts or recurrences of approx. 30%; the optimal dosage remains unclear, but generally a daily dose of 75–100 mg is favored; the most important substance group in hyperlipoproteinemia is the **statins**, which in addition to their lipid lowering properties are also thought to have an anti-arteriosclerotic effect; **β-blockers** can be used intravenously in the setting of an infarct; they lower the blood pressure, heart rate, and diastolic wall tension in the left ventricle and thereby reduce the O_2-consumption of the myocardium; they also prevent the development of arrhythmias by their anti-ischemic action; their early application can minimize the infarct size and the mortality by around 13%; **ACE inhibitors** are important for the management of infarct patients because they inhibit ventricular remodeling and thereby prevent progression to LV dilatation after an infarct; this results in better LV function and a more favorable hemodynamic situation; patients with diabetes mellitus benefit particularly from optimization of their blood pressure values; reduction of the blood pressure can be achieved either with β-blockers or with ACE inhibitors or Ca-antagonists; reduction of the blood pressure in hypertensive patients without accompanying diabetes mellitus has similarly beneficial effects

non-Q wave infarction *s.u. myocardial infarction*

posterior myocardial infarction myocardial infarction in the region of the posterior wall of the heart

posterolateral myocardial infarction myocardial infarction of the posterior and side walls

pulmonary infarction infarction usually of peripheral lung sections due to obstruction of branches of pulmonary arteries [pulmonary embolism]; this is typically a **hemorrhagic pulmonary infarction** [with internal bleeding] and rarely **anemic pulmonary infarction**; **clinical picture**: suddenly onset of local or retrosternal pain, tachypnea, dyspnea, restlessness, anxiety, possibly cyanosis, spitting of blood, fever, and weak, rapid pulse

silent myocardial infarction 15–20% of all patients with infarction [particularly women and diabetics] are not aware of any symptoms; the diagnosis is made based on laboratory tests or on ECG grounds

ST-segment elevation infarction *s.u. myocardial infarction*

infected putrefactive, infective; dirty

infectious *Syn: infective, virulent*; contagious; transmissible

infective → *infectious*

infiltration 1. the act or process of infiltrating **2.** something that infiltrates

calcareous infiltration calcium deposition in tissues, e.g., in hypercalcemia, atherosclerosis and arteriosclerosis, calcinosis, necroses, or inflammations

inflammation localized response to irritation with increased blood flow resulting in swelling, redness, heat, and pain

myocardial inflammation → *myocarditis*

vascular inflammation 1. → *angiitis* **2.** → *vasculitis*

infra- combining form denoting relation to inferior to, below, or beneath

infracardiac below the heart

infrapulmonary → *subpulmonary*

infundibulectomy excision of the infundibulum [conus arteriosus] of the heart

infundibulum of heart → *arterial cone*

inherent → *intrinsic*

inhibitor a substance that interferes with the action of another substance

ACE inhibitors *Syn: angiotensin converting enzyme inhibitors*; inhibitors of angiotensin converting enzyme, which, as part of the renin-angiotensin-aldosterone system, converts angiotensin I into angiotensin II; ACE inhibitors [e.g., captopril, enalapril] are used in arterial hypertension and coronary heart disease to lower the blood pressure

aggregation inhibitors *Syn: platelet aggregation inhibitors*; substances that prevent or inhibit clumping of blood platelets [thrombocytes]; predominantly inhibitors of prostaglandin synthesis that are used to prevent thrombosis

angiotensin converting enzyme inhibitors → *ACE inhibitors*

beta-lactamase inhibitors → *β-lactamase inhibitors*

carbonic anhydrase inhibitor diuretic that inhibits the water and sodium ion exchange in the tubule cells of the kidney; this increases the excretion of potassium, sodium, and bicarbonate ions and decreases that of ammonium ions; the loss of bases leads to acidosis, which can influence the excretion of other drugs

direct renin inhibitor new class of antihypertensive agents that decrease plasma renin activity and inhibit conversion of angiotensinogen to angiotensin I within the renin-angiotensin-aldosterone system

ECE inhibitors *Syn: ECE blockers*; *s.u. endothelins*

fibrinolysis inhibitor *Syn: fibrinolytic, antifibrinolytic agent*; a substance that inhibits fibrinolysis

gyrase inhibitors *Syn: quinolones, quinolone antibiotics*; antibiotics that inhibit the enzyme gyrase; they impair bacterial replication and transcription and therefore have a bactericidal effect; because almost all of them are derived from 4-hydroxyquinoline-3-carboxylic acid [quinolone], they are also called **quinolones** or **quinolone antibiotics**; they are more effective against gram-negative causative agents [staphylococci, streptococci, Neisseria, Escherichia coli, Klebsiella, salmonellas, Shigella] than against gram-positive causative agents; **indications**: respiratory and urinary tract infections, nosocomial infections, problematic bacteria

HMG-CoA reductase inhibitors inhibitors of HMG-CoA reductase inhibit cholesterol synthesis and lead to a reduction in the intracellular cholesterol concentration; they are therefore used as lipid reducers; the increased LDL-receptor count resulting from this leads to activation of LDL breakdown and a fall in the plasma cholesterol level

β-lactamase inhibitors *Syn: beta-lactamase inhibitors*; substances that inhibit β-lactamase; prescribed in combination with β-lactam antibiotics

phosphodiesterase inhibitor substance that inhibits the enzymatic degradation of cyclic-AMP to adenosine monophosphate and thereby increases the intracellular concentration of cyclic-AMP; leads, among other effects, to increased lipolysis and glycolysis, vascular dilatation, and reduction in thrombocyte aggregation

platelet aggregation inhibitors → *aggregation inhibitors*

prostaglandin synthesis inhibitor substance that inhibits the formation of prostaglandins; this includes substances with anti-inflammatory and anti-rheumatic action, such as acetylsalicylic acid and the so-called non-steroidal anti-inflammatories

thrombin inhibitors *Syn: antithrombins*; substances that inhibit the formation or action of thrombin

injection 1. the act of injecting **2.** something that is injected

intra-arterial injection injection into an artery

intracardiac injection injection into the heart

inosemia → *fibrinemia*

insensibility → *unconsciousness*

inspiratory relating to inspiration

insufficiency *Syn: incompetence, incompetency*; functional impairment of an organ or part of an organ

acute adrenocortical insufficiency → *addisonian crisis*

acute respiratory insufficiency based on a rapidly progressive loss of respiratory pump function or gas exchange function and within a very short time leads to a life-threatening condition; the most frequent underlying diseases are pneumonia, asthma attack, pulmonary embolism, pneumothorax, and cardiogenic pulmonary edema; an adult respiratory distress syndrome develops clinically

adrenal insufficiency → *adrenocortical insufficiency*

adrenal cortical insufficiency → *adrenocortical insufficiency*

adrenocortical insufficiency *Syn: adrenal cortical insufficiency, adrenal insufficiency, hypoadrenalism, hypoadrenocorticism, hypocorticism, hypocorticalism*; reduced formation of adrenal hormones; in **primary adrenal insufficiency** all three hormone groups are affected [glucocorticoids, mineralocorticoids, androgens], whereas in **secondary adrenal insufficiency** the formation of mineralocorticoids is at least partly preserved

aortic insufficiency *Syn: aortic regurgitation, aortic valve insufficiency*; valvular heart disease with incomplete closure of the aortic valve; the cause can be a primary disease of the valve or a dilation of the aortic root; the valve insufficiency leads to regurgitation of blood into the left ventricle during the diastole, to a volume overload, and to an increase in the afterload; this combined pressure and volume load leads to hypertrophy and dilation of the left ventricle; hypertrophy and increased systolic wall tension lead to an increased myocardial O_2 demand; **clinical picture**: exertional dyspnea, later paroxysmal nocturnal dyspnea and orthopnea occur in **chronic aortic insufficiency**; angina pectoris occurs primarily at night, when the diastolic flow in coronary vessels declines; typical for the moderately severe to severe insufficiency is a large blood pressure amplitude [quick and strong pulse, possibly water-hammer pulse] with in part extremely low diastolic values; i.e., Korotkoff sounds can at times be heard up to zero values; other signs found during examination: thrusting apex beat, which can be displaced laterally and inferiorly; systolic thrill over the base of the heart; Traube's sign; Duroziez's murmur; Quincke's sign; Hill's sign; de Musset sign; the characteristic sound on auscultation is a high-frequency diastolic murmur, which begins immediately after the aortic closing sound and usually has a decrescendo character; normal to quiet first heart sound, the second heart sound is weakened and can be absent; point of maximal impulse is the left sternal border in the third-fourth intercostal space; in **acute aortic insufficiency**, e.g., in aortic dissection, valve damage, or endocarditis, the ventricle has no time to adjust to the very sudden regurgitation; the prominent **clinical** features are acute dyspnea and profound hypotension to collapse; tachycardia, cyanosis, and peripheral vasoconstriction may indicate pulmonary congestion or incipient pulmonary edema; the typical examination findings listed above are not present in chronic aortic insufficiency, but the auscultatory findings are usually identical; **diagnosis**: because of the hypertrophy, there is a left displacement in the ECG in chronic aortic insufficiency, which is not present in acute insufficiency; the **radiograph** in both insufficiencies shows a typical aortic configuration with an enlargement of the heart silhouette; **two-dimensional echocardiography** and **Doppler echocardiography** are the methods of choice today for noninvasive diagnosis and monitoring; **left heart catheterization** is performed only before valve replacement surgery; **therapy**: in acute aortic insufficiency there is usually a clear indication for urgent valve replacement, because the mortality without replacement is up to 75%; in chronic aortic insufficiency, in the case of mild insufficiency, treatment is limited to conservative therapy; in moderate and severe aortic insufficiency [reflux greater than 50% or greater than 30% with severe symptoms], valve replacement or correction is indicated

basilar insufficiency disordered perfusion in the vascular territory of the basilar artery; in partial occlusion or steal syndrome, the symptoms are those of vertebrobasilar insufficiency, namely dizziness, headache, and possibly cerebellar and cranial nerve deficits

cardiac insufficiency → *heart failure*

cerebrovascular insufficiency *Syn: impaired cerebral blood flow*; underperfusion of the brain mostly caused by arteriosclerosis of the cerebral vessels, which can lead to an ischemic infarct [stroke]

chronic venous insufficiency symptom complex caused by chronic disturbance of venous outflow from a leg consisting of edema, subfascial engorgement, and skin changes; following L. Widmer, three stages can be differentiated: **stage I**: pre- and subfascial edema, dilatation of small veins below the inner ankle [**corona phlebectatica**], **stage II**: induration of the skin, stasis eczema, dermatosclerosis, hyperpigmentation, **stage III**: venous ulcers of the shins [ulcus cruris] or the condition following ulcus cruris; the **cause** is mostly marked varicose insufficiency of the deep veins and perforating veins, disturbances of the muscle pump [after fractures, in paralysis] or a state following deep vein thrombosis [post-thrombotic syndrome]; **diagnosis**: history, clinical findings, Doppler ultrasonography, plethysmography; **therapy**: compression stockings or graduated elastic bandages, which only have a low resting pressure and can therefore be left on at night, treatment of any existing ulcers

coronary insufficiency *Syn: coronarism*; form of coronary heart disease caused by an absolute or relative deficiency of perfusion of the coronary arteries; in acute coronary insufficiency, this leads to an attack of angina pectoris; generally the ischemia is due to primary coronary insufficiency, whose cause is mostly stenosing sclerosis of the coronary vessels; in cases with unremarkably large coronary vessels, other causes include diseases of the small intramural vessels [small vessel disease] or spasm of the coronary vessels; in addition to these morphologic factors, functional changes, such as a fall in the perfusion pressure or the oxygen content of the blood in, e.g., anemia, hypoxemia, which lead to secondary coronary insufficiency, are important

exercise insufficiency *Syn: exertional insufficiency; s.u. heart failure*

exertional insufficiency *Syn: exercise insufficiency; s.u. heart failure*
global insufficiency *Syn: total heart failure, global heart failure; s.u. heart failure*
heart insufficiency → *heart failure*
heart valve insufficiency *Syn: valvular insufficiency, valvular regurgitation; s.u. valvular defect*
mitral insufficiency *Syn: mitral incompetence, mitral regurgitation*; inability of the mitral valve to close with backward flow of blood into the left atrium during systole; clinically divided into acute and chronic mitral insufficiency as well as absolute and relative or functional mitral insufficiency; **acute mitral insufficiency** mostly arises as a result of injury to the valve cusps due to bacterial endocarditis, ischemic/degenerative/traumatic/endocarditic damage of the valve retaining apparatus [chordae, papillary muscles], or failure of or damage to a valve prosthesis; the left atrium and ventricle are not enlarged or only minimally so [except in prosthesis carriers]; **chronic mitral insufficiency** is significantly more common and may be caused by a series of factors; often, there is also a **functional** or **relative mitral insufficiency**, i.e., the mitral valve is too small for the enlarged ventricle and can no longer close adequately; all the diseases, which can cause enlargement of the left ventricle [coronary heart disease, dilated cardiomyopathy, myocarditis, aortic stenosis, and insufficiency], can also cause relative mitral insufficiency; the retrograde flow of blood from the left ventricle to the left atrium during systole [regurgitation] has two consequences: 1. the **regurgitation volume** [also pendular volume] is lost to the systemic circulation and therefore the left ventricle has to increase its output if it is to meet the peripheral needs 2. the retrograde flow of blood under high pressure increases the pressure in the atrium and, by retrograde extension, so does the pressure in the pulmonary circulation; in acute mitral insufficiency, this leads to acute elevation of pressure in the pulmonary capillary bed, which when it exceeds 35 mmHg leads to pulmonary edema; at the same time, the regurgitation also leads to a reduction in the cardiac minute volume; in chronic mitral insufficiency, the combination of pendular blood flow and increased pumping work leads to dilatation and hypertrophy of the left atrium and ventricle that is visible as eccentric hypertrophy; as long as the cardiac minute volume is sufficiently large, this is called **compensated mitral insufficiency**, but if the cardiac minute volume falls below the required amount, then it is called **decompensated mitral insufficien-**

cy; **clinical**: dyspnea [initially exertional, later also resting dyspnea], tachycardia, dry cough, more frequent infections, and reduced exercise tolerance are the cardinal symptoms; in acute mitral insufficiency, lung edema develops, in decompensated mitral insufficiency the signs of cardiac insufficiency; **diagnosis**: history, auscultation [weakened 1. heart sound, 2. heart sound unremarkable or louder, 3. heart sound], inspection [mitral facies, less pronounced than in mitral stenosis], palpation [apex beat displaced to the left, enlarged and heaving], percussion [enlargement to the left]; chest X-ray [enlargement of the left ventricle, splaying of the tracheal bifurcation, signs of lung engorgement or edema], echocardiography, cardiac catheterization; **therapy**: medically by reducing the afterload with ACE-antagonists [captopril, enalapril] or hydralazine; digitalis to improve the left ventricular function; diuretics to treat the pulmonary edema; surgical management [annuloplasty, valve replacement] is indicated in acute mitral insufficiency or severe chronic mitral insufficiency [regurgitation fraction 50% or more]

myocardial insufficiency → *heart failure*

pulmonary insufficiency Syn: *pulmonary valve insufficiency, pulmonary artery insufficiency*; usually acquired inability of the pulmonary valve to close; it is seen primarily in adults as **relative pulmonary insufficiency** resulting from pulmonary hypertension with consecutive expansion of the valve ring; the second most frequent cause is bacterial endocarditis, primarily in i.v.-drug addicts; isolated pulmonary valve insufficiency leads to combined pressure and volume loading and eccentric hypertrophy of the right ventricle; **diagnosis**: Graham Steell murmur in relative pulmonary insufficiency; otherwise, a soft, low-frequency regurgitant murmur in the third and fourth intercostal space parasternal on the left; ECG [signs of right ventricular load, right bundle-branch block], chest X-ray, echocardiography, cardiac catheter; **therapy**: pharmacological with cardiac glycosides and diuretics; possibly valve replacement

pulmonary artery insufficiency → *pulmonary insufficiency*
pulmonary valve insufficiency → *pulmonary insufficiency*
respiratory insufficiency → *respiratory failure*
secondary adrenocortical insufficiency usually begins insidiously with, among others, fatigue, weakness, weight loss, hyperpigmentation of the skin, hypotension with tendency to collapse and abdominal and gastrointestinal pains; since the formation of mineralocorticoids

is mainly controlled by the renin-angiotensin system, it is not affected, in contrast to primary adrenal insufficiency; **therapy**: replacement with glucocorticoids

total heart insufficiency *Syn: total heart failure, global insufficiency, global heart failure, total heart insufficiency; s.u. heart failure*

tricuspid insufficiency → *tricuspid regurgitation*

valvular insufficiency → *valvular regurgitation*

vertebrobasilar insufficiency unilateral narrowing usually remains asymptomatic, while bilateral high-grade stenosis can lead to temporary neurologic symptoms [TIA, dizziness, nystagmus, double vision, loss of tone]

insult seizure, attack

interatrial *Syn: interauricular*; situated between the atria of the heart

interauricular → *interatrial*

intercurrent *Syn: intervening*; accessory, (occurring) in the meantime

intermittent not continuous

interval an intervening period of time

    atrioventricular interval *Syn: auriculoventricular interval, A-V interval, P-Q interval; s.u. electrocardiogram*

    auriculoventricular interval *Syn: atrioventricular interval, A-V interval, P-Q interval; s.u. electrocardiogram*

    A-V interval *Syn: auriculoventricular interval, atrioventricular interval, P-Q interval; s.u. electrocardiogram*

    P-Q interval *Syn: atrioventricular interval, auriculoventricular interval, A-V interval; s.u. electrocardiogram*

    Q-T interval *s.u. electrocardiogram*

intervascular situated between blood vessels

intervening → *intercurrent*

interventricular situated between ventricles

intima *Syn: Bichat's tunic, endangium*; the innermost layer of the wall of arteries or veins consisting of the vascular endothelium and subendothelial connective tissue; controls substance and gas exchange between blood and vessel wall and makes various humoral factors [e.g., nitric oxide]

intimitic relating to or marked by intimitis

intimitis inflammation of the intima of a blood vessel

intolerance **1.** quality or condition of being intolerant; lack of tolerance **2.** abnormal sensitivity or allergy to a food, drug, etc

    analgesic intolerance symptom complex often only distinguished with difficulty from an allergic reaction of immediate type involving skin, mucous membrane, and circulatory reactions [**intolerance triad**] following systemic or local application of acetylsalicylic acid and other non-steroidal anti-inflammatory drugs; probably due to an inhibition of cyclooxygenase and the resulting overproduction of leukotrienes

intoxication → *poisoning*
   cyanide intoxication → *cyanide poisoning*
   septic intoxication → *septicemia*

intra-arterial *Syn: endarterial*; situated within an artery or arteries

intra-atrial *Syn: intra-auricular*; situated within an atrium or atria

intra-auricular → *intra-atrial*

intrabronchial → *endobronchial*

intracardiac *Syn: intracordal, intracordial, endocardiac, endocardial*; situated within the heart

intracordal → *intracardiac*

intracordial → *intracardiac*

intractable → *refractory*

intramyocardial situated within the myocardium

intrapericardiac → *intrapericardial*

intrapericardial *Syn: endopericardiac, intrapericardiac*; situated within the pericardium

intrapulmonary (situated) within the lung, (situated) in the lung parenchyma

intrathoracic → *endothoracic*

intravascular situated within a vessel or vessels

intraventricular situated within a ventricle

intrinsic *Syn: inherent, intrinsical*; inner, arising from or acting within, indwelling, inside; endogenous

intrinsical → *intrinsic*

inversion *Syn: inversion*; **1.** the act of inverting **2.** the state of being inverted
   visceral inversion *Syn: situs inversus, situs transversus*; mirror image inversion of the internal organs; may affect all organs [**situs inversus totalis**] or only some of them [**situs inversus partialis**], e.g., situs inversus cordis [dextrocardia]

irregularity the quality or state of being irregular
   irregularity of pulse → *arrhythmia*

irrigation the flushing or washing out of anything with water or other liquid

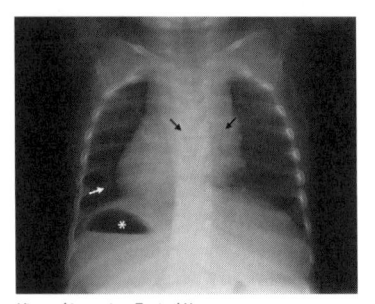

Visceral inversion. Typical X-ray

Ringer's irrigation → *Ringer's mixture*
ischaemia → *ischemia*
ischemia *Syn: hypoemia, ischaemia*; local lack of blood or underperfusion due to a reduction [**relative** or **incomplete ischemia**] or total absence [**absolute** or **complete ischemia**] of arterial blood supply; often the blood supply is sufficient at rest, but during [physical/psychologic] stress clinical symptoms develop [e.g., angina pectoris, intermittent claudication]; **acute ischemia** is, among other things, the cause of heart attacks and strokes
ischemia retinae damage to the retina caused by chronic ischemia in carotid stenosis or occlusion, often with typical punctate hemorrhages
ischemic relating to or affected with ischemia
iso- combining form denoting relation to equal, alike, the same, or uniform
isoagglutinin *Syn: isohemagglutinin*; alloantibody to antigens of the AB0 blood groups
isoamyl nitrite → *amyl nitrite*
isobaric at the same or constant pressure
isochoric → *isovolumetric*
isochronal → *isochronous*
isochronic → *isochronous*
isochronous *Syn: isochronal, isochronic*; lasting equally long, of equal duration
isoconazole antibiotic, antimycotic effective against Candida species, der-

matophytes, and molds

isoelectric *Syn: isopotential*; at or with constant electric potential

isoenzymes *Syn: isozymes*; enzymes that react with the same substrates, but which differ in their structure; they also differ in their activity and their relationship to inhibitory agents and substrate analogs; of particular interest are the isoenzymes of enzymes, which occur in various tissues in different concentrations and whose levels in the tissue or blood plasma permit inferences to be made about illnesses; a classic example is **creatine kinase**, which exists in three isoforms: CK-BB [**brain type**], CK-MM [**skeletal muscle type**], and CK-MB [**heart muscle type**]; CK-MB is used in the diagnosis and monitoring of myocardial infarction

isogeneic *Syn: isogenic*; of the same species and genetically identical

isogenic → *isogeneic*

isohemagglutinin → *isoagglutinin*

isohemolysin isoantibody that leads to disintegration of red blood corpuscles

isologous *Syn: syngeneic, syngenetic*; genetically identical, from the same species

isopotential → *isoelectric*

isosorbide dinitrate organic nitrate; vasodilator; improves cardiac efficiency and reduces the myocardial oxygen demand; **indications**: angina pectoris, myocardial infarction, pulmonary edema, and hypertensive crisis

isosorbide mononitrate organic nitrate; vasodilator; improves cardiac efficiency and reduces the myocardial oxygen demand; **indications**: angina pectoris, myocardial infarction, pulmonary edema, and hypertensive crisis

isotonic with or at the same osmotic pressure (as the blood)

isovolumetric *Syn: isochoric, isovolumic*; at or with constant volume

isovolumia constant blood volume aimed for by the body

isovolumic → *isovolumetric*

isozymes → *isoenzymes*

isthmus narrowing, constriction

    isthmus aortae → *aortic isthmus*

    aortic isthmus *Syn: aortic constriction, isthmus aortae*; narrowing of the aorta between the aortic arch [arcus aortae] and the descending aorta [aorta descendens]

J

joint articulation

    bleeder's joint *Syn: hemophilic arthritis, hemophilic arthropathy, hemophilic joint*; chronic joint disease in hemophiliacs with advanced deformity and restriction of movement

    hemophilic joint → *bleeder's joint*

josamycin oral macrolide antibiotic; it is effective against, for example, staphylococci, chlamydia, mycoplasma, and Bacteroides fragilis

jugular relating to the jugular vein

K

kallidin *Syn: bradykininogen, lysyl-bradykinin*; tissue hormone belonging to the kinins, which reduces blood pressure; part of the kallikrein-kinin system

kallikrein *Syn: callicrein*; protease, which releases kinins from kininogens; the kallikrein that occurs in the plasma is called **plasma kallikrein**; **tissue kallikrein** or **glandular kallikrein** is found in granulocytes, salivary glands, tear glands, sweat glands, kidneys, pancreas, and intestines

khellin furanochrome derived from khella [Ammi visnaga]; **usage**: spasmolytic in disturbances of coronary perfusion, angina pectoris, bronchial asthma

kidney one of a pair of bean-shaped organs situated in the body cavity near the spinal column that excrete waste products of metabolism
  arteriosclerotic kidney most common form of renal cirrhosis caused by sclerosis of the arteries and arterioles

kinemia → *cardiac output*

Kingella kingae *s.u. HACEK group*

kininase II → *angiotensin converting enzyme*

kiss of life → *transanimation*

kymography the recording of variations or undulations
  video kymography kymography that makes the movements of the heart visible on a fluoroscopy screen

L

lack deficiency or absence of something needed
   lack of energy → *asthenia*

β-lactamase *Syn: beta-lactamase*; enzyme that breaks open the β-lactam ring and thereby inactivates β-lactam antibiotics

lactate dehydrogenase enzyme containing zinc, which catalyzes the reduction of pyruvate to lactate in glycolysis; the serum level of lactate dehydrogenase rises sharply in the first 24 hours following a myocardial infarction and then slowly declines

lamina thin plate, coating, layer
   lamina parietalis pericardii → *parietal pericardium*

lamoxactam → *moxalactam*

lanatosides cardiac glycosides [lanatoside A-E] derived from Digitalis lanata

larvaceous → *masked*

larval → *masked*

larvate → *masked*

larvated → *masked*

latamoxef → *moxalactam*

latent *Syn: potential*; concealed, unapparent, invisible, hidden

latex any emulsion in water of finely divided particles of synthetic rubber or plastic
   RF latex *Syn: rheumatoid factor latex agglutination test*; latex test to demonstrate the presence of rheumatoid factors

law rule, principle
   Frank-Starling law *Syn: Starling's law of the heart*; when the diastolic filling increases, the cardiac pumping performance initially increases, but then falls off once a maximum has been reached
   Marey's law reflex increase in the heart rate in response to a drop in the blood pressure in the aorta
   Starling's law of the heart → *Frank-Starling law*

layer a thickness of material laid on or spread over a surface

parietal layer of serous pericardium *Syn: parietal pericardium*; parietal layer of the pericardium, which is firmly attached to the fibrous pericardium; lies opposite the visceral layer; between them lies the pericardial cavity, which is filled with serous fluid [**liquor pericardii**]

subserous layer of serous pericardium tela subserosa of the serous pericardium

visceral layer of pericardium → *epicardium*

lead recording of the electrical activity of the heart from defined surface points by means of electrodes

chest leads *Syn: precordial leads*; ECG recording from the surface of the chest

Einthoven's leads classical ECG technique developed by Einthoven, in which electrodes are attached to the right and left arms and the left leg; the three recordings form an equilateral triangle [**Einthoven's triangle**], with the heart situated in the middle; lead I is recorded between the right and left arm, lead II between the right arm and left leg, and lead III between the left arm and left leg

Goldberger's augmented limb leads ECG recording from the limbs

limb lead *Syn: limb recording*; ECG recording from the extremities after the methods of Einthoven or Goldberger

Nehb's leads bipolar ECG chest lead with a recording point over the right 2nd rib parasternally, the cardiac apex and the left posterior axillary line; rarely used today

precordial leads → *chest leads*

Wilson's precordial leads unipolar ECG tracing from the chest wall; generally 6 electrodes [V_1–V_6] are applied; in addition to these standard leads, there are also left precordial leads [V_7–V_9] and right precordial leads [V_{3R}–V_{5R}]

leak an unintended hole that allows something to enter or escape

capillary leak *s.u. shock*

lecithin → *phosphatidylcholine*

lecithin acyltransferase → *lecithin-cholesterol acyltransferase*

lecithin-cholesterol acyltransferase *Syn: lecithin acyltransferase, phosphatidylcholine-cholesterol acyltransferase, phosphatidylcholine-sterol acyltransferase*; enzyme made in the liver, which catalyzes the formation of cholesterol esters; bound by HDL precursors and catalyzes the reaction cholesterol + phosphatidylcholine → cholesterol ester + lysophosphatidylcholine; this increases the cholesterol content of the HDL, which transports it to the liver [**reverse cholesterol transport**], where it is broken down and excreted in the bile

left-ventricular relating to the left ventricle

left ventricular mass index left ventricular mass as measured by echocardiography or cardiac MRI indexed to body surface area and expressed as g/m^2; complex index often calculated by means of a formula described by Devereux; increased LVMI indicates hypertrophy of the left ventricle usually as a consequence of hypertension and has been shown to be associated with higher mortality

leg either of the two lower limbs

   left leg of av-bundle → *left bundle branch*

   right leg of av-bundle → *right bundle branch*

   smoker's leg *s.u. nicotine*

leiomyolipoma a benign tumor composed of smooth muscular tissue and fat tissue

   vascular leiomyolipoma → *angioleiomyolipoma*

leiomyoma a benign tumor composed of smooth muscular tissue

   vascular leiomyoma → *angiomyoma*

leipo- combining form denoting relation to fat or lipid

leucocytosis → *leukocytosis*

leukemia malignant tumor of blood-forming tissues

   megakaryocytic leukemia *Syn: essential thrombocythemia, hemorrhagic thrombocythemia, idiopathic thrombocythemia, primary thrombocythemia*; rare form of myeloid leukemia with clonal proliferation of atypical megakaryocytes in the bone marrow; the thrombocyte count is usually increased

leukocytal → *leukocytic*

leukocytes *Syn: white blood cells, white blood corpuscles*; umbrella term for all nucleated blood cells containing no hemoglobin; they are divided into granulocytes, lymphocytes, and monocytes; the blood contains 4,000–11,000 leukocytes/μl; all leukocytes exhibit ameboid motility and can actively leave the bloodstream [leukocyte diapedesis]; their main task is to recognize and destroy or kill foreign bodies and pathogens

   granular leukocyte → *granulocyte*

   polynuclear leukocyte → *granulocyte*

leukocytic *Syn: leukocytal*; relating to leukocytes

leukocytopenia reduced leukocyte content of the blood; mostly due to a reduction in the neutrophil granulocytes [neutropenia]

leukocytopoiesis → *leukopoiesis*

leukocytosis *Syn: hypercytosis, leucocytosis*; increase in the leukocyte count in the blood
  lymphocytic leukocytosis → *lymphocythemia*
leukogram blood picture with enumeration of the various types of leukocyte
leukopenia a decrease in the number of white blood cells in the blood
  lymphocytic leukopenia → *lymphopenia*
  neutrophilic leukopenia → *neutropenia*
leukophlegmasia painful white swellings on the thigh, mostly occurring after childbirth and caused by deep venous thrombosis of the leg and pelvic veins; reflex arterial spasm leads to a cool, pale extremity with diminished pulses
leukopoiesis *Syn: leukocytopoiesis*; the formation of granulocytes and monocytes occurs in the bone marrow, that of the lymphocytes in the bone marrow and the thymus [later also in the spleen and the lymph nodes]
leukotoxic destroying leukocytes, damaging to leukocytes
levarterenol → *noradrenalin*
level an extent, measure, or degree of intensity
  blood level *Syn: blood concentration*; concentration of a substance in the blood (plasma)
  blood glucose level *Syn: blood glucose value, glucose level, glucose value*; the glucose content of the blood must be monitored and regulated by the body, since both hyperglycemia and hypoglycemia are pathologic and can lead to serious damage; the goal of regulation is therefore to maintain the blood sugar level in the region of 4.4–6.6 mmol/l; if the blood sugar level falls below the lower value, insulin secretion is inhibited, leading to a reduction in the glucose uptake of muscle and fat tissues; in addition, the secretion of glucagon and catecholamines is increased, which leads to increased release of glucose from the liver; more glucocorticoids are also secreted and inhibit the use of glucose in muscle and fat; if the glucose level rises above the upper value, more insulin is released, while the secretion of glucagon, catecholamines, and glucocorticoids is inhibited; this leads to increased glucose uptake into muscle and fat tissues and stimulation of glycogenesis
  glucose level → *blood glucose level*
levobunolol β-blocker; **usage**: hypertension, treatment of glaucoma
levocardiogram X-ray contrast image of the left heart and start of the aorta

levocardiography X-ray contrast demonstration of the left side of the heart and the start of the aorta; injection of the contrast agent is usually performed using a left heart catheter [**retrograde arterial levocardiography**] or as **trans-septal levocardiography** [right heart catheter with puncture of the atrial septum]

levosimendan calcium sensitizer; has positive inotropic and vasodilator actions; due to its especially long half-life [approx. 80 h], it acts long after the recommended duration of infusion

lidocaine *Syn: lignocaine*; local anesthetic; class IB antiarrhythmic; **usage:** ventricular extrasystoles and arrhythmias [predominantly following myocardial infarction], ventricular fibrillation; surface, infiltration, and regional anesthesia; **side effects:** sinus arrest, AV-block, hypotension, bradycardia, asystole, dizziness, cramps

ligament → *ligamentum*

  ligament of Botallo → *ligamentum arteriosum*

  Luschka's ligaments → *sternopericardiac ligaments*

  sternopericardiac ligaments *Syn: Luschka's ligaments*; connective tissue strands between the posterior surface of the sternum and the pericardium

ligamentum *Syn: ligament, band*; bands consist of firm connective tissue, in which the collagen fibers are arranged in a pattern matching the tensile stress; their task is to strengthen and stabilize true joints and other bony connections [synarthroses]; the anatomical terminology differentiates ligaments that occur within joints [intracapsular ligaments], ligaments of the joint capsule [capsular ligaments], and ligaments located outside the joint capsule [extracapsular ligaments]

  ligamentum arteriosum *Syn: ligament of Botallo*; connective tissue remnant of the ductus arteriosus

  ligamenta sternopericardiaca → *sternopericardiac ligaments*

lignocaine → *lidocaine*

limbus edge, border, fringe, hem

  limbus fossae ovalis → *margin of oval fossa of heart*

limit final, utmost, or furthest boundary or point

  resuscitation limit timescale within which resuscitation may lead to full recovery; heart and brain have a particularly short ischemic time of about 4 minutes [heart] and approx. 8–10 minutes [brain] at normal body temperature; actually, the ischemic time of the resting, i.e., non-beating, heart is several hours, which is why the heart can be taken from a deceased patient and implanted into a recipient; the ischemic times of liver and kidney are approx. 3–4 hours

lincomycin bacteriostatic antibiotic produced by Streptomyces lincolnensis; it is effective against gram-positive causative agents and anaerobes

line strip, streak, mark

central line → *central venous catheter*

Kerley lines linear shadows in chest radiographs, which are usually an indication of a congested lung but also occur in mitral valvular disease, inflammation of the lung, pulmonary fibroma, etc.; these are differentiated further into **Kerley A lines**: hilifugal lines in the upper fields, **Kerley B lines**: horizontal lines in the lower fields, and **Kerley C lines**: diffuse, finely meshed network-like pattern, also called a reticular pattern

venous line → *venous catheter*

Zahn's lines delicate oblique striations on the surface of thrombi formed in vivo; important in differentiating post mortem clots that have a smooth surface

lipacidemia elevation of the free fatty acids in the blood

lipemia *Syn: hyperlipemia, lipohemia, lipoidemia, pionemia*; increased neutral fat content of the blood

lipidemia → *hyperlipidemia*

lipo- combining form denoting relation to fat or lipid

lipoclasis → *lipolysis*

lipodieresis → *lipolysis*

lipohemia → *lipemia*

lipoidemia → *lipemia*

lipoidosis a disorder of fat metabolism especially involving the deposition of fat in an organ

arterial lipoidosis → *atherosclerosis*

lipolysis *Syn: adipolysis, lipoclasis, lipodieresis*; the triglycerides in food are broken down by lipase into free fatty acids and monoacylglycerides; these are taken up by the intestinal mucosa and converted back into triglycerides, which reach the circulation in the form of chylomicrons via the thoracic duct; in extrahepatic tissues, the triglycerides are split by lipoprotein lipase into glycerin and fatty acids; the fatty acids are metabolized by the extrahepatic tissues, the glycerin by contrast is phosphorylated in the liver and channeled into metabolism

lipoma *Syn: fatty tumor, adipose tumor, pimeloma, steatoma*; a benign tumor composed of fat tissue

nevoid lipoma → *angiolipoma*
telangiectatic lipoma → *angiolipoma*
lipomicron → *chylomicron*
lipoprotein molecule consisting of a lipid and a protein moiety [**apolipoprotein**]; lipoproteins are synthesized in the liver and intestinal wall; their main role is the transport of cholesterol, lipids, and fat-soluble vitamins in the blood
lisinopril ACE inhibitor; usage: arterial hypertension, cardiac insufficiency
liver large, reddish-brown, glandular organ located in the upper right side of the abdominal cavity; is active in the formation of certain blood proteins and in the metabolism of carbohydrates, fats, and proteins
cardiac liver → *cardiac cirrhosis*
frosted liver Syn: *Curschmann's disease, icing liver, sugar-icing liver, zuckergussleber*; inflammation leading to typical changes in the liver capsule; generally a result of chronic liver congestion due to right heart insufficiency
icing liver → *frosted liver*
sugar-icing liver → *frosted liver*
losartan angiotensin-II blocker; selectively blocks binding of angiotensin II to the AT1 receptor subtype; has a nephroprotective effect; usage: essential hypertension
lung Syn: *pulmo*; the main task of the lung is gas exchange between the inhaled air and blood; the air enters via the airways [mouth, nose, trachea, bronchi] into the **air vesicles** [pulmonary alveoli] in which the gas exchange occurs; each lung contains about 300 million alveoli, which are separated by pore-containing septa [interalveolar septum]; the alveoli increase the internal lung surface to about 120 m^2; the surface of the lung is covered by the visceral pleura [pleura visceralis], which in the area of the hilum changes into the parietal pleura; both lungs consist of 3 [right lung] or 2 [left lung] **lobes** [lobi pulmoni], which are separated by the **fissura obliqua** and the **fissura horizontalis** [only the right lung]; the lobes of the lung in turn consist of 9 [left lung] or 10 [right lung] wedge-shaped or pyramidal **lung segments** [segmenta bronchopulmonalia]; each segment consists of a lobe section, which is separated from other segments by connective tissue septa [incomplete]; in the middle of the segment, there is a **segmental bronchus** [bronchus segmentalis], which is accompanied by an artery; the corresponding vein occurs within the connective tissue septa; the

lung segments are divided in the periphery by connective tissue septa into **pulmonary lobules** [lobuli pulmonis], which create a distinct polygonal pattern on the lung surface; this division does not occur in the lobe center

artificial lung → *oxygenator*

wet lung → *pulmonary edema*

lunula *Syn:* lunule; a crescent-shaped area

lunulae of semilunar cusps of aortic valve semilunar rim of the cusps of the aortic valve [valva aortae]; consists of sickle-shaped inclusions of collagen fibers with nodular thickening in the center [**noduli valvularum semilunarium valvae aortae**]

lunulae of semilunar cusps of pulmonary valve semilunar rim of the cusps of the pulmonary valve [valva trunci pulmonalis]; consists of sickle-shaped inclusions of collagen fibers with nodular thickening in the center [**noduli valvularum semilunarium valvae trunci pulmonalis**]

lunulae valvularum semilunarium valvae aortae → *lunulae of semilunar cusps of aortic valve*

lunulae valvularum semilunarium valvae trunci pulmonalis → *lunulae of semilunar cusps of pulmonary valve*

lusitropic influencing the rate of relaxation of the heart musculature during diastole

LVMI → *left ventricular mass index*

lycine → *betaine*

lymphaden → *lymph node*

lymphatics → *lymphatic system*

lymphedema *Syn:* lymphatic edema; edema caused by disordered outflow of lymph; mostly **secondary lymphedema** after occlusion of the lymph vessels by inflammation, infection [filariasis], tumors, operations, or irradiation; **primary lymphedema** occurs in aplasia or hypoplasia of the lymphatics; **therapy**: lymph drainage, compression bandages

lymphocytes white blood corpuscles consisting of two groups [B-lymphocytes and T-lymphocytes], whose main role is to fight pathogens and destroy abnormal cells

thymus-dependent lymphocytes *Syn:* T-cells; rarely used term for T-lymphocytes

thymus-independent lymphocytes → *B-lymphocytes*

lymphocythemia *Syn:* lymphocytic leukocytosis, lymphocytosis; increase in the lymphocytes in the blood beyond the normal range

lymphocythemic relating to or marked by lymphocythemia
lymphocytic relating to or characterized by lymphocytes
lymphocytopenia → *lymphopenia*
  acute lymphocytopenia massive reduction in the lymphocytes in peripheral blood; prognostically unfavorable sign in severe infective diseases
lymphocytopoiesis *Syn:* *lymphopoiesis*; B-lymphocytes are initially made in the bone marrow and later in the lymphatic tissues; they migrate through the blood from the bone marrow to the secondary lymphatic organs [spleen, lymph nodes]; T-lymphocytes are primarily made in the thymus [which is why they are also called thymus-dependent lymphocytes or thymolymphocytes], later in the lymphatic tissues
lymphocytosis → *lymphocythemia*
lymphoglandula → *lymph node*
lymphonodus → *lymph node*
lymphopenia *Syn:* hypolymphemia, lymphocytic leukopenia, lymphocytopenia, sublymphemia; reduction in the lymphocyte count in the peripheral blood; if the leukocyte count is increased, this is **relative lymphopenia**; in **absolute lymphopenia**, the lymphocyte count is less than $1 \times 10^9/l$
lymphopoiesis → *lymphocytopoiesis*
lypressin antidiuretic, vasoconstrictor
lysine basic amino acid
  lysine acetylsalicylate water-soluble salt of acetylsalicylic acid; analgesic, anti-rheumatic, inhibitor of thrombocyte aggregation
lysyl-bradykinin → *kallidin*

M

macro- combining form denoting relation to large, or of abnormal size or length

macroangiopathy *Syn: angiopathy of great vessels;* disease of larger vessels, e.g., in diabetic macroangiopathy

   diabetic macroangiopathy *s.u. diabetic angiopathy*

macroelectrode *s.u. electrode*

macroglobulinemia elevation of the macroglobulins in the blood

macrophage any mononuclear phagocytic cell

   blood macrophages → *monocytes*

magnesemia *Syn: hypermagnesemia;* increased magnesium content of the blood

magnetocardiograph apparatus for magnetocardiography

magnetocardiography description of the biomagnetic fields of the heart

maladie illness, disease

   maladie de Roger → *Roger's disease*

malfunction → *dysfunction*

maneuver manipulation; operation

   Valsalva's maneuver compression against a closed glottis leads to increase in the pressure in the chest and to changes in the blood pressure and pulse

mannite → *mannitol*

mannitol *Syn: mannite;* hexavalent alcohol derived from mannose; used as a sweetener and an osmotic diuretic

manometer *Syn: pressometer;* pressure gage, pressure gauge

   catheter tip manometer manometer attached to the tip of a catheter for direct pressure measurement in vessels or hollow organs [heart, bladder]

margin border, edge, boundary

   margin of oval fossa of heart muscle bulge, which surrounds the fossa ovalis in the right atrium

   right margin of heart right heart border

masked *Syn: concealed, larvaceous, larval, larvate, larvated*; hidden
mass a number or quantity
    renin mass → *plasma renin concentration*
massage kneading and rubbing parts of the body
    cardiac massage *Syn: heart massage*; rhythmic compression of the heart in order to maintain or restore the blood circulation; achieved either by compression of the chest wall [**extrathoracic** or **closed cardiac massage**] or by direct compression [**intrathoracic** or **open cardiac massage**] after opening the chest cavity
    closed cardiac massage *Syn: extrathoracic cardiac massage*; the helper kneels or stands at chest height on the right side close to the patient; the ball of one hand is placed on the lower third of the sternum; the other hand is placed palm down on the first hand without the fingers touching the chest wall; the arms are stretched out straight and brought directly above the hands; the sternum is depressed briefly with a force of 30–40 kp over a distance of about 5 cm; the frequency of compressions should be approx. 80/min

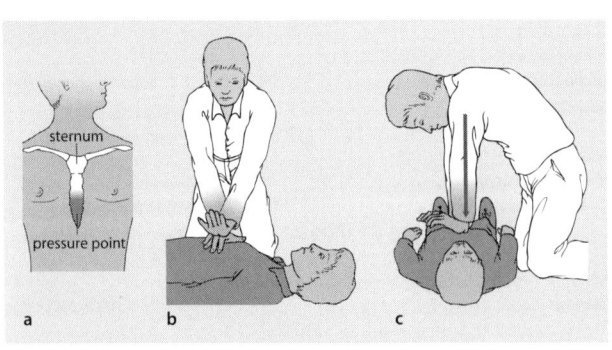

Closed cardiac massage

    open cardiac massage *Syn: intrathoracic cardiac massage*; direct cardiac massage after opening the chest cavity
mechanism bodily process or function
    Goldblatt's mechanism *Syn: Goldblatt's hypertension, Goldblatt's phenomenon*; restriction of the renal perfusion leads in animal experiments to stimulation of the renin-angiotensin system and to elevated

blood pressure

pressoreceptive mechanism → *carotid sinus syndrome*

mechanocardiogram graphical representation obtained by mechanocardiography

mechanocardiography description of mechanically assessable heart functions, e.g., cardiac apex beat

media middle layer of a vessel; consists in arteries almost exclusively of circular and spirally arranged smooth muscle fibers; the media of veins contains smooth muscle fibers and elastic nets, which are loosened by collagenous connective tissue

mediastinopericarditic relating to or marked by mediastinopericarditis

mediastinopericarditis *Syn: pericardiomediastinitis*; inflammation of the pericardium and adjacent connective tissue of the mediastinal space

mediastinum *Syn: mediastinal cavity, mediastinal space, interpulmonary septum*; space in the chest cavity lying between the two pleural cavities; it is limited by the sternum anteriorly and by the vertebral column posteriorly; it ends on the diaphragm inferiorly, and superiorly it extends continuously into the connective tissue space of the neck; the thymus, esophagus, heart, and the large vessels lie within or pass through the mediastinum

anterior mediastinum → *mediastinum anterius*

mediastinum anterius *Syn: anterior mediastinal cavity, anterior mediastinum*; portion of the inferior mediastinum [mediastinum inferius] situated between the sternum and pericardium

mediastinum inferius *Syn: inferior mediastinal cavity, inferior mediastinum*; portion of the mediastinum situated below the tracheal bifurcation; it consists of three divisions: mediastinum anterius, mediastinum medium, and mediastinum posterius

mediastinum medium *Syn: middle mediastinal cavity, middle mediastinum*; portion of the inferior mediastinum [mediastinum inferius] which is coterminus with the pericardium

middle mediastinum → *mediastinum medium*

posterior mediastinum → *mediastinum posterius*

mediastinum posterius *Syn: posterior mediastinal cavity, posterior mediastinum, postmediastinum*; portion of the inferior mediastinum [mediastinum inferius] situated below the pericardium

mediastinum superius *Syn: superior mediastinal cavity, superior mediastinum*; portion of the mediastinum situated above the tracheal bifurcation;

medionecrosis Syn: *medial necrosis*; necrosis of the tunica media
  medionecrosis of aorta → *Erdheim-Gsell medial necrosis*
mefruside saluretic, antihypertensive
mega- combining form denoting relation to large, or of abnormal size or length
megacardia → *cardiomegaly*
megalo- combining form denoting relation to large, or of abnormal size or length
megalocardia → *cardiomegaly*
membrana → *membrane*
  membrana bronchopericardiaca → *bronchopericardial membrane*
membrane Syn: *membrana*; thin skin
  bronchopericardial membrane connective tissue sheet, which runs from the front of the tracheal bifurcation to the back of the pericardium and on to the diaphragm
  external elastic membrane *s.u. artery*
  Held's limitting membrane → *blood-brain barrier*
  internal elastic membrane *s.u. artery*
meningioma a benign tumor of the meninges
  angioblastic meningioma → *hemangioblastoma*
meningococcemia the presence of meningococci in the blood
  acute fulminating meningococcemia → *Friderichsen-Waterhouse syndrome*
meningovascular relating to the meninges and the blood vessels
mepindolol β-blocker, antihypertensive
meproscillarin cardiac glycoside
meropenem carbapenem antibiotic with a broad spectrum of activity
mesaortitis Syn: *meso-aortitis*; inflammation of the muscular coat of the aorta
  luetic mesaortitis Syn: *Döhle's disease, Döhle-Heller aortitis, Döhle-Heller disease, Heller-Döhle disease, syphilitic aortitis, luetic aortitis, syphilitic mesaortitis*; inflammation of the aorta and aortic media occurring in the setting of late syphilis
  syphilitic mesaortitis → *luetic mesaortitis*
mesarteritic relating to or marked by mesarteritis
mesarteritis arterial inflammation with predominant involvement of the media
  Mönckeberg's mesarteritis → *Mönckeberg's sclerosis*
meso-aortitis → *mesaortitis*

mesocardia anomalous position of the heart in which the apex points forwards toward the sternum

mesodiastolic *Syn: mid-diastolic*; (occurring in) mid-diastole

mesophlebitic relating to or marked by mesophlebitis

mesophlebitis venous inflammation with predominant involvement of the media

mesosystolic *Syn: midsystolic*; in mid-systole

mesothelioma any tumor derived from mesothelial tissue

    pleural mesothelioma tumor of the mesothelial cells of the pleura; the **fibrous pleural mesothelioma** is usually benign or semimalignant and can be cured by resection [possibly with the adjacent lung tissue]; the **diffuse pleural mesothelioma** is malignant and is caused in half of cases by asbestos; the malignant neoplasm can occur even 20 years after exposure; it can be an epithelial, sarcomatous, or mixed form histologically; the epithelial form is said to have a more favorable prognosis, but the average life expectancy overall at the time of diagnosis is only 7–14 months; **clinical picture**: chest pain, pleural effusion, weight loss, cough, and dyspnea; because of the nonspecific and few acute symptoms, patients usually consult a physician rather late; **diagnosis**: chest X-ray, CT, pleural biopsy; **therapy**: with unilateral involvement, surgical removal of the lung together with the pleura [**pleuropneumonectomy**], possibly portions of the pericardium and the diaphragm; in extensive tumor infiltration, a palliative parietal and visceral pleurectomy is performed; in some cases, intrapleural chemotherapy or radiotherapy have also been tried, but thus far the results are not very positive

metachysis → *blood transfusion*

metapneumonic *Syn: postpneumonic*; (occurring) after a lung inflammation/pneumonia

methenamine *Syn: aminoform, hexamethylenamine, hexamethylentetramine, hexamine*; splits in acidic solution into ammonia and formaldehyde; **usage**: antiseptic [mainly in urine infections], diuretic

method procedure, means, technique

    Duke's method *Syn: Duke's test*; determination of the bleeding time by pricking the ear lobe and wiping away the exiting blood with filter paper until the bleeding stops [normal 2–5 min]

    dye dilution method *Syn: indicator-dilution method, indicator-dilution technique*; method of determining blood volumes, e.g., cardiac minute volume; **principle**: a water-soluble dye is injected at one point in the circulation and after a defined interval a blood sample is taken at the same point or elsewhere; the concentration of the dye measured in it permits conclusions to be drawn about various volumes

Einthoven's method *Syn: Einthoven's triangle*; *s.u. Einthoven's leads*

Fick's method → *Fick's principle*

indicator-dilution method *Syn: indicator-dilution technique*; method of determining the magnitudes of circulatory parameters [e.g., blood volume, cardiac output] by injection or inhalation of an indicator [dye, cold solution, radioactive isotope]

Quick's method → *Quick's value*

Riva-Rocci method indirect blood pressure measurement by means of an inflatable cuff; the measurement is usually performed on the upper arm of the seated patient; the site of measurement should lie roughly at heart height; the arm is bent slightly, the stethoscope is applied loosely over the brachial artery, and the cuff [12 cm wide, 30 cm long] is rapidly inflated until the pressure is about 30 mmHg higher than the systolic pressure; the pressure in the cuff is then slowly released until pulse-synchronous sounds can be heard over the artery [**Korotkoff sounds**]; the pressure on the manometer corresponds to the systolic blood pressure; with further release of air, the sounds become very quiet or disappear altogether; this pressure corresponds to the diastolic blood pressure; in obese patients or patients with extremely strong upper arms, high values are often measured; after physical or emotional stress, or in hyperthyroidism, anemia, and aortic insufficiency, the sounds are often audible right down to a cuff pressure of zero and determination of the diastolic value is difficult; measurement of the blood pressure in the thigh requires a special large cuff [18 cm wide, 60–80 cm long]; the measurement is performed in a lateral or prone position; the values are 10–30 mmHg higher than in the arms

single vessel method *s.u. exchange transfusion*

two vessel method *s.u. exchange transfusion*

Westergren method *s.u. erythrocyte sedimentation rate*

Wintrobe method *s.u. hematocrit*

methyldopa antisympathotonic; its metabolites [α-methyldopamine and α-methylnoradrenaline] act as pseudoneurotransmitters and displace noradrenaline from its receptor; **usage:** antihypertensive; **side effects:** heavy sedation, orthostatic hypotension; sleepiness, reduced libido, and potency

metildigoxin cardiac glycoside; **usage:** early and long-term treatment of cardiac insufficiency

metipranolol β-blocker; antihypertensive

metolazone saluretic, antihypertensive

metoprolol selective $β_1$-blocker; **usage:** coronary heart disease, angina pectoris, supraventricular tachycardia, tachycardic heart rhythm disturbances, myocardial infarction, migraine prophylaxis

metronidazole nitroimidazole derivative; antibiotic effective against trichomonads, amebas, clostridia, and protozoa; it is the most effective agent in rosacea

mexiletine class IB antiarrhythmic; **usage:** tachycardic heart rhythm disturbances, ventricular tachycardias, ventricular extrasystoles

mezlocillin acylaminopenicillin with a broad action spectrum against gram-positive and gram-negative pathogens

micrangiopathy → *microangiopathy*

micro- combining form denoting relation to small size

microaerophil *Syn:* microaerophile, microaerophilic, microaerophilous; growing at reduced oxygen tension

microaerophile → *microaerophil*

microaerophilic → *microaerophil*

microaerophilous → *microaerophil*

microanastomosis operative connection of small vessels or nerves

microaneurysm aneurysmal dilatation of the smallest vessels

microangiopathic relating to or marked by microangiopathy

microangiopathy *Syn:* micrangiopathy; non-inflammatory changes in the small and smallest arteries, e.g., in diabetes mellitus

    diabetic microangiopathy *s.u.* diabetic angiopathy

    thrombotic microangiopathy *Syn:* microangiopathic anemia, microangiopathic hemolytic anemia, Moschcowitz disease, Moszkowicz's disease, thrombotic thrombocytopenic purpura; purpura of unknown etiology [possibly autoimmune disease, allergy] with multiple thromboses, hemolytic anemia, and neurologic deficits

microangioscopy → *capillaroscopy*

microbial *Syn:* microbian, microbic, microbiotic; relating to or caused by a microbe or microbes

microbian → *microbial*

microbic → *microbial*

microbicidal *Syn:* microbicide; disinfectant

microbicide an agent which kills microbes/microorganisms; antibiotic

microbiotic → *microbial*

microcirculation blood circulation in the capillary bed; the total surface area for exchange is approx. 300 m^2; substance exchange between the blood or intravascular space and the interstitial space mainly occurs by diffusion; the exchange of lipid-soluble substances, such as, e.g., the respiratory gases, occurs over the entire surface, i.e., it depends predominantly upon the perfusion [**perfusion limited exchange**]; water-soluble substances can only diffuse through pores or intercellular clefts, i.e., there is **diffusion limited exchange**; perfusion limited exchange is substantially more prone to external influences, which cause reduced perfusion, whereas diffusion limited exchange is only restricted following extensive capillary damage

microemboli embolization of the smallest vessels

microthrombosis *Syn: microthrombus formation*; thrombosis of the smallest vessels, e.g., capillaries

microthrombus microthrombus of capillaries

mid-diastolic → *mesodiastolic*

midodrine sympathomimetic; **usage**: antihypotensive, orthostatic hypotension

midsystolic → *mesosystolic*

mineralocorticoids steroid hormones synthesized in the zona glomerulosa of the adrenal cortex, which influence water and mineral homeostasis; the two most important are deoxycortisone and aldosterone, which are both derivatives of cholesterol; their secretion depends upon the blood volume and the electrolyte content of the blood; a drop in the sodium concentration, rise in the potassium concentration and reduction in the blood volume are the strongest stimuli for secretion, whereas sodium retention, a fall in the potassium level and an increase in the blood volume lead to a reduction in formation and secretion; mineralocorticoids increase the reabsorption of sodium and chloride ions in the proximal and distal tubules and lead to increased excretion of potassium, hydrogen, and ammonium ions; the sodium retention leads to a corresponding water retention

minoxidil antihypertensive agent

miocardia → *systole*

mitral relating to the mitral valve

mixture something that consists of diverse elements

    Ringer's mixture *Syn: Ringer's irrigation, Ringer's solution*; physiologic salt solution; contains sodium, potassium, calcium chlorides and sodium bicarbonate

M-mode *Syn: time-motion, TM-mode*; *s.u. sonography*

molsidomine coronary therapeutic; works by producing venous vasodilatation, improvements in heart work, and reduction of the oxygen requirements; inhibits thrombocyte aggregation; **usage**: coronary heart disease, angina pectoris in the acute stages of a myocardial infarct

monalazone disodium disinfectant for skin disinfection

monitoring the act of continually checking, observing, recording or testing

    ambulatory blood pressure monitoring a procedure where an automated electronic device is worn by the patient usually for a period of 24 hours; it measures blood pressure at regular intervals throughout the day and the night

    Holter monitoring *s.u. electrocardiogram*

monoacylglycerols *s.u. fat*

monobactams β-lactam antibiotic with monocyclic ring structure, e.g., aztreonam

monocytes *Syn: blood macrophages*; large mononuclear leukocytes of the peripheral blood, which are capable of phagocytosis and migration; the monocyte granules are rich in hydrolyses and peroxidases; monocytes constitute 4–8% of the total leukocyte count; in the blood they have a diameter of 12–20 µm; as soon as they migrate into the surrounding tissues, they enlarge and the number of granules increases; mature monocytes in the tissues are called histiocytes or tissue macrophages

monomer a molecule that can combine with others to form a polymer

    fibrin monomers *s.u. fibrin*

monotherapy therapy using only one pharmaceutical

    individualized sequential monotherapy *s.u. arterial hypertension*

morbific → *pathogenic*

morbigenous → *pathogenic*

morbus → *disease*

moxalactam *Syn: lamoxactam, latamoxef*; cephalosporin with a broad action spectrum

moxonidine antihypertensive agent

multi- combining form denoting relation to many or much

multifactorial caused by many factors

multifocal relating to or arising from many locations

murmur → *sound*

    arterial murmur sound of flowing blood heard over an artery; usually relates to the sound over an area of stenosis, which is caused by turbulent flow

atriosystolic murmur → *presystolic murmur*
Austin Flint murmur → *Austin Flint phenomenon*
bronchial murmur → *bronchial breathing*
Carey Coombs murmur → *Coombs' murmur*
Coombs' murmur *Syn: Carey Coombs murmur*; mid-diastolic heart sound in relative stenosis in mitral insufficiency
diastolic murmur (heart) sound occurring during diastole
distant murmur loud heart sound, which can be heard without applying the stethoscope; most commonly found in a low-lying ventricular septal defect [maladie de Roger]
Duroziez's murmur *Syn: Duroziez's sign, Duroziez's symptom*; audible bruit over the femoral artery when the stethoscope is applied more firmly; consists of a short, high-frequency systolic sound; found mainly in aortic insufficiency and patent ductus arteriosus
early diastolic murmur heart sound in the early phase of diastole
early systolic murmur heart sound in the early phase of systole
ejection murmurs *Syn: ejection clicks, ejection sounds*; sounds that can be auscultated over the heart during the ejection phase [systole]
Flint's murmur *Syn: Austin Flint murmur, Austin Flint phenomenon*; heart sound in aortic insufficiency due to the accompanying functional mitral stenosis; late-diastolic, low-frequency sound over the cardiac apex; only occurs in severe aortic insufficiency
friction murmur → *friction sound*
Graham Steell's murmur *Syn: Steell's murmur*; early diastolic heart sound in relative pulmonary insufficiency; decrescendo sound in the left parasternal 3. intercostal space
heart murmurs murmurs occurring between the main heart sounds, which are caused by turbulent blood flow; time of occurrence, duration, and character [crescendo, decrescendo] of the noises, as well as the loudest point, allow them to be attributed to certain causes; **diastolic sounds** are found in, for example, mitral valve stenosis and aortic or pulmonary valve insufficiency, while **systolic sounds** indicate mitral or tricuspid valve insufficiency or aortic or pulmonary valve stenosis
holosystolic murmur *Syn: pansystolic murmur*; (heart) sound which can be heard throughout systole
humming-top murmur → *bruit de diable*

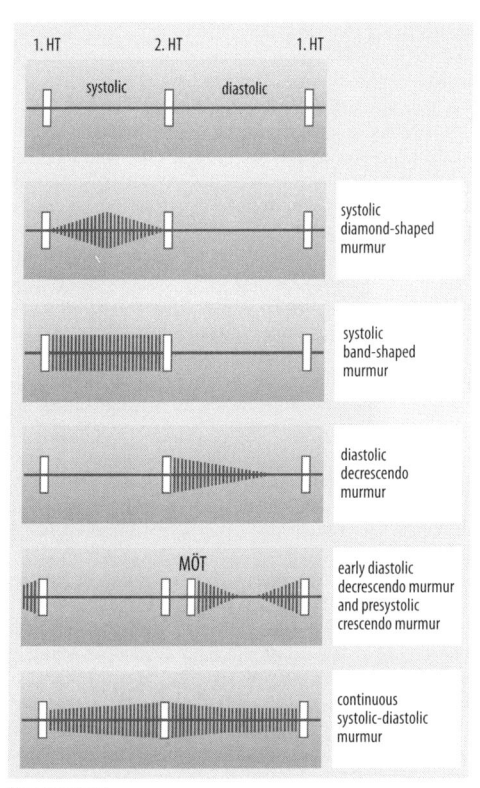

Heart murmurs

late diastolic murmur heart murmur in the late stages of diastole
late systolic murmur heart murmur in the late stages of systole
machinery murmur typical sound in patent ductus arteriosus; systolic-diastolic sound over the left 2. intercostal space; continuous sound that gets louder during systole and quieter during diastole
middiastolic murmur heart sound in mid-diastole

midsystolic murmur heart sound in mid-systole

nun's murmur → *bruit de diable*

pansystolic murmur → *holosystolic murmur*

pericardial murmur → *pericardial friction sound*

presystolic murmur *Syn: atriosystolic murmur, late diastolic murmur*; (heart) sound occurring before systole

Steell's murmur *Syn: Graham Steell's murmur*; early diastolic murmur in relative pulmonary insufficiency; decrescendo murmur in the left parasternal 3. intercostal space

stenosal murmur 1. vascular murmur over a narrowed vessel section **2.** heart murmur due to a stenotic cardiac valve murmur over a narrowed vessel section **3.** audible breath sound in constriction in the laryngeal or tracheal region

Still's murmur accidental, low-frequency precordial heart sound in children and juveniles

systolic murmur *Syn: systolic bruit*; heart sound arising during systole

Traube's murmur → *gallop*

tricuspid murmur early diastolic murmur heard in tricuspid valve stenosis

vascular murmur flow murmur heard on auscultation over vessels; mostly a sound due to stenosis

vesicular murmur → *vesicular breathing*

muscle → *muscle tissue*

cardiac muscle the heart muscle tissue in many respects resembles striated muscle tissue of the skeletal muscles, but it also has many peculiarities: heart muscle cells are approx. 100 µm long and branch irregularly; all the heart muscle cells form a large network, in which the individual cells are connected sequentially via intercalated discs; heart muscle cells cannot regenerate after injury, and instead are replaced by scar tissue; a part of the heart muscle tissue is specialized for conduction of excitation and together this forms the excitation conduction system of the heart

papillary muscles *Syn: musculi papillares cordis*; conical muscles in the right and left ventricle, from which the chordae tendineae pass to the valve cusps; the right ventricle contains three papillary muscles [**anterior, posterior, septal papillary muscles**], the left two [**anterior, posterior papillary muscles**]

pectinate muscles *Syn: pectinate bundles, musculi pectinati*; muscle

ridge in the right and left atria
musculus muscle
   musculi papillares cordis → *papillary muscles*
   musculus papillaris anterior ventriculi dextri anterior papillary muscle of the right ventricle
   musculus papillaris anterior ventriculi sinistri anterior papillary muscle of the left ventricle
   musculus papillaris posterior ventriculi dextri posterior papillary muscle of the right ventricle
   musculus papillaris posterior ventriculi sinistri posterior papillary muscle of the left ventricle
   musculus papillaris septalis ventriculi dextri septal papillary muscle of the right ventricle
   musculi pectinati → *pectinate muscles*
mushroom-shaped → *fungiform*
mycethemia → *fungemia*
mycostatic → *fungistatic*
myelogram quantitative evaluation of cells in a bone marrow smear
myocardiac → *myocardial*
myocardial *Syn:* myocardiac; relating to the myocardium
myocardiopathy 1. disease of the heart muscle 2. → *cardiomyopathy*
myocardiorrhaphy → *cardiorrhaphy*
myocardiosis → *myocardosis*
myocarditic relating to myocarditis
myocarditis *Syn: myocardial inflammation;* inflammation of the heart muscle; most commonly as **infective myocarditis** due to viruses, bacteria, fungi, or parasites; **non-infective myocarditis** is significantly rarer; it occurs in the setting of collagenoses, granulomatoses, Kawasaki syndrome, and in the immunologic diseases; **clinical**: dyspnea, reduced exercise capacity, fatigue, tachycardia, or bradycardia; **diagnosis**: history, physical examination [edema, signs of cardiac insufficiency, new heart murmurs, enlargement of the heart], chest X-ray, ECG, echocardiography, cardiac catheterization; **therapy**: antibiotics in bacterial, mycotic, or parasitic myocarditis; rest, salt, and water restriction, symptomatic treatment with β-blockers, in advanced cardiac insufficiency diuretics, ACE inhibitors and digitalis; possibly antiarrhythmics or pacemaker therapy
   acute isolated myocarditis → *Fiedler's myocarditis*
   bacterial myocarditis acute inflammation of the heart muscle, mostly

in the setting of pyemia; relatively rare

diphtheritic myocarditis now rare, toxic inflammation of the heart muscle during infection [diphtheria toxin] with marked confluent necrosis

Fiedler's myocarditis *Syn: acute isolated myocarditis, idiopathic myocarditis*; idiopathic myocarditis with numerous multinucleated giant cells; leads to flaccid dilatation of the ventricle and pericardial effusion; mostly leads to acute fatal heart failure between the ages of 20 and 50

giant cell myocarditis *Syn: tuberculoid myocarditis*; myocarditis characterized by the formation of giant cells

granulomatous myocarditis giant cell myocarditis accompanied by the formation of granulomas, with which it is often equated

idiopathic myocarditis → *Fiedler's myocarditis*

infectious-allergic myocarditis heart muscle inflammation caused by a hypersensitivity reaction [type IV]

infectious-toxic myocarditis damage to the heart muscle caused by pathogenic toxins; classic examples include diphtheroid myocarditis and the myocarditis of scarlet fever

interstitial myocarditis form of myocarditis primarily affecting the interstitial connective tissues

rheumatic myocarditis heart muscle inflammation that occurs commonly in the setting of rheumatic fever [approx. 50% of patients]

scarlet fever myocarditis infective/toxic myocarditis as a late complication of scarlet fever

toxic myocarditis inflammatory myocardial damage caused by the action of toxins [medications, irradiation]

tuberculoid myocarditis → *giant cell myocarditis*

viral myocarditis most common form of infective myocarditis; mostly caused by enteroviruses or coxsackie viruses; other viruses known to cause it include mumps virus, influenza A or B virus, adenoviruses, cytomegalovirus, varicella zoster virus, flaviviruses, measles virus, poliovirus, toga viruses

myocardium *Syn: cardiac muscle*; working musculature of the heart wall built up from cardiac muscle tissue, from which the papillary muscles and the trabeculae carneae arise; in the atria, the myocardium is smooth, in the ventricles it forms macroscopically visible bundles, which surround the left ventricle in three layers [**outer oblique layer, middle circular layer, inner longitudinal layer**]; at the apex of the heart, the steeply angled fibers of the outer oblique layer bend upwards; in both ventricles, the myocardium contains 1 capillary per muscle fiber; however, since the muscle fibers of the left ventricle are significantly thicker, the relationship between muscle fiber surface area and capillary surface area is approx. 1:2.9 and is therefore significantly less favorable than in the right ventricle [1:2]; the worse oxygen supply this results in is one reason for the more frequent involvement of the left ventricle in myocardial infarction

myocardosis *Syn: myocardiosis*; generic term for non-inflammatory heart muscle diseases

myocyte *Syn: muscle cell*; *s.u. muscle tissue*

Anichkov's myocyte *Syn: Anichkov's body, Anichkov's cell, Anitschkow's body, Anitschkow's cell, caterpillar cell, Anitschkow's myocyte*; typical cells occurring in rheumatic myocarditis

Anitschkow's myocyte → *Anichkov's myocyte*

myoglobin *Syn: muscle hemoglobin, myohematin, myohemoglobin*; a protein in the muscle tissue related to hemoglobin, which serves as an oxygen store in the skeletal and cardiac muscles; consists of 153 amino acids and the oxygen binding moiety heme; myoglobin has a significantly higher oxygen affinity than hemoglobin

myoglobinuria myoglobin excretion in the urine, e.g., in rhabdomyolysis, myocardial infarction

myohematin → *myoglobin*

myohemoglobin → *myoglobin*

myopericarditic relating to or marked by myopericarditis

N

nadolol beta-blocker

naftidrofuryl vasodilator, sympatholytic; **usage**: disturbances of peripheral and cerebral perfusion

nail fingernail or toenail

   hippocratic nails *Syn:* *watch-crystal nails*; convex arched fingernails in chronic oxygen deficiency [pulmonary or cardiac cyanosis]; can also occur as an autosomal dominant form

   watch-crystal nails → *hippocratic nails*

Na$^+$-K$^+$-ATPase *Syn:* *sodium-potassium adenosinetriphosphatase, sodium-potassium-ATPase*; membrane-bound enzyme, which transports potassium ions into the cell in exchange for sodium ions; present in the membrane of all cells and responsible for the setting and maintenance of the different sodium and potassium concentrations of the intracellular and extracellular spaces; cardiac glycosides work by inhibiting the sodium-potassium pump

nalidixic acid chinolone; gyrase inhibitor; acts against Gram-negative bacteria [predominantly Escherichia coli, Salmonella, Shigella, Proteus, Brucella]

narrowing → *stenosis*

natremia → *hypernatremia*

natriemia → *hypernatremia*

natrium → *sodium*

natriuresis *Syn:* *natruresis*; sodium excretion in the urine

natriuretic *Syn:* *natruretic*; **1.** an agent with natriuretic properties **2.** promoting the excretion of sodium in the urine

natrum → *sodium*

natruresis → *natriuresis*

natruretic → *natriuretic*

necro- combining form denoting relation to death or to a dead body, cells, or tissue

necrosis *Syn:* *sphacelation*; local cell or tissue death in a living organism;

possible causes are physical [rays, heat], chemical [acids, bases], and mechanical [trauma] damage, pathogens [septic necrosis], or oxygen deficiency [avascular necrosis]

arteriolar necrosis → *arteriolonecrosis*

cardiac muscle necrosis → *myocardial necrosis*

cystic medial necrosis → *Erdheim-Gsell medial necrosis*

Erdheim's cystic medial necrosis → *Erdheim-Gsell medial necrosis*

Erdheim-Gsell medial necrosis *Syn: cystic medial necrosis, Erdheim's cystic medial necrosis, medionecrosis of aorta, mucoid medial degeneration*; idiopathic necrosis of the aortic media, which can cause spontaneous aortic rupture or dissecting aneurysm

ischemic necrosis necrosis caused by ischemia

myocardial necrosis *Syn: cardiac muscle necrosis, cardionecrosis*; generally localized necrosis of the heart muscle; mostly due to ischemic necrosis following myocardial infarction

necrotic relating to or characterized by necrosis, sphacelated, dead

necrotizing *Syn: necrotic*; converting to necrosis, causing necrosis, becoming necrotic

needle sharp pointed implement

recording needle in recording electrical potentials, the electrode that has a potential relative to a neutral electrode

neocytosis occurrence of immature cell precursors in the peripheral blood

nephric → *renal*

nephritic → *renal*

nephritis inflammation of the renal parenchyma

arteriosclerotic nephritis age- or hypertension-related kidney inflammation with progressive sclerosis and scarring

nephro- combining form denoting relation to the kidney(s)

nephrocardiac *Syn: cardionephric, cardiorenal*; relating to kidney and heart

nephrogenic → *renal*

nephrogenous → *renal*

nephropathy any disease of the kidney(s)

hypertensive nephropathy kidney disease resulting from long-standing arterial hypertension

nephrosclerosis sclerosis of the arteries and arterioles in the kidney(s); leads to the development of renal hypertension and renal insufficiency

arterial nephrosclerosis → *arterionephrosclerosis*
hyperplastic arteriolar nephrosclerosis → *Fahr-Volhard disease*
malignant nephrosclerosis → *Fahr-Volhard disease*
senile nephrosclerosis → *arterionephrosclerosis*

nerve bundle of specialized fibers that conveys impulses from the central nervous system to the periphery or vice versa

carotid sinus nerve → *Hering's sinus nerve*

depressor nerve Syn: *right/left aortic nerve*; clinical description of the superior cervical cardiac branches of the right [**nervus depressor dexter**] or left vagus nerve [**nervus depressor sinister**], which exert negative chronotropic and inotropic effects upon the heart

Hering's nerve → *Hering's sinus nerve*

Hering's sinus nerve Syn: *carotid sinus branch of glossopharyngeal nerve, carotid sinus nerve, Hering's nerve*; branch of the glossopharyngeal nerve to the carotid sinus

inferior cardiac nerve → *inferior cervical cardiac nerve*

inferior cervical cardiac nerve Syn: *inferior cardiac nerve*; sympathetic cardiac branch of the inferior cervical ganglion

middle cardiac nerve → *middle cervical cardiac nerve*

middle cervical cardiac nerve Syn: *middle cardiac nerve*; sympathetic cardiac branch of the middle cervical ganglion

phrenic nerve → *nervus phrenicus*

right/left aortic nerve clinical description of the superior cervical cardiac branches of the right [**nervus depressor dexter**] or left vagus nerve [**nervus depressor sinister**], which exert negative chronotropic and inotropic effects upon the heart

superior cardiac nerve → *superior cervical cardiac nerve*

superior cervical cardiac nerve Syn: *superior cardiac nerve*; sympathetic cardiac branch of the superior cervical ganglion

vagus nerve → *nervus vagus*

vasomotor nerves can cause dilatation [vasodilator] or constriction [vasoconstrictor]; an important part of the central and peripheral control of perfusion

nerves of vessels nerves supplying vessels

nervus nerve

nervus cardiacus cervicalis inferior → *inferior cervical cardiac nerve*
nervus cardiacus cervicalis medius → *middle cervical cardiac nerve*
nervus cardiacus cervicalis superior → *superior cervical cardiac nerve*
nervus phrenicus Syn: *phrenic nerve, diaphragmatic nerve*; mixed

nerve from the cervical plexus [C₄]; it passes along the anterior scalene muscle into mediastinum; the right phrenic nerve passes in front of the root of the lung and between mediastinal pleura and pericardium to the diaphragm; the left phrenic nerve crosses below the left subclavian vein and above the vagus nerve, before it passes through the diaphragm near the cardiac apex; the motor portion supplies the diaphragm; the pericardiac branch [**ramus pericardiacus**] is a sensory branch to the pericardium, and the phrenicoabdominal branches [**rami phrenicoabdominales**] contain the sensory fibers for the mediastinal and diaphragmatic pleura, parietal peritoneum, and celiac plexus

nervus vagus mixed cranial nerve with motor, sensory, and parasympathetic fibers; among others, it innervates the muscles of the palate, pharynx, upper esophagus, and larynx; it supplies the sensory fibers to the pharynx, larynx, trachea, esophagus, and chest and abdominal organs; the nerve leaves the mesencephalon in the posterolateral sulcus and the posterior cranial fossa through the jugular foramen; within the foramen it forms the superior vagal ganglion [**ganglion superius**], and below it the inferior vagal ganglion [**ganglion inferius**]; it then passes between the internal carotid artery and the internal jugular vein downward through the thoracic inlet; the **left vagus nerve** passes in front of the aortic arch [arcus aortae] and behind the left primary bronchus to the anterior surface of the esophagus, where, together with the right vagus nerve, it forms the esophageal plexus and continues through the diaphragm; below the diaphragm the fibers continue as **anterior vagal trunk** to the anterior surface of the stomach; the **right vagus nerve** passes over the right subclavian artery, between the right brachiocephalic vein and brachiocephalic trunk and behind the right primary bronchus to the posterior surface of the esophagus; its fibers join the fibers from the left vagus nerve in forming the esophageal plexus, before continuing in the **posterior vagal trunk** to the posterior surface of the stomach; important branches of the vagus nerve are: rami pharyngei [sensory, motor, and secretory fibers to the pharynx, which form the pharyngeal plexus], nervus laryngeus superior, nervus laryngeus recurrens, and the rami bronchiales [sensory, motor, and secretory fibers to the bronchi]

nervi vasorum → *nerves of vessels*

nesiritide recombinant natriuretic peptide type B [brain natriuretic peptide]; synthesized endogenously in the ventricular myocardium;

it causes vasodilatation of the arteries and veins, including the coronary vessels, increases the excretion of sodium in the kidney, acts as a diuretic, and suppresses the renin-angiotensin-aldosterone system; endogenous production and secretion of BNP is stimulated by increased wall tension, as well as by hypertrophy and volume loading of the heart; correspondingly, the concentration of BNP in the plasma increases in the course of the development of cardiac insufficiency; **usage**: reduction in the preload and afterload in decompensated cardiac insufficiency; **side effects**: hypotension, worsening of renal function

netilmicin aminoglycoside antibiotic; **indications**: administered parenterally in gram-negative problematic microorganisms

network net-like combination of vessels or nerves

    arterial network *Syn: arterial rete, arterial rete mirabile*; arterial plexus

    lymphocapillary network → *lymphocapillary rete*

    subendocardial terminal network *Syn: rami subendocardiales*; s.u. *cardiac conducting system*

    Trolard's network → *venous plexus of hypoglossal canal*

    venous network → *venous plexus*

neurocardiac relating to the nervous system and heart

neurocirculatory relating to the nervous system and circulation

neurosis *Syn: psychoneurosis*; a mental or personality disturbance not attributable to any known neurological or organic dysfunction

    cardiac neurosis *Syn: cardioneurosis*; pattern of illness belonging to the organ neuroses, with cardiac symptoms independent of the degree of exertion, combined with anxiety and insecurity

neurovascular relating to the nervous system and vascular system

neutrocytopenia → *neutropenia*

neutropenia *Syn: granulocytopenia, granulopenia, neutrocytopenia, neutrophilic leukopenia*; relative or absolute reduction in the neutrophil granulocytes in the peripheral blood

nicardipine calcium channel blocker; **usage**: essential hypertension, angina pectoris

nicotine exceptionally poisonous alkaloid derived from the tobacco plant; initially has excitatory actions on the autonomic ganglia, but after longer exposure it acts as a blocker; the initially increased blood pressure is then replaced by a drop in blood pressure, which is increased by the vasopressin release it provokes; chronic nicotine intake [smoking, chewing tobacco] leads to an increased risk of coronary heart disease and disturbances of perfusion, mainly affecting the lower extremities [smoker's leg]; the discussion as to whether or not nicotine can lead to addiction [physical/psychologic] is not yet decided; it has been shown that giving up smoking is significantly more successful when nicotine is given [transdermal or as chewing gum] than abrupt cessation, which suggests addiction or dependence

nifedipine calcium antagonist; **usage**: hypertensive crisis, angina pectoris, hypertension, coronary heart disease

nimodipine calcium antagonist; **usage**: arterial hypertension, subarachnoid hemorrhage

nisoldipine calcium antagonist of nifedipine type; **usage**: coronary heart disease, angina pectoris

nitrate salt of nitric acid

    organic nitrates umbrella term for esters of nitric acid, such as, e.g., nitroglycerin, isosorbide dinitrate, and isosorbide mononitrate; **action**: they lower the mean pulmonary pressure, aortic pressure, peripheral resistance, and left and right ventricular filling pressure; they cause vasodilatation, lower the oxygen consumption by the myocardium, and improve cardiac efficiency; **indications**: angina pectoris, myocardial infarction, coronary spasms, hypertensive crisis, acute left ventricular failure, and cardiac pulmonary edema; **side effects**: headache, flush, drop in blood pressure, reflex tachycardia, hypotension, nausea, and orthostatic circulatory disorders; tolerance development after repeated administration

nitrendipine calcium antagonist; **usage**: arterial hypertension, hypertensive relapse

nitroglycerin *Syn: glyceryl trinitrate, trinitroglycerin, trinitrin, trinitroglycerol*; organic nitrate; **indications**: angina pectoris, myocardial infarction, coronary spasm, hypertensive crisis, and acute left ventricular failure

nitroprusside sodium *Syn: sodium nitroprusside, sodium nitroferricyanide*; potent vasodilator which reduces the preload and afterload, antihypertensive; **indications**: hypertensive crisis, malignant and essential hypertension

nocturia → *nycturia*

node a circumscribed swelling or mass of tissue; knob, nodosity

    Aschoff's node → *Aschoff-Tawara's node*

    Aschoff-Tawara's node *Syn: Aschoff's node, atrioventricular node, AV-node, av-node, Koch's node, node of Tawara*; node situated at the atrioventricular border that consists of specialized muscle fibers, which transmit excitation from the atrium to the ventricle; part of the excitation conduction system of the heart; takes over the pacemaker function as a secondary center of excitation if the sinoatrial node fails

atrioventricular node → *Aschoff-Tawara's node*

brachiocephalic lymph nodes lymph nodes in the upper mediastinum; **inflow:** thymus, pericardium, right half of the heart

Flack's node → *Keith-Flack's node*

Keith's node → *Keith-Flack's node*

Keith-Flack's node *Syn:* atrionector, Flack's node, Keith's node, sinoatrial node, sinus node, sinuatrial node; primary center of excitation in the heart in the wall of the right atrium; part of the excitation conduction system of the heart; since no direct connection between the sinoatrial node and the atrioventricular node has been found, the excitation must be transmitted along the contracting muscles [myocardium] to the atrioventricular node

Koch's node → *Aschoff-Tawara's node*

lateral aortic lymph nodes lymph nodes belonging to the left lumbar lymph node group

lateral pericardial lymph nodes small lymph nodes along the pericardial vessels, which drain the pericardial lymph

lymph node *Syn:* lymph gland, lymphatic gland, lymphonodus, lymphaden, lymphoglandula; bean-shaped bodies incorporated into the lymph vessels; they filter the lymph and remove pathogens, toxins, cell fragments, and the like; they are the storage and proliferation depot for B and T lymphocytes

Osler's nodes *Syn:* Osler's sign; small, painful, reddish nodules mainly on the knuckles of the fingers and toes as well as in the thenar and hypothenar areas caused by microemboli in subacute endocarditis due to Streptococcus viridans

sinoatrial node → *Keith-Flack's node*

sinuatrial node → *Keith-Flack's node*

sinus node → *Keith-Flack's node*

node of Tawara → *Aschoff-Tawara's node*

tracheobronchial lymph nodes *Syn:* nodi lymphoidei tracheobronchiales; large lymph nodes below [**nodi lymphoidei tracheobronchiales inferiores**] and above [**nodi lymphoidei tracheobronchiales superiores**] the tracheal bifurcation; **supply:** nodi lymphoidei bronchopulmonales, heart; **drainage:** nodi lymphoidei paratracheales

nodule small node
  Aschoff's nodules *Syn: rheumatic nodule, rheumatoid nodule*; nodular granuloma developing in rheumatic fever, predominantly in the interstitial tissues of the heart muscle
  rheumatic nodule → *Aschoff's nodules*
  rheumatoid nodule → *Aschoff's nodules*
nodulus → *nodule*
  noduli valvularum semilunarium valvae aortae *s.u. lunulae of semilunar cusps of aortic valve*
  noduli valvularum semilunarium valvae trunci pulmonalis *s.u. lunulae of semilunar cusps of pulmonary valve*
nodus node, nodule, nodular structure
  nodi lymphoidei aortici laterales → *lateral aortic lymph nodes*
  nodi lymphoidei brachiocephalici → *brachiocephalic lymph nodes*
  nodi lymphoidei pericardiaci laterales → *lateral pericardial lymph nodes*
  nodi lymphoidei tracheobronchiales → *tracheobronchial lymph nodes*
nonbacterial → *abacterial*
nonhemolytic → *gamma-hemolytic*
nonpathogenetic → *nonpathogenic*
nonpathogenic *Syn: nonpathogenetic*; (micro-organisms) not provoking disease
nonvalvular → *avalvular*
noradrenalin *Syn: arterenol, levarterenol, noradrenaline, norepinephrine*; neurotransmitter formed in the adrenal medulla and the sympathetic nervous system; in part has the same actions as adrenaline, in part the opposite actions; acts on α and $β_2$ receptors, less strongly on $β_1$ receptors; increases the blood pressure [vasoconstrictor] and provokes uterine contraction; in contrast to adrenaline, it has hardly any effect on metabolism; **therapeutically**, noradrenaline is used in arterial hypotension, severe shock, and as a vasoconstricting additive to local anesthetics
noradrenaline → *noradrenalin*
norepinephrine → *noradrenalin*
norfenefrine vasoconstrictor, α-sympathomimetic; **usage**: arterial hypotension, circulatory collapse
normocalcemia normal calcium content of the blood
normocalcemic relating to normocalcemia
normocholesterolemia normal cholesterol content of the blood

normokalemia *Syn: normokaliemia*; normal potassium content of the blood

normokalemic relating to normokalemia

normokaliemia → *normokalemia*

normotensive *Syn: normotonic*; with normal blood pressure

normotonia *Syn: orthoarteriotony*; normal blood pressure

normotonic 1. with normal blood pressure **2.** with normal tone

normovolemia normal blood volume

normovolemic relating to or characterized by normovolemia

nosogenic → *pathogenic*

nosopoietic → *pathogenic*

nucleus a mass of nerve cells in the brain or spinal cord

    nucleus dorsalis nervi vagi → *dorsal nucleus of vagus nerve*

    dorsal vagal nucleus → *dorsal nucleus of vagus nerve*

    dorsal nucleus of vagus nerve *Syn: dorsal vagal nucleus, posterior nucleus of vagus nerve*; nucleus of the vagus nerve in the floor of the rhomboid fossa; the parasympathetic nucleus, from which efferent fibers to the thoracic organs, upper abdominal organs, and intestines as far as the Cannon-Böhm point run

    posterior nucleus of vagus nerve → *dorsal nucleus of vagus nerve*

number numeral or group of numerals

    erythrocyte number → *red blood count*

nycturia *Syn: nocturia*; increased nocturnal urination; symptom of, among others, cardiac insufficiency, diabetes mellitus, benign prostatic hypertrophy

O

occlusion complete closure

acute arterial occlusion acute occlusion of a peripheral artery; the pelvic and leg arteries are the most commonly involved [80%], the large arteries of the upper extremities [subclavian, axillary, brachial arteries] accounting for the rest; in 75–80%, the cause is arterial embolism, acute thromboses account for 15–20%; the source of the embolus is predominantly the heart [80–90%; aneurysms, valve replacement, valve failure, endocarditis, disturbances of rhythm] and upstream arteries [10–15%; atheromatous plaques, aneurysms]; the **clinical** features are mostly acute, although there can be a more muted course, if the occlusion affects a previously damaged artery with good collateral supply; usually, one finds the **6-Ps symptom complex** of Pain, Pallor, Pulselessness, Paresthesias, Paralysis in the affected extremity as well as symptoms of shock [Prostration]; **therapy**: embolectomy is the method of choice; in incomplete ischemia syndromes, local or systemic thrombolysis can be tried

arterial occlusion occlusion of the arterial lumen from the inside [arteriosclerosis, arterial embolism, thrombosis] or outside [compression by tumor, hematoma, etc.]; the symptoms depend mainly on the acuteness of the closure [acute arterial occlusion, occlusive arterial disease] and the localization of the ischemic area [peripheral, central]

coronary occlusion *Syn:* coronary; acute occlusion of one or more coronary vessels; causes acute myocardial infarction

occult hidden, cryptic, concealed, larvate

octopamine sympathomimetic, antihypertensive

dextrothyroxine sodium sodium salt of the D-isomer of the thyroid hormone thyroxine; **usage**: to reduce lipid levels

oligemia → *hypovolemia*

oligemic → *hypovolemic*

oligocardia → *bradycardia*

oligocythemia *Syn:* oligocytosis; reduction in the cells in the blood or

oligocytosis

[more particularly] the erythrocyte count

oligocytosis → *oligocythemia*

oligohemia → *hypovolemia*

opening hole, passage, gap, aperture

aortic opening *Syn: aortic orifice, aortic ostium*; opening in the left ventricle, in which the aortic valve sits

opening of coronary sinus opening of the coronary sinus into the right atrium

opening of inferior vena cava orifice for the inferior vena cava in the right atrium

left atrioventricular opening *Syn: mitral orifice*; opening between the left atrium and ventricle; closed by the mitral valve

right atrioventricular opening *Syn: tricuspid orifice*; opening between the right atrium and ventricle; closed by the tricuspid valve

opening of superior vena cava orifice for the superior vena cava in the right atrium

operation surgery, surgical procedure

arterial switch operation *Syn: arterial switch; s.u. transposition of the great vessels*

Blalock-Taussig operation → *Blalock-Taussig anastomosis*

Fontan's operation operation performed for tricuspid atresia; the pulmonary trunk is divided and anastomosed to the right atrium or the right pulmonary artery

Glenn's operation *Syn: cavopulmonary anastomosis, bidirectional cavopulmonary anastomosis*; end-to-end anastomosis of the right pulmonary artery and the inferior vena cava created in tricuspid atresia with septal defect; it improves pulmonary blood flow

Leriche's operation *Syn: periarterial sympathectomy*; removal of the periarterial sympathetic nerve fibers to treat disturbances of perfusion

Meredino's operation annuloplasty of the annulus fibrosus of the mitral valve in mitral insufficiency

Trendelenburg's operation → *pulmonary embolectomy*

orciprenaline β-sympathomimetic, bronchodilator; **usage**: bradycardic disturbances of heart rhythm, Stokes-Adams attacks, 2. degree AV-block, antidote in α-blocker overdose

organ any part of the body exercising a specific task

glomus organ → *glomiform body*

respiratory organs → *respiratory tract*

orifice opening, aperture
  aortic orifice → *aortic opening*
  mitral orifice → *left atrioventricular opening*
  tricuspid orifice → *right atrioventricular opening*

orthoarteriotony → *normotonia*

orthodromic (running) in the normal direction

orthopnea dyspnea occurring in a supine position, which disappears in an upright position; it is typical for left ventricular failure

orthostatic relating to an erect position/orthostatism

oscillograph apparatus for demonstrating rapidly changing processes, e.g., blood pressure, pulse

oscillometer apparatus for measuring pulsatile changes in blood pressure

oscillometry measurement of pulsatile changes in blood pressure

osmodiuretic osmotic diuretic

osmotherapy intravenous infusion of hyperosmolar solutions to increase the osmotic pressure in the circulation

osmotic relating to osmosis

ostium orifice, opening, mouth
  ostium aortae → *aortic opening*
  aortic ostium → *aortic opening*
  ostium atrioventriculare dextrum → *right atrioventricular opening*
  ostium atrioventriculare sinistrum → *left atrioventricular opening*
  ostium sinus coronarii opening of the coronary sinus into the right atrium
  ostium trunci pulmonary opening of the pulmonary trunk in the right ventricle; it is closed by the pulmonary valve [valva trunci pulmonalis]
  ostium venae cavae inferioris orifice for the inferior vena cava in the right atrium
  ostium venae cavae superioris orifice for the superior vena cava in the right atrium
  ostia venarum pulmonarium opening of the two pulmonary veins [venae pulmonales] in the left atrium

output the quantity or amount produced
  cardiac output *Syn:* kinemia; blood volume ejected per unit time
  minute output → *minute volume*

overhydration → *hyperhydration*

oxacillin penicillinase-resistant penicillin **indications**: primarily infections with penicillinase-producing staphylococci

oxedrine → *synephrine*

oxilofrine sympathomimetic, anti-hypotonic

oximetry → *oxymetry*

oxprenolol β-blocker, antihypertensive; **usage**: angina pectoris, disturbances of heart rhythm

oxyfedrine coronary remedy

oxygenation oxygen saturation of the venous blood; also a description of oxygen administration

    apneic oxygenation → *diffusion respiration*

oxygenator *Syn: artificial lung*; device for oxygen saturation of the blood; part of the heart-lung machine; today only **membrane oxygenators** are still used in practice, in which the gas and blood phases are separated by a membrane and the gas exchange occurs by diffusion

    membrane oxygenator *s.u. oxygenator*

oxymetry *Syn: oximetry*; spectroscopic measurement of the oxygen saturation of the blood

    exercise oxymetry *Syn: oxymetric ergometry*; *s.u. ergometry*

    pulse oxymetry non-invasive measurement of the arterial oxygen saturation by means of transcutaneous measurement with a probe, which is generally placed on the ear lobe or a finger; has proven its worth in the Intensive Care Unit and in anesthesia in recent years

oxyneurine → *betaine*

oxytetracycline antibiotic made by various **Streptomyces** species with a broad spectrum of activity

P

pacemaker 1. the sinoatrial node in the atrium of the heart **2.** *Syn: cardiac pacemaker*; in principle, there are two types of pacemaker, **demand cardiac pacemakers**, which are guided by the electrical activity of the heart and only work if required, and **fixed rate cardiac pacemakers**, which fire at constant frequency; the demand pacemakers are further subdivided into **ventricular** and **atrial demand pacemakers**; fixed rate pacemakers are hardly used any more; generally, **single chamber systems**, which stimulate either the atrium or ventricle, or **dual chamber systems**, with bifocal stimulation, are used; these systems permit as close as possible a matching to the cause of the disorder and thereby the best possible improvement in function and the patient's quality of life; every pacemaker is identified by a 5-letter code, which summarizes its stimulation site, the triggering chamber(s) [detection point], the operation mode, programmability, and anti-tachycardia functions; the most common systems are: **VVI-stimulation**: triggered and stimulated chamber: right ventricle; supraventricular excitation or extrasystoles inhibit the pacemaker, i.e., this is a demand-triggered cardiac pacemaker, **AAI-stimulation**: triggered and stimulated chamber: right atrium; increase in the sinus rate and supraventricular extrasystoles inhibit the pacemaker, **DDD-stimulation**: programmable system for sequential stimulation of atrium and ventricle, which is also triggered from the atrium or ventricle **DDI-stimulation**: demand cardiac pacemaker, which stimulates atrium and ventricle, if the atrial or ventricular rate falls below a chosen base rate

artificial pacemaker *s.u. pacemaker*

atrial demand pacemaker *Syn: atrial triggered demand pacemakers*; *s.u. demand pacemaker*

atrial triggered demand pacemaker *Syn: atrial demand pacemaker*; *s.u. demand pacemaker*

cardiac pacemaker →*pacemaker*

demand pacemaker cardiac pacemaker, which is controlled by the electrical activity of the heart and only fires on demand; divided into **ventricular triggered** and **atrial triggered demand pacemakers**

fixed-rate pacemaker constant frequency cardiac pacemaker now hardly ever used

ventricular demand pacemaker *Syn: ventricular triggered demand pacemakers; s.u. demand pacemaker*

ventricular triggered demand pacemakers *Syn: ventricular demand pacemaker; s.u. demand pacemaker*

painful → *algetic*

painless → *indolent*

pairing → *bigeminy*

palpable appreciated by touch/palpation, tangible

palpation important part of the clinical examination; permits assessment of pulsation, hardening, temperature differences, fluctuation, etc.; the size, shape, position, surface characteristics, and mobility of organs can be determined by palpation

palpatory relating to palpation

palpitation stronger and faster heartbeat, which is perceived as unpleasant

panangiitic relating to or marked by panangiitis

panangiitis inflammation of a vessel affecting all the wall layers

panarteritic relating to or marked by panarteritis

panarteritis *Syn: diffuse arterial disease, polyarteritis*; arterial inflammation affecting all the wall layers

panarteritis nodosa → *Kussmaul's disease*

pancarditic relating to or marked by pancarditis

pancarditis *Syn: endoperimyocarditis, perimyoendocarditis*; inflammation of all the ventricular wall layers [endocardium, myocardium, pericardium]; *s.a. endocarditis, myocarditis, pericarditis*

pancytopenia *Syn: panhematopenia, hematocytopenia*; an abnormal deficiency in all blood cells

congenital pancytopenia → *Fanconi's anemia*

Fanconi's pancytopenia → *constitutional infantile panmyelopathy*

pang sudden, brief, sharp pain or physical sensation

breast pang → *angina pectoris*

panhypogammaglobulinemia → *hypogammaglobulinemia*

panmyelopathia → *panmyelopathy*

panmyelopathy *Syn: panmyelopathia*; disease of the blood formation system, which affects all cell series in the bone marrow and is characterized by a reduction in the amount of blood forming marrow; clinically it is usually a severe aplastic anemia with granulocytopenia and thrombocytopenia; if only two cell series are affected, it is called **bi-cytopenia**, otherwise **tri-cytopenia**

constitutional infantile panmyelopathy *Syn: congenital aplastic anemia, congenital hypoplastic anemia, congenital pancytopenia, Fanconi's anemia, pancytopenia-dysmelia syndrome, Fanconi's pancytopenia*; inherited disorder of hematopoiesis affecting all series in the bone marrow, i.e., it causes anemia, granulocytopenia, and thrombocytopenia; in addition, there are malformations [microcephaly, hypogonadism, hypo- or aplasia of the forearm or wrist]; bone marrow transplantation can cure the panmyelopathy, but most patients die from malformations of the internal organs or common malignancies [e.g., leukemia] before reaching adulthood

panmyelophthisis → *aplastic anemia*

pansystolic → *holosystolic*

pantoprazole irreversible proton pump inhibitor; **usage**: gastric or duodenal ulcer, reflux esophagitis, Zollinger-Ellison syndrome

panzerherz → *armored heart*

papulosis the occurrence of numerous papular lesions
  malignant atrophic papulosis → *Degos' syndrome*

paracardiac situated beside the heart

paracentesis surgical puncture or tapping of a fluid-filled body cavity
  paracentesis of heart → *cardiocentesis*

parafunction → *dysfunction*

paraganglion *Syn: chromaffin body, pheochrome body*; epithelial cell clusters arising from sympathetic or parasympathetic nerve cells, which produce hormones [adrenaline, noradrenaline]
  jugular paraganglion *Syn: jugular body, tympanic body*; parasympathetic paraganglion in the wall of the superior jugular bulb

parahemophilia → *factor V deficiency*

paramyloidosis → *primary amyloidosis*

paranephros → *adrenal gland*

parasympathicotonia → *vagotonia*

parasympatholytic → *anticholinergic*

parasympathoparalytic → *anticholinergic*

parasystole → *parasystolic rhythm*

parasystolic relating to parasystole

paravascular situated beside a vessel

Pardee Q *s.u. myocardial infarction*
pars part, portion
    pars atlantica *Syn: atlantic part of vertebral artery; s.u. vertebral artery*
    pars cavernosa arteriae carotidis internae portion of the internal carotid artery running in the cavernous sinus
    pars cerebralis arteriae carotidis internae intradural/cerebral portion of the internal carotid artery
    pars cervicalis arteriae carotidis internae cervical portion of the internal carotid artery
    pars cervicalis arteriae vertebralis *Syn: cervical part of vertebral artery; s.u. vertebral artery*
    pars intracranialis *Syn: intracranial part of vertebral artery; s.u. vertebral artery*
    pars intracranialis arteriae vertebralis *Syn: intracranial part of vertebral artery; s.u. vertebral artery*
    pars membranacea septi interventricularis upper, membranous part of the interventricular septum
    pars muscularis septi interventricularis lower, muscular part of the interventricular septum
    pars petrosa arteriae carotidis internae petrosal portion of the internal carotid artery
    pars prevertebralis *Syn: prevertebral part of vertebral artery; s.u. vertebral artery*
    pars transversaria *Syn: transverse part of vertebral artery; s.u. vertebral artery*
part division, portion
    abdominal part of aorta → *abdominal aorta*
    ascending part of aorta *Syn: aorta ascendens; s.u. aorta*
    atlantic part of vertebral artery *Syn: pars atlantica; s.u. vertebral artery*
    cavernous part of internal carotid artery portion of the internal carotid artery running in the cavernous sinus
    cerebral part of internal carotid artery intradural portion of the internal carotid artery
    cervical part of vertebral artery *Syn: pars cervicalis arteriae vertebralis; s.u. vertebral artery*
    descending part of aorta *Syn: aorta descendens; s.u. aorta*
    intracranial part of vertebral artery *Syn: pars intracranialis arteriae*

vertebralis; *s.u. vertebral artery*

membranous part of interventricular septum upper, membranous part of the interventricular septum

parasympathetic part of autonomic nervous system → *parasympathetic nervous system*

prevertebral part of vertebral artery *Syn:* pars prevertebralis; *s.u. vertebral artery*

thoracic part of aorta → *thoracic aorta*

transverse part of vertebral artery *Syn:* pars transversaria; *s.u. vertebral artery*

passage channel, duct; opening, pore

respiratory passages → *respiratory tract*

patho- combining form denoting relation to disease

pathogen microorganism, which causes infection

pathogenic *Syn: morbific, morbigenous, nosogenic, nosopoietic, peccant*; causing disease, causing sickness

pathway path, course, route; a bundle of myelinated nerve fibers following a path through the brain

extrinsic pathway *s.u. fibrinolysis*

extrinsic pathway of coagulation *s.u. blood coagulation*

intrinsic pathway *s.u. fibrinolysis*

intrinsic pathway of coagulation *s.u. blood coagulation*

peccant → *pathogenic*

pefloxacin synthetic chinolone antibiotic; gyrase inhibitor with a broad spectrum of activity against Gram-positive and Gram-negative organisms

peliosis → *purpura*

penbutolol beta-blocker

pengitoxin digitalis glycoside

penicillin antibiotic from Penicillium notatum discovered by Alexander Fleming in 1928; the term is used today for all natural or synthetic antibiotics that are derived from penicillin; a feature common to all penicillins is a main skeleton [**6-aminopenicillanic acid**] containing a β-lactam ring; the bacteriostatic action of penicillin is based on inhibition of murein synthesis in the bacterial wall by irreversible complex formation with glycopeptide transpeptidase

benzathine penicillin G poorly soluble depot penicillin for intramuscular injection

benzyl penicillin → *penicillin G*

clemizole penicillin depot form of benzylpenicillin

depot penicillins penicillins whose absorption is delayed by the formation of poorly soluble salts, e.g., benzathine penicillin G

penicillin G *Syn: benzylpenicillin, benzyl penicillin, penicillin II*; penicillinase-sensitive penicillin; **indications**: gram-positive and gram-negative causative agents [streptococci, pneumococci, gonococci, meningococci, treponemas, leptospiras, and spirochaetes]

penicillin G benzathine → *benzylpenicillin benzathine*

penicillin II → *penicillin G*

penicillin V *Syn: phenoxymethylpenicillin*; acid-fast oral penicillin; it is more effective against gram-positive than gram-negative bacteria, especially against β-hemolytic group A streptococci

penicillin amide-β-lactamhydrolase → *penicillinase*

penicillinase *Syn: penicillin amide-β-lactamhydrolase, penicillin beta-lactamase*; enzyme produced by bacteria; it cleaves the beta-lactam ring and as a result makes penicillin ineffective

pentalogy a combination of five simultaneous defects or symptoms

pentalogy of Cantrell malformation syndrome of unexplained etiology with abdominal wall defects [rectus diastasis up to omphalocele], cleft sternum, median diaphragmatic defect, partial pericardial defect and heart defects

pentalogy of Fallot tetralogy of Fallot with additional atrial septal defect

peptide compound consisting of two or more amino acids in which the carboxyl group of one acid is linked to the amino group of the other

brain natriuretic peptide *Syn: B-type natriuretic peptide*; polypeptide produced mainly in the ventricular muscle cells and released in response to excessive stretching of the myocardium; binds to and activates atrial natriuretic factor receptors [NPRA, NPRB]; decreases systemic vascular resistance and central venous pressure thus increasing cardiac output and natriuresis, leading to a decreased blood volume

B-type natriuretic peptide → *brain natriuretic peptide*

peracute *Syn: fulminant, fulminating, superacute*; (*course, reaction*) extremely acute, hyperacute

percussion tapping of the body surface; this external action causes tissues to vibrate; the resulting percussion sound depends substantially on the air content in tissues or organs; this makes it possible to distinguish, e.g., air-containing tissues [e.g., lung] from tissues that do not contain air [e.g., liver, heart]; in **direct** or **immediate percussion**, the

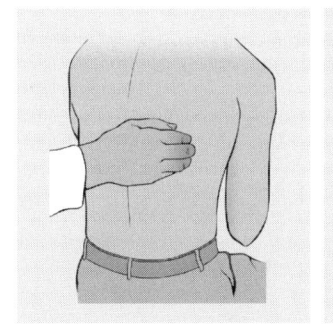

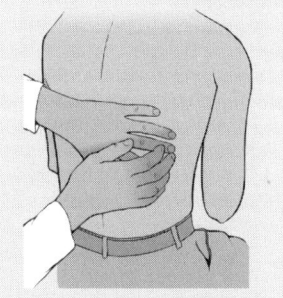

Percussion. Direct percussion [left]; indirect percussion [finger percussion] [right]

fingers [held together] of one hand are used to tap directly on the wall of the abdomen, chest, etc.; the sound is relatively quiet; in **indirect** or **mediate percussion**, a finger or a pleximeter is placed on the skin and then tapped; the percussion sound is much louder than with the direct method

perfusion 1. blood flow through an organ or tissue **2.** perfusion of an organ or a tissue with fluid

impaired perfusion *Syn: disturbance of perfusion*; reduced perfusion of an organ or tissue

peri- combining form denoting relation to around

periadventitial around the adventitia

periangiitis *Syn: periangitis, perivasculitis*; inflammation of the tissue surrounding a vessel

periangitic relating to or marked by periangiitis

periangitis → *periangiitis*

periaortic around the aorta

periaortitic relating to or marked by periaortitis

periarterial around an artery

periarteritic relating to or marked by periarteritis

periarteritis *Syn: exarteritis*; inflammation of the arterial adventitia and the surrounding connective tissue

periatrial *Syn: periauricular*; around the atrium

periauricular → *periatrial*

pericardectomy → *pericardiectomy*
pericardiac → *pericardial*
pericardial *Syn:* *pericardiac*; relating to the pericardium
pericardicentesis → *pericardiocentesis*
pericardiectomy *Syn:* *pericardectomy*; partial or complete removal of the pericardium, e.g., in constrictive pericarditis
pericardiocentesis *Syn:* *pericardicentesis*; puncture of the pericardial sac to relieve pressure in pericardial effusion or pericardial tamponade
pericardiolysis operative release of the adherent pericardium
pericardiomediastinitis *Syn:* *mediastinopericarditis*; inflammation of the pericardium and adjacent connective tissue of the mediastinal space
pericardiopleural relating to or associated with the pericardium and pleura
pericardiorrhaphy suture of the pericardium
pericardiostomy operative fenestration of the pericardium, e.g., to evacuate an effusion
pericardiotomy *Syn:* *pericardotomy*; operative opening of the pericardium
pericarditic relating to or marked by pericarditis
pericarditis infective or sterile inflammation of the pericardial sac, which often leads to involvement of the myocardial layers adjacent to the epicardium and always results in the formation of an effusion [**pericardial effusion**]; in at least half of the pericardial inflammations, no

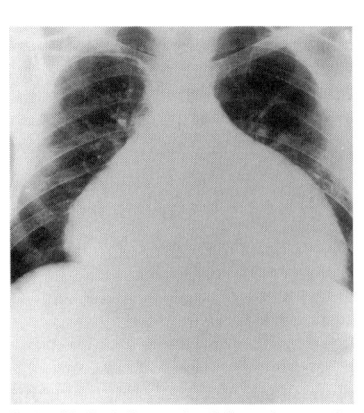

Pericarditis. Typical water-bottle heart due to pericardial effusion cause can be found [idiopathic pericarditis], the rest is made up of infective pericarditis as well as pericarditides as accompaniments to diseases affecting adjacent organs [e.g., myocardial infarction, myocarditis], in metabolic disorders [predominantly uremia], tumors, etc.; the clinical course can be used to differentiate acute pericarditis, chronic pericarditis and constrictive pericarditis, with each acute pericarditis, regardless of cause, having the capacity to change from an acute to a chronic relapsing course; the relapses are generally sterile, post-infective autoimmune disorders; **clinical signs** of pericarditis or a pericardial effusion include a pericardial rub, muffled heart sounds, engorgement of the neck veins, peripheral edema, ascites, arterial hypotension, and pulsus paradoxus; in the **ECG** there is usually elevation of the ST-segments, low voltage peripherally, and centrally and possibly electrical alternans; the **X-ray** shows a typical **bent box shape** with large effusions; **echocardiography**; **pericardial tap** and microbiologic/serologic/biochemical/cytologic/immunologic examination of the aspirate helps to identify the cause; the **therapy** depends heavily upon the etiology and genesis; it is the mainstay of treatment of pericardial effusions or the pericardial tamponade that they cause; further therapy is then aimed at the cause

acute pericarditis in most of the acute forms, there is formation of fibrinous coverings, which, by friction, produce significant precordial pain and presystolic, systolic, and early diastolic pericardial friction rubs; the rapid development of a pericardial effusion leads to compression of the ventricle and possibly the atria; ventricular filling is impaired with engorgement of the neck veins and a reduction in cardiac minute volume and blood pressure; **clinical** and **therapy** *s.a. pericarditis*

acute fibrinous pericarditis acute inflammation of the pericardium with precipitation of fibrin, which presents as dry pericarditis [without effusion] or serous pericarditis [with effusion]

adhesive pericarditis *Syn: adherent pericardium*; pericardial inflammation leading to adhesions

amebic pericarditis inflammation of the pericardial sac in the context of extra-intestinal amebiasis

bacterial pericarditis usually purulent pericarditis mostly caused by staphylo-, strepto-, or pneumococci; follows the clinical course of sepsis with high fever and rigors; the mortality is up to 50%; **therapy**: surgical opening of the pericardium and insertion of a suction/irrigation drain; high-dose antibiotics

carcinous pericarditis → *pericardial carcinomatosis*

chronic pericarditis inflammation of the heart sac, which lasts for more than three months; progresses as either a **chronic non-constrictive pericarditis** or a **chronic constrictive pericarditis**; since the effusion generally develops slowly, the pericardium stretches and in extreme cases can contain up to 2 l of effusion without signs of pericardial tamponade; both primary chronic pericarditis and chronic pericarditis developing from an initial acute pericarditis are due to autoimmune inflammations; **therapy** therefore generally consists of anti-inflammatories as well as corticosteroids and azathioprine in severe or refractory cases

chronic constrictive pericarditis *s.u. chronic pericarditis*

chronic non-constrictive pericarditis *s.u. chronic pericarditis*

constrictive pericarditis inflammation of the heart sac with fibrotic constriction and adhesion of the two layers of the pericardium [concretio pericardii]; leads to a restriction in diastolic ventricular filling, which can no longer adjust to loads but rather remains more or less constant; the performance of the heart can therefore only be adjusted by an increase in the heart rate and in the late stages this leads to compensatory tachycardia even at rest; otherwise, the features are typical of right heart failure [peripheral edema, ascites] and liver engorgement; **therapy**: (partial) resection of the pericardium

dry pericarditis *s.u. fibrinous pericarditis*

external pericarditis → *pleuropericarditis*

fibrinous pericarditis initial phase of acute pericarditis with fibrin deposition and resultant severe precordial pain and presystolic, systolic, and early diastolic pericardial rub; as long as no effusion develops, this is called **dry pericarditis**

hemorrhagic pericarditis pericarditis with bloody pericardial effusion; mostly occurs in viral or tuberculous pericarditis, more rarely in idiopathic pericarditis

idiopathic pericarditis most common form [> 50%] of pericarditis; caused by primary and secondary [postinfective] autoimmune processes; progresses as a sterile, serous, or fibrinous, or more rarely a hemorrhagic inflammation; it has a high tendency to recur and can easily convert to a chronic pericarditis; **therapy**: anti-inflammatories; in severe or refractory cases corticosteroids and azathioprine

infectious pericarditis caused for the most part by viruses [coxsackie-, echo-, measles-, mumps-, rubella-, cytomegalovirus] [30–50%]; bacteria [staphylo-, strepto- or pneumococci] and fungi [mainly in immunocompromised patients] generally cause purulent pericarditis, while viral pericarditis runs a course of serous, fibrinoid, or hemorrhagic inflammation; pericarditis caused by protozoa [Amoebas, Toxoplasma] is practically only encountered in patients with seriously compromised immune systems [predominantly HIV Infection]

obliterating pericarditis adhesive pericarditis leading to obliteration of the pericardial sac

postinfarction pericarditis pericarditis in transmural myocardial infarction; caused by necrosis and the inflammatory response; mostly progresses as fibrinous or hemorrhagic pericarditis

purulent pericarditis → *pyopericarditis*

rheumatic pericarditis involvement of the pericardium in the setting of rheumatic fever; mostly a pancarditis

serofibrinous pericarditis exudative pericarditis with serofibrinous effusion

serous pericarditis pericardial inflammation with pericardial effusion

tuberculous pericarditis now rare form of pericarditis, characterized by a serohemorrhagic exudate

uremic pericarditis involvement of the pericardium presenting as fibrinous pericarditis in the setting of acute or chronic renal failure with uremia

pericardium → *pericardial sac*
  adherent pericardium → *adhesive pericarditis*
  cardiac pericardium → *epicardium*
  parietal pericardium parietal layer of the pericardium, which is firmly attached to the fibrous pericardium; lies opposite the visceral layer; between them lies the pericardial cavity, which is filled with serous fluid [**liquor pericardii**]
  visceral pericardium → *epicardium*

pericardotomy → *pericardiotomy*

pericyte connective-tissue cells about capillaries or other small blood vessels
  capillary pericytes → *Rouget's cells*

pericytes → *adventitial cells*

peridiastole → *prediastole*

peridiastolic → *prediastolic*

perimyocarditic relating to or marked by perimyocarditis
perimyoendocarditis → *pancarditis*
perindopril ACE inhibitor, antihypertensive
period a particular stage or point of advancement in a cycle, phase
  ejection period the second half of systole, during which the bloodstreams out of the heart into the systemic and pulmonary circulations
  relaxation period *s.u. cardiac cycle*
  Wenckebach period type 1 2. degree AV-block
periphlebitic relating to periphlebitis
periphlebitis inflammation of the tissue surrounding a vein
peripneumonia → *pleuropneumonia*
peripneumonitis → *pleuropneumonia*
perisystole → *presystole*
peritoneopericardial relating to peritoneum and pericardium
perivascular *Syn: circumvascular*; situated around a vessel
perivasculitic relating to or marked by perivasculitis
perivasculitis *Syn: periangiitis, periangitis*; inflammation of the tissue surrounding a vessel
periventricular around a ventricle
petechia *Syn: petechial bleeding, petechial hemorrhage*; point bleeding, punctate bleeding
petechial (*bleeding*) punctuate, patchy
phagocyte *Syn: carrier cell*; cell that can take up animate or inanimate particles and break them down, e.g., monocytes, granulocytes, histiocytes; also a description of osteoclasts or macrophages
pharmacoradioangiography X-ray contrast demonstration of vessels with simultaneous administration of pharmaceuticals [e.g., vasoconstrictors]
phase a particular stage or point of advancement in a cycle, period
  contraction phase *s.u. cardiac cycle*
  deformation phase *s.u. cardiac cycle*
  depolarization phase *s.u. action potential*
  filling phase *Syn: filling phase; s.u. diastole*
  pressure-increase phase *s.u. cardiac cycle*
  rapid filling phase *s.u. diastole*
  repolarization phase *s.u. action potential*
phenomenon sign, symptom
  Ashley's phenomenon → *Aschner's reflex*

Austin Flint phenomenon *Syn: Austin Flint murmur, Flint's murmur*; heart sound in aortic insufficiency caused by an accompanying functional mitral stenosis; late diastolic, low-frequency sound at the cardiac apex; only occurs in severe aortic insufficiency

blue toe phenomenon blue discoloration of one or more toes in acute ischemia, e.g., in arterial embolism or peripheral arterial occlusive disease

Doppler phenomenon → *Doppler effect*

Goldblatt's phenomenon → *Goldblatt's mechanism*

Hecht phenomenon *Syn: Leede-Rumpel phenomenon, Rumpel-Leede phenomenon, Rumpel-Leede sign, bandage sign*; s.u. *Rumpel-Leede test*

Leede-Rumpel phenomenon *Syn: Rumpel-Leede phenomenon, Rumpel-Leede sign, bandage sign, Hecht phenomenon*; s.u. *Rumpel-Leede test*

Raynaud's phenomenon *Syn: Raynaud's disease*; secondary Raynaud's disease

R-on-T phenomenon collision of the R waves of an early ventricular extrasystole with the T wave of the preceding heartbeat; can lead to ventricular tachycardia or fibrillation; occurs more frequently in the early stages of a myocardial infarction

Rumpel-Leede phenomenon *Syn: Rumpel-Leede sign, bandage sign, Hecht phenomenon, Leede-Rumpel phenomenon*; s.u. *Rumpel-Leede test*

steal phenomenon *Syn: steal*; symptoms caused by diversion or deflection of blood; can be caused by, e.g., stenosis, occlusion, anastomosis, or collateral circulation

T-P phenomenon ECG change that develops in metabolic or respiratory alkalosis with relative prolongation of the ST-interval in sinus tachycardia; this places the P-wave of the next contraction immediately after the T-wave of the previous heartbeat

walk-through phenomenon in peripheral arterial occlusive disease with intermittent claudication [Fontaine stage II], exertion leads initially to pain, which disappears if the patient keeps going, i.e., the patients can "walk through" the pain

phenoxymethylpenicillin *Syn: penicillin V*; acid-fast oral penicillin; it is more effective against gram-positive than gram-negative bacteria, especially against β-hemolytic group A streptococci

α-phenoxypropylpenicillin → *propicillin*

phentolamine α-blocker; **indications**: severe acute heart failure with pulmonary edema

phenytoin → *diphenylhydantoin*

phlebalgia pain in or along a vein or varicose vein, e.g., in thrombophlebitis

phlebectasia *Syn: phlebectasis, venectasia*; uniform dilatation of a vein; in contrast to varices, the wall is unchanged and the typical tortuosity is absent

phlebectasis → *phlebectasia*

phlebectomy *Syn: venectomy*; operative (partial) removal of a vein, e.g., in varicose veins

phlebemphraxis → *venous thrombosis*

phlebexairesis inflammation of veins (phlebitis) that have undergone varicose change

phlebitic relating to phlebitis

phlebitis inflammation of the vein wall; can affect parts of or the whole wall [panphlebitis]

    iron wire phlebitis venous inflammation predominantly affecting the legs with hardening of the vein wall, although this does not lead to thickening of the vessels

    migrating phlebitis recurrent, multifocal inflammation of the small and medium sized [subcutaneous] veins, e.g., in thromboangiitis obliterans, Behçet's disease or systemic lupus erythematosus; if there is recurrent superficial and deep thrombosis with emboli in combination with malignancy [mostly mesothelioma] this is referred to as **Trousseau's syndrome** [thrombophlebitis migrans]

    productive phlebitis → *phlebosclerosis*

phlebo- combining form denoting relation to a vein or veins

phlebodynamometry measurement of the venous pressure at rest and during exertion

phlebofibrosis connective tissue fibrosis in the wall of a vein

phlebogenous arising from a vein, deriving from a vein

phlebogram *Syn: venogram*; X-ray contrast image of veins

phlebograph apparatus for phlebography

phlebography *Syn: venography*; X-ray contrast demonstration of veins following direct [i.v. injection, venous catheter] or indirect [injection into an upstream artery] application of contrast agent; the main area of use is in the diagnosis of thrombosis, embolism, post-thrombotic syndrome, and venous insufficiency

phleboid → *venous*

phlebolite → *phlebolith*

phlebolith *Syn: calcified thrombus, phlebolite, vein stone*; concretion arising from calcification of a thrombus; mostly a chance finding of no clinical significance

phlebolithiasis asymptomatic occurrence of phleboliths

phlebology study of the veins and their diseases

phlebophlebostomy *Syn: venovenostomy*; operative connection of two veins or two sections of vein

phleboplasty plastic surgery on veins, e.g., Palma operation

phleborrhagia → *venous bleeding*

phleborrhaphy *Syn: venesuture, venisuture*; suturing of a vein after traumatic or operative division or incision

phleborrhexis tear in or rupture of the wall of a vein

phlebosclerosis *Syn: productive phlebitis, proliferative endophlebitis, venosclerosis*; thickening and hardening of the vein wall; usually combined with phlebectasia; therapeutically following sclerosant treatment of varices

phleboscopy phlebography under fluoroscopic control

phlebostasia → *phlebostasis*

phlebostasis *Syn: phlebostasia*; reduction of the venous return by congestion of the extremities for a maximum of 30 minutes; a procedure only rarely performed in pulmonary edema; superseded nowadays by rapidly acting diuretics

phlebothrombosis *Syn: venous thrombosis*; non-inflammatory thrombosis affecting the deep veins with occlusion of the lumen; thrombosis of superficial veins is called thrombophlebitis

phlebothrombosis of the leg → *leg vein thrombosis*

phlebotomy 1. operative exposure and opening of a vein **2.** incision into a vein

phonoangiography eliciting of sound phenomena over vessels

phonocardiogram graphical representation obtained by phonocardiography

phonocardiograph apparatus for phonocardiography

phonocardiographic relating to phonocardiography

phonocardiography eliciting of sound phenomena over the heart

phosphatidylcholine *Syn: choline phosphatidyl, choline phosphoglyceride, lecithin*; basic module of the cell membrane made from choline, glycerin, phosphoric acid, and fatty acids

phosphatidylcholine-cholesterol acyltransferase → *lecithin-cholesterol acyl-*

transferase

phosphoglyceride amphiphilic lipid, which contains glycerophosphoric acid; among others, phosphatidylcholine, phosphatidylserine, phosphatidylethanolamine, phosphatidylinositol, cardiolipin, lysophosphatidylcholine, and their plasma analogs belong to the group

phosphonomycin → *fosfomycin*

photometer an instrument for measuring a property of light, especially luminous intensity or flux

flow photometer *s.u. flow cytometry*

photoscan photographic representation of radioactive impulse density with a **photoscanner**

photoscanner *s.u. photoscan*

phrenocardia → *neurocirculatory asthenia*

phrenopericarditic relating to or marked by phrenopericarditis

phrenopericarditis pericarditis with extension into the surrounding diaphragm; can lead to adhesion of the cardiac apex and diaphragm

pi- combining form denoting relation to fat or lipid

piesis → *blood pressure*

pigment a substance that produces a color in tissue

blood pigment → *hemoglobin*

pill small pellet or tablet of medicine, often coated, taken by swallowing whole or by chewing

water pill → *diuretic*

pimelo- combining form denoting relation to fat or lipid

pimobendan calcium sensitizer; acts as a positive inotrope and inhibits phosphodiesterase III in the myocardium

pindolol β_1- and β_2-blocker, antihypertensive; **usage**: sinus tachycardia, supraventricular tachycardia, atrial fibrillation, essential tremor

pio- combining form denoting relation to fat or lipid

pionemia → *lipemia*

pipamperone butyrophenone derivative; neuroleptic; **usage**: disturbances of sleep-wake cycle, sleep disorders, confusion, psychomotor agitation, mood lability

pipemidic acid gyrase inhibitor, antibiotic; acts mainly against Gram-negative organisms

piperacillin acylaminopenicillin with a broad action spectrum against gram-positive and gram-negative pathogens; at present, it is one of the strongest antibiotics

pirenzepine parasympatholytic; **usage**: gastric or duodenal ulcers, stress ulcers, gastritis

piretanide loop diuretic

pivampicillin semisynthetic penicillin with a broad action spectrum

plaque plate-like embossment of the skin or mucous membrane

plasm → *plasma*

plasma *Syn: blood plasma, plasm*; the cell-free blood fluid makes up approx. 54–56% of the blood volume; 1 kg of plasma consists of 900–910 g of water, 65–80 g of plasma proteins and 20 g small molecules [mainly electrolytes, glucose, urea]; the specific gravity is around 1.025–1.029 and the pH value in the region of 7.37–7.43; the majority of the more than 100 plasma proteins are synthesized in the liver and the lymphatic tissues; most compounds are not pure proteins, rather they contain sugar or lipid moieties [glycoprotein, lipoprotein]; the separation technique generally used, electrophoresis, produces five fractions, of which the albumins form the largest fraction at 55–70%; since they are primarily formed in the liver, their concentration is a measure of liver function; the globulins are a heterogenous group, which differ from the albumins in their shape and lower worse water solubility; they are subdivided into α_1-, α_2-, β- and γ-globulins depending upon their electrophoretic speed; the main roles of the plasma proteins are the maintenance of a constant blood volume and pH value, their function as transporters for water-insoluble substances [bilirubin, cholesterol], metals [iron], hormones [cortisol], and vitamins [vitamin B_{12}], their involvement in blood clotting and hemolysis, defense against pathogenic organisms and toxins, as well as their involvement in the acute phase reaction of inflammation

blood plasma → *plasma*

citrated plasma plasma prevented from clotting by the addition of citrate

plasmapheresis separation of the blood plasma from the blood cells; the plasma can be cleaned and then reinfused together with the cells or the cells can be reinfused together with foreign plasma, plasma substitute, etc.; used, for example, to promote perfusion in disturbances of arterial perfusion, rapidly progressive glomerulonephritis, hemolytic-uremic syndrome, or autoimmune diseases

plasma renin activity *Syn: plasma renin assay*; the rate at which renin cleaves angiotensinogen to form angiotensin I per unit time; expressed in nanograms per milliliter per hour (ng/ml/hr); the normal adult value is 0.2 to 4 ng/ml/hr, depending on salt intake and the time the patient has been in an upright position before the test [an upright position raises production of renin, and a high salt intake lowers it]; PRA may be used to screen for renal hypertension or in the diagnosis of primary aldosteronism; it is also an independent predictor of cardiovascular morbidity and mortality

plasma renin assay → *plasma renin activity*

plasma renin concentration *Syn: renin mass*; a direct measure of the level of the renin in the plasma; determines the concentration of renin molecules, both active and inactive, whereas plasma renin activity measures the enzymatic activity of activated renin only; expressed in pg/ml or ng/l

plasmatherapy therapy/treatment with (blood) plasma

plasmin → *fibrinolysin*

plasmokinin → *factor VIII*

plasmozyme → *prothrombin*

plateletpheresis → *thrombapheresis*

platelets → *thrombocytes*

   blood platelets → *thrombocytes*

pleio- combining form denoting relation to many or much

pleo- combining form denoting relation to many or much

plethora overfilling (with blood), i.e., elevation of the blood volume due to increased plasma [**plethora serosa**], elevation of the cell count [**plethora polycythaemica**], or elevation of both components [**plethora vera** or **sanguis**]

pleura glossy, smooth serous membrane lining the thoracic cavity [**parietal pleura/pleura parietalis**] and investing the lung [visceral pleura/pleura pulmonalis]; the capillary space between the parietal pleura and visceral pleura forms the **pleural cavity** [cavitas pleuralis]; so-called reserve spaces [recessus pleurales] are found at the junctions of the different portions of the pleura; these can expand during deep inspiration and enlarge the pleural cavity; the **tela subserosa** of the pleura lies on the surface of the chest wall and lung; the mesothelium of the **epithelial lamina** [lamina epithelialis] changes its form depending on the breathing position; during inhalation it is flat and becomes cubic during exhalation; the **pleural borders** diverge from the lung borders only in the area of the pleural recesses; they move downward during inhalation and upward during exhalation

pleura pericardiaca → *pericardial pleura*

pericardial pleura *Syn: pleura pericardiaca*; the portion of the pleura

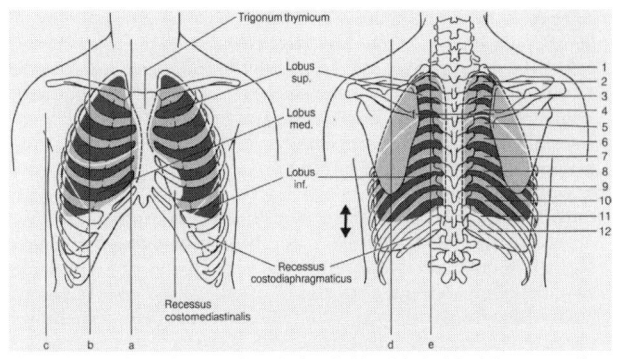

Pleura. Pleura and pleural margins from the front [left] and the back [right]. a = sternal line; b = midclavicular line; c = axillary line; d = scapular line; e = paravertebral line

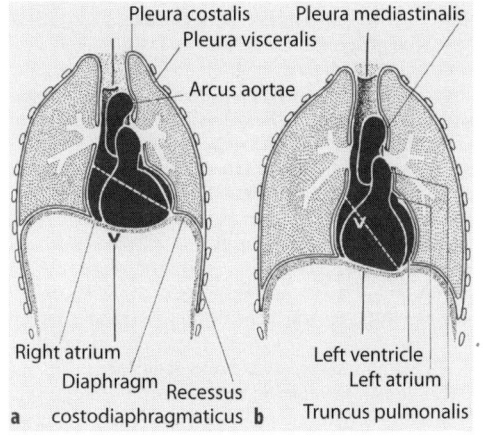

Pleura. Pleura and pleural spaces during maximum expiration [**a**] and maximum inspiration [**b**]

adjacent to the pericardium

pleura pulmonalis → *pulmonary pleura*

pulmonary pleura *Syn: visceral pleura, pleura visceralis, pleura pulmonalis*; the pleura investing the lung externally [exception: hilum]; it extends between the lobes up to the root of the lung [radix pulmonis]

visceral pleura → *pulmonary pleura*

pleura visceralis → *pulmonary pleura*

pleuracotomy → *thoracotomy*

pleurisy *Syn: pleuritis*; inflammation of the parietal or visceral pleura; depending on the localization, it is called **parietal pleurisy** [parietal pleura], **pulmonary pleurisy** [pulmonary pleura], or **costal pleurisy** [costal pleura]; there are also forms affecting the diaphragmatic pleura [**diaphragmatic pleurisy**] or mediastinal pleura [**mediastinal pleurisy**]; the most frequent causes of pleurisy are bacterial pneumonia, pulmonary tuberculosis, pulmonary infarction, viral infections, bronchiectases, and lung abscesses; almost all forms of pleurisy begin as dry pleurisy [pleuritis sicca] with deposition of fibrin on the pleura; sharp, respiration-dependent chest pain, hacking cough, fever, and shallow breathing with guarding and pleural friction rub are seen **clinically**; in the second phase, exudate formation [exudative pleurisy] occurs, which improves the clinical symptomatology; the exudate is usually serous but can also be serosanguineous or purulent [pleural empyema]; dyspnea may occur with massive effusions; **diagnosis**: chest X-ray, CT, exploratory puncture with ultrasound monitoring; **therapy**: in aseptic pleurisy, analgesics and treatment of the primary illness; the effusion can be removed by puncture and aspiration

costal pleurisy *Syn: pleuritis*; *s.u. pleurisy*

pulmonary pleurisy *Syn: visceral pleurisy*; *s.u. pleurisy*

visceral pleurisy → *pulmonary pleurisy*

pleuritis → *pleurisy*

pleuropericardial relating to or associated with the pleura and pericardium

pleuropericarditic relating to or marked by pleuropericarditis

pleuropericarditis *Syn: external pericarditis*; inflammation of the pericardium [pericarditis] and the adjacent pleura [pleurisy]; the inflammation can originate primarily in the pericardium and then spread to the pleura or vice versa

pleuropneumonectomy surgical removal of a lung together with the pleura

pleuropneumonia *Syn: peripneumonia, peripneumonitis, pneumopleuritis,* *pneumonopleuritis, pleuritic pneumonia*; pneumonia accompanied by pleurisy [**secondary pleurisy**]

pleuropneumonolysis surgical separation of adhesions between the lung and pleura [costal pleura]

pleuropneumopericardiectomy →*pleuropneumo-pericardiectomy*

pleuropneumo-pericardiectomy *Syn: pleuropneumopericardiectomy; s.u. pleural mesothelioma*

pleuropneumo-pericardio-diaphragmectomy *Syn: pleuropneumopericardiophrenectomy; s.u. pleural mesothelioma*

pleuropneumopericardio-phrenectomy →*pleuropneumo-pericardio-diaphragmectomy*

pleuropulmonary relating to or associated with the pleura and lung(s)

pleurorrhea →*pleural effusion*

pleurotomy →*thoracotomy*

plexus a network (of nerves or vessels)

anterior cardiac plexus →*superficial cardiac plexus*

cardiac plexus autonomic plexus lying between the aorta and pulmonary trunk, whose fibers run to the working muscles, but particularly to the sinoatrial node and AV-node

plexus cardiacus →*cardiac plexus*

plexus cardiacus profundus →*deep cardiac plexus*

plexus cardiacus superficialis →*superficial cardiac plexus*

deep cardiac plexus *Syn: great cardiac plexus*; posterior, larger part of the cardiac plexus

great cardiac plexus →*deep cardiac plexus*

internal carotid venous plexus venous plexus in the carotid canal

periarterial plexus autonomic plexus that surrounds arteries

plexus periarterialis →*periarterial plexus*

superficial cardiac plexus *Syn: anterior cardiac plexus*; anterior, smaller part of the cardiac plexus

Trolard's plexus →*venous plexus of hypoglossal canal*

vascular plexus **1.** network built from blood or lymphatic vessels **2.** autonomic nerve plexus; mostly as a peri-arterial plexus

plexus vascularis →*vascular plexus*

plexus venosus →*venous plexus*

plexus venosus canalis hypoglossi *Syn: Trolard's net, Trolard's network, Trolard's plexus*; venous plexus in the hypoglossal canal

plexus venosus caroticus internus →*internal carotid venous plexus*

venous plexus *Syn: venous network, venous plexus*; network built from veins

venous plexus of hypoglossal canal *Syn: Trolard's net, Trolard's network, Trolard's plexus*; venous plexus in the hypoglossal canal

plica fold; mucosal fold

plica venae cavae sinistrae → *fold of left vena cava*

pluri- combining form denoting relation to many or much

pneumal → *pulmonary*

pneumathemia → *air embolism*

pneumato- combining form denoting a relationship to **1.** air/gas **2.** breath/breathing

pneumatocardia occurrence of free air in the heart

pneumatohemia → *air embolism*

pneumatosis gas or air collection in the tissues, organs, or body cavities

pneumatothorax → *pneumothorax*

pneumo- combining form denoting a relationship to **1.** air/gas **2.** breath/breathing **3.** lung **4.** lung inflammation/pneumonia

pneumocardial *Syn: cardiopulmonary*; relating to or associated with the lung(s) and heart

pneumococcemia *Syn: pneumococcal sepsis*; presence of pneumococci in the blood

pneumococcus → *Streptococcus pneumoniae*

pneumohemia → *air embolism*

pneumohemopericardium *Syn: hemopneumopericardium*; collection of air and blood in the pericardium

pneumohydropericardium → *hydropneumopericardium*

pneumonedema → *pulmonary edema*

pneumonia *Syn: lung inflammation*; inflammation of the lung parenchyma with involvement of the alveoli [**alveolar pneumonia**] and the interstitium [**interstitial pneumonia**], which can be caused by chemical, physical, or infectious factors or allergic reactions, with infectious pneumonia being by far the most frequent; pneumonia can be subdivided by anatomical/histological aspects [e.g., focal pneumonia, lobular pneumonia] or according to its clinical course [acute or chronic pneumonia]; in the case of infectious pneumonias, a distinction is made between **typical pneumonia** [i.e., bacterial pneumonia] and **atypical** or **nonbacterial pneumonia**, but this term is used more and more often only for Mycoplasma pneumoniae pneumonia; many physicians today prefer to differentiate **nosocomial pneumonia** [hospital-acquired pneumonia] and **community-acquired pneumonia**, because these differ considerably in their pathogen spectrum and treatment

pleuritic pneumonia → *pleuropneumonia*

viral pneumonia atypical pneumonia caused by viruses; viral pneumonias are found rarely in adults outside of epidemics [e.g., influenzal pneumonia]

pneumonic → *pulmonary*

pneumonococcus → *Streptococcus pneumoniae*

pneumonopleuritis → *pleuropneumonia*

pneumopericardium air collection in the pericardium

pneumophagia → *aerophagy*

pneumopleuritis → *pleuropneumonia*

pneumopyopericardium air and pus collection in the pericardium

pneumoradiography X-ray demonstration using air as a negative contrast agent

pneumothorax *Syn: pneumatothorax*; collection of air in the pleural space with partial or total lung collapse; in **open pneumothorax** there is a connection to the airways of the lung or to the outside; a **closed pneumothorax** is present when there is no connection to the external air;

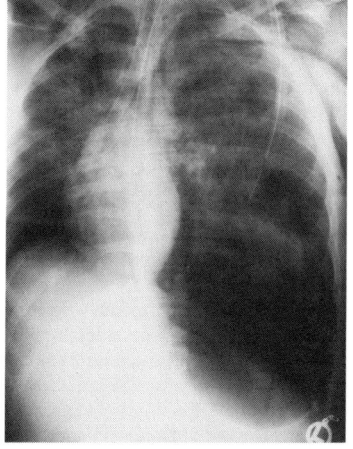

Pneumothorax. Tension pneumothorax on the left side

it becomes life-threatening acutely, when a highly positive pressure forms due to valve action or positive pressure breathing; this so-called **tension pneumothorax** displaces the heart and mediastinum to the opposite side and impedes venous reflux in the inferior and superior vena cava; this results in hypotension, tachycardia, and dyspnea; a drain must be placed in the fourth intercostal space in the anterior axillary line as **emergency treatment**

pressure pneumothorax → *tension pneumothorax*

spontaneous pneumothorax pneumothorax occurring spontaneously, i.e., without injury; it either has no apparent cause [**idiopathic spontaneous pneumothorax**] or, as **symptomatic spontaneous pneumothorax,** is the result of a progressing disease or prior damage, especially in bronchiectasis

tension pneumothorax *Syn: pressure pneumothorax; s.u. pneumothorax*

pocket any pouch-like receptacle, compartment, hollow, or cavity

Zahn's pocket pocket-like outpouching of the parietal endocardium in the wall of the left ventricle beneath the aortic valve; develops due to the increased pressure in aortic stenosis or the retrograde blood flow in aortic valve insufficiency

point the precise location of something; a spatially limited location

auscultation point point on the body surface at which a particular heart sound or murmur is best heard

upper reversal point beginning of the final negative deflection in the ECG, i.e., the interval from the start of the Q-wave to the peak of the R-wave

poisoning *Syn: intoxication*; disease caused by intake of poisonous substances [**exogenous intoxication**] or the formation of a toxin in the body [**autointoxication**]; **clinical features** and **therapy** depend upon the nature of the poisoning; however, the mainstay is always securing the vital functions [breathing, circulation] and prevention of further intake of poison [e.g., gases]; it is important to begin decontamination as soon as possible, although in uncertain cases this can be delayed until hospital admission; inappropriate measures [e.g., induced vomiting in alkaline or acid burns] can worsen the existing injuries or even produce a life-threatening situation

blood poisoning → *septicemia*

cyanide poisoning *Syn: cyanide intoxication*; poisoning characterized by a pink color, bitter almond-like odor in the breath, and shortness of breath; possible suffocation by inhibition of intracellular respiratory enzymes; **therapy**: sodium thiosulfate i.v., assisted ventilation with oxygen

poly- combining form denoting relation to many or much
polyangiitic relating to or marked by polyangiitis
polyangiitis inflammation of several blood vessels
polyarteritic relating to or marked by polyarteritis
polyarteritis inflammation affecting multiple arteries
    benign cutaneous polyarteritis nodosa special form of periarteritis nodosa restricted to the skin; typically there are pressure-sensitive, reddish-livid nodes up to the size of a plum, which ulcerate and heal with scarring; predominantly localized to the extensor surfaces of the legs; **therapy**: glucocorticoids orally or topically; in severe cases immunosuppression with azathioprine, methotrexate, or cyclophosphamide
polyarthritis inflammation of several joints
    acute rheumatic polyarthritis → *rheumatic fever*
polycardia → *tachycardia*
polycythemia *Syn: erythrocythemia*; increased numbers of red blood corpuscles in the blood; often used synonymously with polycythemia
    benign polycythemia → *Gaisböck's syndrome*
polygeminy disturbance of heart rhythm with variable numbers of extrasystoles
polymer a compound formed from two or more compounds
    fibrin polymers *s.u. fibrin*
polyp any mass of tissue protruding from a mucous membrane
    cardiac polyp organized thrombus sitting on the endocardium
polyplasmia → *dilution anemia*
polythiazide thiazide diuretic; **usage**: saluretic, antihypertensive
position a bodily posture or attitude
    squatting position → *squatting*
post-acute (occurring) after the acute stage of an illness
postapoplectic (occurring) after an apoplectic attack
postcava → *inferior vena cava*
postdiastolic (occurring) after diastole
postextrasystolic occurring after an extrasystole, following an extrasystole
posthemorrhagic (occurring) after bleeding
postinfectious *Syn: postinfective*; (occurring) after an infection or infec-

tious disease
postinfective → *postinfectious*
postischemic (occurring) after ischemia
postpneumonic *Syn: metapneumonic*; (occurring) after pneumonia
post-thrombotic (occurring) after thrombosis
potassium *Syn: kalium*; silvery-white metallic element
  potassium canrenoate aldosterone antagonist, antihypertensive diuretic
potential → *latent*
  action potential brief changes in membrane potential during excitation; in principle, this involves rapid depolarization from a resting potential to a positive potential and an automatic return [repolarization] to the resting potential; the course of repolarization is typical for different cells; an action potential is triggered if the membrane is depolarized from the resting potential up to about -50 mV; as soon as the **threshold potential** is reached, the excitation begins and the action potential proceeds in stereotypic fashion [all-or-none law of excitation]; the first phase of the action potential, the **depolarization phase** lasts approx. 0.2–0.5 msec and is therefore significantly shorter than the **repolarization phase**, which can last up to 200 msec [heart muscle]
  resting potential the potential difference between the inner and outer surface of a membrane at rest; depending upon the cell type, it lies between -120 mV and -40 mV; determined by the difference in the intra- and extracellular concentration of sodium, potassium, and chloride ions, of which the K^+-equilibrium is the most important; the activity of the Na^+/K^+-ATPase in the cell membrane is of great importance for the stability of the membrane potential; if it fails, the resting potential approaches zero, because the intracellular Na^+-concentration increases and the K^+-concentration falls
PRA → *plasma renin activity*
prajmalium bitartrate membrane-stabilizing antiarrhythmic; **usage**: ventricular extrasystoles
prazosin selective α_1-blocker, antihypertensive; **usage**: arterial hypertension, cardiac insufficiency, Raynaud's disease
PRC → *plasma renin concentration*
preaortic in front of or anterior to the aorta
precardiac *Syn: precordial*; in front of or anterior to the heart
precava → *superior vena cava*

precordial *Syn: precardiac*; in front of or anterior to the heart
precordialgia pain in the region of the heart
precursor *Syn: progenitor, precursor cell; s.u. blood formation*
  angiotensin precursor → *angiotensinogen*
prediastole *Syn: late systole, peridiastole*; the phase immediately before diastole
prediastolic *Syn: peridiastolic*; (occurring) before diastole
preexcitation premature excitation of parts of the ventricular muscle
  ventricular preexcitation → *preexcitation syndrome*
preload the preload on the heart muscle before it contracts caused by stretching during filling
presbycardia heart disease due to the physiologic reduction in exercise capacity of the heart with aging
presso- combining form denoting relation to weight or pressure
pressoreceptive *Syn: pressosensitive*; reflecting changes in pressure
pressoreceptor *Syn: pressosensor*; receptor in the vessel wall sensitive to pressure and volume changes; the **arterial pressure receptors** sit at the junction between the media and adventitia of the large thoracic and cervical arteries; they are important limbs in the reflex loop controlling the arterial blood pressure; if the arterial pressure increases, the pressure receptors send inhibitory impulses to the neurons in the medulla oblongata, which control the circulation; this leads to a reflex reduction in the cardiac minute volume and total peripheral resistance and thereby a drop in arterial blood pressure
pressosensitive → *pressoreceptive*
pressosensor → *pressoreceptor*
pressure force per unit area
  blood pressure *Syn: arteriotony, hematopiesis, piesis*; the pressure prevailing in the vessels of the systemic and pulmonary circulation; the rhythmic activity of the heart makes the blood pressure value fluctuate between high values for the **systolic blood pressure** and low values for the **diastolic blood pressure**; the **arterial blood pressure** differs significantly from the **venous blood pressure**; the changing perfusion requirements of the individual organs, which often oppose each other or concur with each other, demand constant control and adjustment of the whole circulation, and above all of the mean arterial pressure; while acute regulation of the arterial pressure is mainly mediated by the baroreceptors of the carotid sinus and aorta, the long-term regulation depends upon adjustment of the blood volume by changes in

water excretion in the kidney; the blood pressure values depend upon the position of the patient, their level of activity, the mental state, etc.; to exclude all of these factors as far as possible, the **resting blood pressure** is measured in the sitting or lying position; in healthy adults between the ages of 20 and 40 years, the average value for the systolic blood pressure is around 120 mmHg and for the diastolic blood pressure around 80 mmHg; these values increase somewhat with increasing age, with the systolic pressure increasing more steeply than the diastolic; according to the WHO the normal value for the systolic pressure is less than 140 mmHg and for the diastolic pressure less than 90 mmHg; resting values of 160 mmHg systolic and 95 mmHg diastolic characterize hypertension

capillary pressure blood pressure in the capillaries; approx. 6–12 mmHg at heart level at rest

carbon dioxide partial pressure → CO_2 *partial pressure*

central aortic pressure blood pressure within the aorta; considered to be a stronger indicator of cardiovascular risk in hypertensive patients than blood pressure in peripheral arteries, such as brachial blood pressure

central venous pressure average pressure in the right atrium or superior vena cava; measured by central venous catheter with a catheter manometer or a riser; the normal value lies between 4 and 12 cm H_2O

colloid osmotic pressure the osmotic pressure exerted by macromolecules in colloidal solutions; due to the size of the molecules, it is relatively small; in the blood plasma, it is around 25 mmHg, in the interstitium, 5–8 mmHg; it is important for capillary filtration and reabsorption in the tissues and the kidney

CO_2 partial pressure *Syn: carbon dioxide partial pressure, pCO_2 partial pressure*; partial pressure of carbon dioxide in a gas mixture; in the alveolar gas mixture and the arterial blood, it is around 40 mmHg, in the venous blood around 46 mmHg

high blood pressure → *arterial hypertension*

intraventricular pressure pressure in a cardiac ventricle

low blood pressure reduction in the arterial blood pressure to values below 105/60 mmHg; hypotension itself is not a disease, rather it only needs to be treated if it gives rise to symptoms [e.g., dizziness, tinnitus, autophony, tunnel vision] and the impaired state of health or performance that these cause; in most countries, hypotension is not recognized as a disease; division into **non-postural hypotension** [found in volume deficiency or cardiac diseases with hypotension] and **orthostatic hypotension**, which develops on standing, is more important than a division into essential and secondary hypotension; it may also be further divided into **non-autonomic-neurogenic** or **sympathicotonic hypotension** and **autonomic-neurogenic** or **asympathicotonic hypotension**; the Schellong standing test is the decisive diagnostic test; **therapy**: treatment of the cause in non-postural hypotension; in **sympathicotonic hypotension** no therapy is generally required; physical activity, possibly physiotherapy and morning exercises in bed before standing up, alternating hot and cold showers, massage, swim therapy, dosed administration of caffeine, etc., are usually sufficient; asympathicotonic hypotension can be treated with a combination of dihydroergotamine, fludrocortisone, and sympathomimetic therapy, although the effect is often insufficient

mean filling pressure *Syn: static blood pressure*; pressure in the entire circulation during acute cardiac standstill; it lies 6–7 mmHg above the central venous pressure

O_2 partial pressure → *oxygen partial pressure*

oxygen partial pressure *Syn: O_2 partial pressure*; proportion of oxygen with respect to the total pressure of the gas in blood or alveolar gas; at sea level, the **inspiratory oxygen partial pressure** is 150 mmHg and the **oxygen partial pressure of alveolar air** 100 mmHg; **arterial oxygen partial pressure** is 90 mmHg in adolescents, 80 mmHg at age 40, and 70 mmHg at age 70; the decline is likely due to the increasing distribution irregularities in the lung; **venous oxygen partial pressure**, on the contrary, is more or less constant and constitutes 40 mmHg

pCO_2 partial pressure → *CO_2 partial pressure*

precordial pressure feeling of pressure and tightness in the region of the heart, combined with ill-defined fear

pulmonary capillary wedge pressure → *wedge pressure*

static blood pressure → *mean filling pressure*

venous pressure pressure in the venous limb of the circulation

wedge pressure *Syn: pulmonary capillary wedge pressure*; the pressure in the pulmonary capillaries, which is measured with a pulmonary artery catheter; normally it is between 5 and 15 mmHg

presystole *Syn: perisystole*; the phase immediately before systole

presystolic relating to the beginning of the systole, just before the systole, late diastolic

primary 1. present from the outset, first, originally, primarily **2.** (arisen) without identifiable cause, independent of other diseases

principle rule, law

Doppler principle → *Doppler effect*

Fick's principle *Syn: Fick's method*; the amount of a specific substance that is taken up from or released into the blood in an organ or tissue can be calculated from the arteriovenous concentration difference of the substance and the perfusion volume per unit time

proaccelerin → *accelerator globulin*

procainamide *Syn: procaine amide*; local anesthetic of amide type [less powerful than procaine]; antiarrhythmic

procaine amide → *procainamide*

procedure method, technique; operation

Astrup procedure indirect determination of the carbon dioxide partial pressure in arterial blood or capillary blood; the sample is equilibrated with 2 gas mixtures of known composition, which have different CO_2 partial pressure; in both samples, the pH value is measured and entered into a nomogram; if one then measures the actual pH value, then this value can be equated to an actual CO_2 partial pressure; in addition, one can also read off the base excess and the concentration of buffer bases

proconvertin → *factor VII*

product something produced

fibrin degradation products → *fibrinolytic split products*

fibrinogen degradation products → *fibrinolytic split products*

fibrinolytic split products *Syn: fibrin degradation products, fibrinogen degradation products*; breakdown products of fibrin and fibrinogen, which have partial inhibitory actions on blood clotting; an elevation in the fibrin degradation products is a sign of increased fibrinolysis and is found in, e.g., hyperfibrinolysis, septic shock, pre-eclampsia, and missed abortion

progenitor *Syn: precursor, precursor cell*; *s.u. blood formation*

progressive *Syn: advancing*; increasing, developing further, worsening

prolonged → *protracted*

propafenone class IC antiarrhythmic; **usage**: ventricular extrasystoles and tachycardias, therapy-resistant atrial tachycardia

prophylactic *Syn: preventive, preventative, synteretic*; **1.** an agent with prophylactic properties **2.** relating to prophylaxis, preventing or warding off disease

prophylaxis prevention, preventive treatment
   antibiotic prophylaxis *Syn: prophylactic antibiotics*; prevention of illness by early prescription of antibiotics [e.g., pre-operative]
   chemical prophylaxis → *chemoprophylaxis*
   embolism prophylaxis measures to prevent embolism or thromboembolism, predominantly following trauma, operations, birth, or in bedbound patients [mainly patients with a history of cardiac insufficiency, varicose veins, thrombophlebitis, or thromboses]
propicillin *Syn: α-phenoxypropylpenicillin*; acid-fast oral penicillin; it is more effective against gram-positive than gram-negative bacteria, especially against β-hemolytic group A streptococci
Propionibacterium type of Gram-positive, immobile bacterial rods, which form the majority of the skin flora; are the cause of acne, endocarditis, and SAPHO syndrome
propranolol non-selective β-blocker; **usage**: arterial hypertension, atrial tachycardia, tachycardia in absolute arrhythmia, angina pectoris, coronary heart disease, migraine prophylaxis, essential tremor
proscillaridin cardiac glycoside; generally only used if digitalis cannot be tolerated
prostaglandin any of a group of hormone-like substances produced in various tissues that are derived from amino acids
   prostaglandin E_1 → *alprostadil*
prosthesis replacement
   bifurcated prosthesis *Syn: bifurcation prosthesis*; vascular prosthesis of the aortic bifurcation
   bifurcation prosthesis → *bifurcated prosthesis*
   Starr-Edwards prosthesis heart valve prosthesis in the form of a ball valve
   vascular prosthesis vessel replacement made from plastic
protein any of a group of complex organic macromolecules composed of one or more chains of amino acids
   protein C vitamin K-dependent inhibitor of blood clotting; made as an inactive proenzyme in the liver, which is activated on the endothelial surface under the influence of thrombomodulin
   channel protein proteins incorporated into membranes, which permit diffusion of molecules, particularly anions and cations, along a concentration gradient; the most common are ion channels for sodium, calcium, potassium, and chloride ions
   ion channel protein proteins incorporated into membranes, which

permit diffusion of anions and cations along a concentration gradient; the most common are ion channels for sodium, calcium, potassium, and chloride ions

plasma protein the majority of more than 100 plasma proteins is synthesized in the liver and the lymph tissues; most compounds are not pure proteins but rather contain sugar or lipid moieties [glycoprotein, lipoprotein]; the total protein content of the plasma is between 60 and 80 g/l; together with the proteins of the extracellular space, which are in dynamic equilibrium with the blood plasma proteins, the total protein content of the intra- and extra-vascular spaces is approx. 400 g; since many internal and external factors, congenital and acquired diseases, and diagnostic and therapeutic measures influence the qualitative and quantitative composition of the plasma proteins, quantitative determination of the proteins and the separation of the plasma proteins into individual fractions play an important role; the separation technique generally used, electrophoresis, produces five fractions, of which the albumins form the largest fraction at 55–70%; since they are primarily formed in the liver, their concentration is a measure of liver function; the globulins are a heterogenous group, which differ from the albumins in their shape and lower worse water solubility; they are subdivided into α_1-, α_2-, β- and γ-globulins depending upon their electrophoretic speed; the main roles of the plasma proteins are the maintenance of a constant blood volume and pH value, their function as transporters for water-insoluble substances [bilirubin, cholesterol], metals [iron], hormones [cortisol], and vitamins [vitamin B_{12}], their involvement in blood clotting and hemolysis, defense against pathogenic organisms and toxins, as well as their involvement in the acute phase reaction of inflammation

proteinemia an excess of protein in the blood

broad-beta proteinemia → *type III familial hyperlipoproteinemia*

floating-beta proteinemia → *type III familial hyperlipoproteinemia*

proteinuria *Syn: albuminuria, serumuria*; increased loss of protein in the urine (> 150 mg/24 h) or disturbance of the pattern of distribution of the physiologically excreted proteins; since albumin represents approx. 60% of the excreted proteins, it is generally referred to as albuminuria

cardiac proteinuria *Syn: cardiac albuminuria*; prerenal proteinuria in renal engorgement due to circulatory disorders

prerenal proteinuria *Syn: prerenal albuminuria*; proteinuria as a result of a cause lying (physiologically) before the kidney, e.g., in cardiac insufficiency

prothrombin *Syn: factor II, plasmozyme, serozyme, thrombogen*; factor made in the liver; inactive precursor of thrombin; also belongs to the acute phase proteins

prothrombinopenia → *factor II deficiency*

prothrombokinase → *factor VII*

protodiastolic *Syn: early diastolic*; at the start of diastole

protoheme → *heme*

protopathic → *idiopathic*

protracted *Syn: prolonged*; (acting or maintained) over a prolonged timescale, delayed, prolonged, deferred

pseudocirrhosis → *cardiac cirrhosis*

pseudohemophilia → *von Willebrand's syndrome*

  hereditary **pseudohemophilia** → *von Willebrand's syndrome*

pteropterin → *folic acid*

pteroylglutamic acid → *folic acid*

pulmo- combining form denoting a relationship to lung/pulmo

pulmonal → *pulmonary*

pulmonary *Syn: pulmonal, pulmonic, pneumal, pneumonic*; relating to the lungs

pulmonic → *pulmonary*

pulmono- combining form denoting a relationship to lung/pulmo

pulsatile *Syn: pulsative, pulsatory, throbbing*; (rhythmically) percussive or tapping, thumping, pulsating

pulsating → *systaltic*

pulsative → *pulsatile*

pulsatory → *pulsatile*

pulse the rhythmic ejection of blood from the heart into the aorta and the pulmonary artery produces pulse waves, which propagate right to the capillaries; they consist of a **pressure pulse, flow pulse**, and **sectional pulse** [also **volume pulse**]; as long as the pulse waves only run in one direction, all three pulse types have the same waveform; in places where the wave resistance varies [e.g., branching points, changes in diameter, wall thickness, or elasticity], the pulse wave reflects, causing partial superposition of the reflected wave and peripherally running ones, which leads to an increase in the pressure pulse amplitude and a decrease in the flow pulse amplitude; pressure pulse, flow pulse, and sectional pulse all increase at the start of systole and reach their maximal value approximately at the end of the first third of systole; the maximal flow amplitude of the aorta is then about 500–600 ml/s and the maximal flow velocity is approx. 120 cm/s; in the second half of systole, the pressure pulse, flow pulse, and sectional pulse all reduce; at the beginning of systole, there is a brief period of retrograde flow toward the heart in the vessels near the heart, which is shown on the pressure pulse as an inflection

alternating pulse *Syn: pulsus alternans*; alternatively stronger and weaker pulse, mainly in cardiac insufficiency

bigeminal pulse *Syn: bigeminus, coupled beat, paired beat, coupled pulse, coupled rhythm; s.u. bigeminy*

capillary pulse → *Quincke's pulse*

carotid pulse palpable pulse of the common carotid artery in the neck

contracted pulse small, firm pulse, e.g., in arteriosclerosis

coupled pulse *Syn: coupled rhythm, bigeminal pulse, bigeminus, coupled beat, paired beat; s.u. bigeminy*

cross-sectional pulse *Syn: sectional pulse, volume pulse; s.u. pulse*

dicrotic pulse double peak in the peripheral pulse wave

dropped-beat pulse → *intermittent pulse*

equal pulse *Syn: pulsus aequalis*; equally strong pulse

filiform pulse *Syn: thready pulse*; fine, thready pulse, mainly in circulatory collapse or shock

flow pulse *s.u. pulse*

frequent pulse fast/frequent pulse, e.g., in tachycardia

hard pulse hard, tight pulse, mainly in arterial hypertension

infrequent pulse → *rare pulse*

intermittent pulse *Syn: dropped-beat pulse*; missed pulse; pulse deficit

irregular pulse physiologic in association with breathing in/out [pulsus irregularis respiratorius], pathologic in disturbances of rhythm

Kussmaul's pulse → *paradoxical pulse*

Kussmaul's paradoxical pulse → *paradoxical pulse*

ladder pulse *s.u. Mahler's sign*

long pulse creeping pulse with slow rise, e.g., in aortic stenosis

nail pulse *s.u. Quincke's pulse*

paradoxical pulse *Syn: Kussmaul's paradoxical pulse, Kussmaul's pulse*; reduction of the blood pressure amplitude by more than 10 mmHg during inspiration [normally less than 5 mm]; mainly found in constrictive pericarditis and accretio pericardii

pressure pulse slower, wider pulse due to raised intracranial pressure

Quincke's pulse *Syn: capillary pulse, Quincke's sign*; visible pulsation of capillaries [e.g., **nail pulse**] in aortic insufficiency or other diseases with increased blood pressure amplitude

radial pulse radial artery pulse; felt proximal to the wrist and lateral to the tendon of the flexor carpi radialis muscle

rare pulse *Syn: infrequent pulse, slow pulse*; slow pulse, e.g., in bradycardia

sectional pulse *Syn: cross-sectional pulse, volume pulse*; s.u. pulse

short pulse accelerating pulse due to a sudden increase in pressure and a rapid pressure reduction, e.g., in aortic insufficiency

slow pulse → *rare pulse*

soft pulse easily compressed pulse, mainly in hypotension

strong pulse *Syn: pulsus magnus*; large amplitude pulse with strong pulse wave, e.g., in aortic insufficiency

thready pulse → *filiform pulse*

trigeminal pulse → *trigeminy*

vibrating pulse pulse with a thrill over the artery

volume pulse *Syn: cross-sectional pulse, sectional pulse*; s.u. pulse

weak pulse small pulse amplitude, in aortic and mitral stenosis

wiry pulse clinical description of a very hard pulse with small amplitude, which is caused by simultaneous increase in the systolic and diastolic blood pressure values

pulselessness *Syn: acrotism*; absence of or inability to register the pulse

pulsus → *pulse*

   pulsus aequalis → *equal pulse*
   pulsus alternans → *alternating pulse*
   pulsus celer → *short pulse*
   pulsus contractus → *contracted pulse*
   pulsus dicrotus → *dicrotic pulse*
   pulsus durus → *hard pulse*
   pulsus filiformis → *filiform pulse*
   pulsus frequens → *frequent pulse*
   pulsus intermittens → *intermittent pulse*
   pulsus irregularis → *irregular pulse*
   pulsus irregularis respiratorius s.u. irregular pulse
   pulsus magnus → *strong pulse*
   pulsus mollis → *soft pulse*
   pulsus paradoxus → *paradoxical pulse*
   pulsus parvus → *weak pulse*

pulsus rarus → *rare pulse*
pulsus regularis regular pulse
pulsus tardus → *long pulse*
pulsus vibrans → *vibrating pulse*
pump-oxygenator → *heart-lung machine*
punctum → *point*
punctum maximum → *auscultation point*
purpura *Syn: peliosis*; reddening of the skin and mucous membranes that cannot be made to blanch by compression using a glass slide and that can be seen in bleeding [e.g., thrombocytopenic purpura] and injuries to the vessel wall [e.g., necrotizing vasculitis]; depending upon the configuration and depth of the bleeding, one can differentiate petechiae and suggillations [small macules], ecchymoses [large macules], suffusions [larger areas], vibices [stripes], and hematomas [deep]

idiopathic thrombocytopenic purpura *Syn: essential thrombocytopenia, land scurvy, thrombocytopenic purpura, thrombopenic purpura, Werlhof's disease*; purpura that runs a chronic course or one progressing in acute pulses and that is caused by transient thrombocyte deficiency, which in 60–80% of cases is due to the development of autoantibodies against thrombocytes; in the **acute form**, there are skin and mucous membrane hemorrhages, nosebleeds, oral bleeds and pharyngeal bleeds, melena, and hematuria; the **chronic form** is more impressive for its gum bleeding, prolonged and increased menses, nosebleeds, petechiae on the lower legs, and circumscribed cutaneous and mucous membrane bleeds

thrombocytopenic purpura → *idiopathic thrombocytopenic purpura*
thrombopenic purpura → *idiopathic thrombocytopenic purpura*
thrombotic thrombocytopenic purpura → *thrombotic microangiopathy*
pyemic relating to or suffering from pyemia
pyopericarditic relating to or marked by pyopericarditis
pyopericarditis *Syn: purulent pericarditis*; acute suppurative inflammation of the pericardium by bacteria or, more rarely, fungi
pyopericardium *Syn: empyema of the pericardium*; pus collection in the pericardial sac
pyopneumopericardium pus and air collections in the pericardial sac
pyridostigmine cholinergic drug
pyridostigmine bromide reversible cholinesterase inhibitor; parasympathomimetic; **usage**: myasthenia gravis, glaucoma, bladder or intestinal atonia, meteorism, paroxysmal tachycardia

Q

quality character, nature
  pulse qualities one assesses frequency [e.g., rapid or slow pulse], rhythm [e.g., regular, irregular], strength [e.g., strong, weak], amplitude [e.g., high, low], and pressure rise [e.g., fast or slow rising]

quinidine *Syn: betaquinine, conquinine*; alkaloid derived from chinchona; classic antiarrhythmic, which stabilizes the membrane of the heart cells and thereby has negative chronotropic, dromotropic, and inotropic actions; **usage**: atrial flutter, atrial fibrillation, prophylaxis of paroxysmal supraventricular tachycardia; **side effects**: allergic reactions, gastrointestinal pains, tinnitus, double vision, disturbances of color vision, allergic thrombocytopenia, tachycardia, psychotic reactions; **contraindications**: 2. and 3. degree AV-block, cardiac insufficiency, hyperkalemia, digitalis intoxication

quinolones → *gyrase inhibitors*

quotient the number obtained by dividing one quantity by another
  blood quotient *Syn: color index, globular value*; quotient derived from the hemoglobin and erythrocyte count; replaced nowadays by the pigmentation coefficient

R

radiocardiogram image obtained by radiocardiography

radiocardiography cardiography using radionuclides; permits the assessment of important cardiac parameters [cardiac minute volume, stroke volume, residual volume, wall mobility, circulation time]

radioelectrocardiography → *telelectrocardiography*

radiography the process of making a radiograph; producing an image on a radiosensitive surface by radiation

   double-contrast radiography *Syn: air-contrast barium enema, double-contrast barium technique, mucosal relief radiography*; X-ray contrast demonstration of hollow organs, body or joint cavities by simultaneous use of a contrast agent and gas or air; the positive contrast agent [barium, iodine] spreads over the wall, while the gas or air serves as a negative contrast agent and unfolds the object under study

   mucosal relief radiography → *double-contrast radiography*

radiokymography recording of the movement of an organ on an image; mostly by demonstration of heart wall and vessel pulsation

radiotelemetry → *biotelemetry*

rales *Syn: crackles, rhonchi, adventitious sounds*; sounds heard over the lung on auscultation, which have their origin in the large or small bronchi

   bronchial rales → *bronchial breathing*

   bubbling rales *Syn: coarse crepitations; s.a. moist rales*

   coarse bubbling rales *Syn: gurgling rales; s.u. moist rales*

   crackling rales *Syn: fine bubbling rales, fine crepitations; s.u. moist rales*

   dry rales *Syn: dry adventitious sounds, sibilant and sonorous rhonchi*; sounds that arise due to obstruction of the airways, e.g., by bronchial spasms, mucosal swelling, secretions, or air trapping, and are audible primarily during exhalation; the dry rales arising in the large bronchi are low in frequency and give the impression of snoring or buzzing [**sonorous rhonchi**]; they are loud sounds, which can be heard over the chest wall and orally; they are typical for chronic obstructive bronchitis in emphysema or bronchial asthma, smoker's bronchitis, and acute tracheobronchitis; the dry rales of the small bronchi are high in frequency and are called wheezing and whistling [**sibilant rhonchi**]; they are soft sounds that are audible only over the chest wall and are usually heard in bronchial asthma [caution: the more severe the asthma, the fewer the sibilant rhonchi!]

fine bubbling rales *Syn: crackling rales; s.u. moist rales*

gurgling rales *Syn: coarse bubbling rales; s.u. moist rales*

medium bubbling rales *Syn: subcrepitant rales; s.u. moist rales*

moist rales *Syn: moist adventitious sounds*; rales caused by the accumulation of secretions in the bronchi; they are divided by type into **coarse bubbling**, **medium bubbling**, and **fine bubbling rales**; they are divided by tone into **sonorous** [high-pitched, high frequency] or **nonsonorous rales** [low-pitched, low frequency]; moist rales arising in the large bronchi are medium to coarse bubbling and low-frequency [**deep bubbling**]; they are loud sounds, which can be heard over the chest wall and orally; they occur primarily early during inspiration but rarely also during a combination of inspiration/expiration; they are typical for chronic obstructive bronchitis in emphysema or bronchial asthma, bronchiectases, and acute bronchitis; moist rales of the small bronchi are fine to medium bubbling and high-frequency [**fine crackling**]; they are soft sounds that are audible only over the chest wall; because they arise with the sudden expansion of previously closed airways during inhalation, they are heard only late in inspiration; they are typical for restrictive lung diseases [e.g., fibrosis, fibrosing alveolitis, scleroderma], pneumonia, and pulmonary congestion in heart failure

non-sonorous rales *s.u. moist rales*

sibilant rales *Syn: sibilant rhonchi; s.u. dry rales*

sonorous rales *Syn: sonorous rhonchi; s.u. dry rales, moist rales*

subcrepitant rales *Syn: medium bubbling rales; s.u. moist rales*

ramipril ACE inhibitor, antihypertensive

ramus branch, branching; division, twig

rami atriales arteriae coronariae dextrae *Syn: atrial branches of right coronary artery; s.u. right coronary artery of heart*

rami atriales arteriae coronariae sinistrae *Syn: atrial branches of left coronary artery; s.u. left coronary artery of heart*

ramus atrialis anastomoticus arteriae coronariae sinistrae *Syn: anastomotic atrial artery; s.u. left coronary artery of heart*

ramus atrialis intermedius arteriae coronariae dextrae *Syn: intermediate atrial branch of right coronary artery*; *s.u. right coronary artery of heart*

ramus atrialis intermedius arteriae coronariae sinistrae *Syn: intermediate atrial branch of left coronary artery*; *s.u. left coronary artery of heart*

rami atrioventriculares arteriae coronariae dextrae *Syn: atrioventricular branches of right coronary artery*; *s.u. right coronary artery of heart*

rami atrioventriculares arteriae coronariae sinistrae *Syn: atrioventricular branches of left coronary artery*; *s.u. left coronary artery of heart*

rami bronchiales aortae thoracicae → *bronchial arteries*

rami cardiaci thoracici nervi vagi thoracic cardiac branches of the vagus nerve

ramus circumflexus arteriae coronariae sinistrae *Syn: circumflex branch of left coronary artery*; *s.u. left coronary artery of heart*

ramus coni arteriosi arteriae coronariae dextrae *Syn: right conal artery, right conus artery, third conus artery*; branch of the right coronary artery to the conus arteriosus

ramus coni arteriosi arteriae coronariae sinistrae *Syn: left conal artery, left conus artery*; branch of the left coronary artery to the conus arteriosus

ramus interventricularis anterior *Syn: anterior interventricular branch*; *s.u. left coronary artery of heart*

ramus interventricularis posterior arteriae coronariae dextrae *Syn: posterior interventricular branch of right coronary artery*; *s.u. right coronary artery of heart*

ramus lateralis interventricularis anterior arteriae coronariae sinistrae *Syn: lateral branch of anterior interventricular branch of left coronary artery*; *s.u. left coronary artery of heart*

ramus marginalis dexter *Syn: right marginal artery*; *s.u. right coronary artery of heart*

ramus marginalis sinister *Syn: left marginal artery*; *s.u. left coronary artery of heart*

rami mediastinales arteriae thoracicae internae *Syn: anterior mediastinal arteries*; mediastinal branches of the internal thoracic artery

rami mediastinales partis thoracicae aortae mediastinal branches of the thoracic aorta [aorta thoracica]

ramus nodi atrioventricularis arteriae coronariae dextrae *Syn: atrio-*

ventricular nodal artery; branch of the right coronary artery to the atrioventricular node

ramus nodi atrioventricularis arteriae coronariae sinistrae *Syn: atrioventricular nodal artery*; branch of the left coronary artery to the atrioventricular node

ramus nodi sinuatrialis arteriae coronariae dextrae *Syn: nodal artery, sinoatrial nodal artery, sinuatrial nodal artery, sinus node artery*; branch of the right coronary artery to the sinoatrial node

ramus nodi sinuatrialis arteriae coronariae sinistrae *Syn: nodal artery, sinoatrial nodal artery, sinuatrial nodal artery, sinus node artery*; branch of the left coronary artery to the sinoatrial node

rami pericardiaci aortae thoracicae *Syn: posterior pericardiac arteries*; pericardial branches of the thoracic aorta

rami subendocardiales *Syn: subendocardial terminal network*; s.u. cardiac conducting system

RAAS renin-angiotensin-aldosterone system

rate a measure of the frequency

decay rate loss of efficacy of a pharmaceutical per day, mainly the cardiac glycosides; for example, for digitoxin it is approx. 7%, for digoxin approx. 30%, and for strophanthin approx. 40%

erythrocyte sedimentation rate determination of the sedimentation rate of erythrocytes in blood rendered unclottable; in a healthy man, it is 3–6 mm in the first hour, in a woman 8–10 mm; the blood corpuscle sedimentation is a non-specific parameter, which can be elevated in inflammation and tumors; the blood corpuscle sedimentation rate is mainly influenced by the constitution of the blood plasma; an increase in the albumin concentration reduces the blood corpuscle sedimentation, whereas an increase in the levels of fibrinogen, acute phase proteins, and immunoglobulins leads to an increase in sedimentation; a reduction in the hematocrit as well as various drugs [e.g., acetylsalicylic acid] and steroid hormones increase the blood corpuscle sedimentation; the measurement is usually performed using the **Westergren method**: 1.6 ml of blood is sampled from the antecubital vein using a 2 ml syringe containing 0.4 ml Na-citrate solution; the blood, which has been rendered unclottable, is placed into a **Westergren tube** that has a 200 mm graduated scale and the tube is positioned vertically; the sedimentation is read off after 1 h and 2 h

heart rate number of heartbeats per minute; normally the same as the pulse rate

pulse rate pulse in beats per minute; usually the same as the heart rate

urinary albumin excretion rate *Syn: urine albumin excretion rate*; the amount of albumin excreted in urine in a pre-specified time interval, usually 24 hours; studies have shown that albuminuria is predictive of increased renal and cardiovascular morbidity and mortality

urine albumin excretion rate → *urinary albumin excretion rate*

ratio a relationship between two quantities

LDL/HDL ratio relationship between LDL-cholesterol and HDL-cholesterol in the blood; values of > 5 [LDL-cholesterol > 135 mg/dl, HDL-cholesterol < 35 mg/dl] are associated with increased risk of arteriosclerosis

sodium-potassium ratio ratio of sodium to potassium in the urine; normally 1.0–2.0; lowered in sodium retention with edema, NaCl-poor diet, corticosteroid therapy and hyper-aldosteronism; increased in Addison's disease, laxative abuse, acute polyuric renal failure, and chronic diarrhea

urinary albumin/creatinine ratio → *urine albumin-to-creatinine ratio*

urine albumin-to-creatinine ratio *Syn: urinary albumin/creatinine ratio*; estimates 24-hour urine albumin excretion; as a ratio between two measured substances it is unaffected by variation in urine concentration; reducing urine albumin to the normal or near-normal range can improve the prognosis of renal and cardiovascular diseases

reaction 1. response, counteraction **2.** conversion of two or more reactants with the creation of new end products **3.** response of cells, tissues, and organs to chemical or physical stimuli

Eisenmenger's reaction hardening of the vessel wall and thereby an increase in vascular resistance in pulmonary circulation occur in the long term in a left-to-right shunt; if the pulmonary vascular resistance exceeds that of the systemic circulation, there is a shunt reversal, i.e., a right-to-left shunt forms with cyanosis

hemagglutination-inhibition reaction → *hemagglutination-inhibition assay*

hemolytic transfusion reaction hemolysis caused by antibodies against the donor erythrocytes; correct performance of a cross-match test before the transfusion practically excludes it; **clinical**: during or shortly after the transfusion, fever, rigors, malaise, chest pain, and shortness of breath may develop; this may be followed by shock, acute renal failure, and consumptive coagulopathy; in addition to this classic, acute, hemolytic **immediate reaction**, there are also rare **late reac-**

tions, which can develop after a latency of a few days to up to three weeks; they are mostly caused by antigens of the Kidd or Duffy blood groups and run a relatively mild course [fever, reduced hemoglobin, mild jaundice]

non-immunologic transfusion reactions *s.u. transfusion reactions*

transfusion reactions undesired side effects of the transfusion of blood or blood products; in addition to the mostly acute hemolytic transfusion reactions, there is a series of **non-immunologic transfusion reactions** that may run an acute or chronic course; these include fever and rigors due to pyrogens, transfusion acidosis and hyperkalemia, hypocalcemia due to the citrate used as a stabilizing agent, hypocoagulability due to dilution of the clotting factors, thrombocytopenia, infections [HIV, hepatitis], hypervolemia, and transfusion siderosis

reanastomosis operative reconnection of divided hollow organs, vessels or nerves

rebound sudden cessation of a medication after taking it for long periods can lead to an overshooting of the action the drug suppressed, e.g., tachycardia and blood pressure rise following cessation of beta-blockers

receptor 1. structure for sensing mechanical [**mechanoreceptor**], chemical [**chemoreceptor**], thermal [**thermoreceptor**], etc., stimuli **2.** defined binding point for molecules on a membrane surface

β **receptors** *Syn: β-adrenergic receptors, beta receptors, beta-adrenergic receptors*; receptors that respond to adrenergic transmitters [catecholamines] in the sympathetic system; they are subdivided into β_1-receptors [heart, kidney] and β_2-receptors [bronchi, vessels, fat tissue]

β-**adrenergic receptors** →β *receptors*

beta receptors →β *receptors*

beta-adrenergic receptors →β *receptors*

vascular receptors vessel receptors, e.g., chemoreceptors

recess →*recessus*

phrenicomediastinal recess *Syn: phrenicomediastinal sinus*; space between the diaphragmatic pleura and mediastinal pleura; it is part of the so-called reserve spaces [recessus pleurales]

pleural recesses *Syn: pleural sinus, reserve spaces, complemental spaces, recessus pleurales*; spaces occur at the junctions of the different sections of the visceral pleura, which expand during deep inhalation and thereby enlarge the pleural cavity

recessus *Syn: recess*; hollow, cavity, niche

recessus pleurales → *pleural recesses*
recording → *lead*
    limb recording → *limb lead*
reentry model to explain the development of extrasystoles by circular excitation
    AV nodal reentry s.u. *reentrant tachycardia*
reflex involuntary reaction in response to a stimulus
    aortic reflex → *depressor reflex*
    Aschner's reflex *Syn:* Aschner's sign, Ashley's phenomenon, *eyeball compression reflex, eyeball-heart reflex, oculocardiac reflex;* pressure over the eye leads to bradycardia, skin pallor, and nausea; found in childhood and in 50% of adults; can be used therapeutically in paroxysmal tachycardia
    Bainbridge reflex elevation of the heart rate and increase in the blood pressure in response to elevation of the pressure in the right atrium
    Bezold-Jarisch reflex reduction in the heart rate and diameter of the blood vessels following stimulation of certain heart muscle receptors; acts as a **protective reflex** in myocardial infarction
    carotid sinus reflex drop in blood pressure and heart rate following a blow over the carotid sinus
    depressor reflex *Syn: aortic reflex;* reflex arising in the pressure receptors, which regulates the blood pressure by reducing the arterial tone, e.g., Bezold-Jarisch reflex
    eyeball compression reflex → *Aschner's reflex*
    eyeball-heart reflex → *Aschner's reflex*
    Gauer-Henry reflex *Syn: Henry-Gauer reflex;* volume regulatory reflex controlling the renal excretion of water via stretch receptors in the atria; increase in the blood volume leads to a drop in the secretion of ADH and thereby to increased diuresis, while reduction in the blood volume produces increased secretion of ADH and reduces excretion of fluid through the kidney
    Henry-Gauer reflex → *Gauer-Henry reflex*
    oculocardiac reflex → *Aschner's reflex*
    physiologic reflex the majority of reflexes operate continuously and unnoticed and are parts of physiologic control loops, which regulate, e.g., muscle tone, cardiac output, blood pressure, carbon dioxide partial pressure
    pressoreceptor reflex → *carotid sinus syndrome*
    silver-wire reflexes → *silver-wire arterioles*

visceral reflex reflex affecting the internal organs, e.g., oculocardiac reflex

refractory *Syn: intractable*; not responding to therapy

regeneration restoration, reconstitution

    blood regeneration description of the physiologic breakdown of old erythrocytes and their replacement by new erythrocytes from the blood-forming tissues; the breakdown occurs in the cells of the reticuloendothelial system, mainly the spleen; increased breakdown, e.g., in hemoglobinopathies, therefore often leads to enlargement of the spleen [splenomegaly]

regurgitation backward flow, back-damming of blood due to insufficiency of a valve

    aortic regurgitation → *aortic insufficiency*

    mitral regurgitation → *mitral insufficiency*

    tricuspid regurgitation *Syn: tricuspid incompetence, tricuspid insufficiency*; mostly acquired inability of the tricuspid valve to close, mainly as functional tricuspid insufficiency due to dilatation of the valve ring in right ventricular enlargement due to pulmonary hypertension; rarely occurs in isolation, rather almost always combined with mitral valve defects; leads to systolic retrograde flow of blood into the right ventricle, obstruction to venous inflow and hepatomegaly; **clinical**: jugular venous pulse, liver enlargement with systolic pulsation, ascites and peripheral edema; on auscultation, possibly a pansystolic, high-frequency retrograde flow murmur with the maximum point at the right sternal border at the level of the 6. rib; **therapy**: surgical correction by annulorrhaphy or valve replacement

    valvular regurgitation *Syn: incompetence of the cardiac valves, regurgitant disease, valvular incompetence, valvular insufficiency*; congenital or acquired inability to close leads to retrograde blood flow during systole [insufficiency of the atrioventricular valves] or diastole [insufficiency of the aortic or pulmonary valve]; **relative** or **functional heart valve insufficiency** is caused by overdistension of a ventricle; the valve is no longer able to close completely and retrograde flow develops; *s.a. mitral insufficiency, aortic insufficiency, tricuspid insufficiency, pulmonary insufficiency*

reinfarction each infarction following the first myocardial infarct

remediable → *curative*

remedial → *curative*

remedy treatment, cure

coronary remedy agent for the treatment or palliation of coronary vascular diseases, in particular coronary heart disease and angina pectoris; these include, among others, organic nitrates, calcium antagonists, β-sympatholytics, and coronary vasodilators

renal *Syn: renogenic, nephric, nephritic, nephrogenous, nephrogenic*; relating to the kidney

renicapsule → *adrenal gland*

renin tissue hormone produced by the juxtaglomerular cells of the kidney; part of the renin-angiotensin-aldosterone system; stimulates the formation of angiotensin II in blood and tissues, which in turn stimulates the release of aldosterone from the adrenal cortex and causes vasoconstriction

renin-angiotensin-aldosterone system major regulatory system keeping the blood volume, osmolality, and pressure constant; is closely connected with atrial natriuretic peptide and brain natriuretic peptide; hypovolemia, reduced pressure in the afferent glomerular arteriole and reduction in the sodium concentration in the serum lead to increased renin secretion, which leads to increased formation of angiotensin II and stimulation of aldosterone secretion and vasoconstriction

renin mass → *plasma renin concentration*

reno- combining form denoting relation to the kidney(s)

renogenic → *renal*

renovascular relating to the renal vessels

reptilase enzyme [protease] made by the poisonous snake Bothrops atrox; formerly used as a hemostyptic; nowadays only used to determine the reptilase time

rescinnamine rauwolfia alkaloid; antihypertensive

reserpine rauwolfia alkaloid; inhibits dopamine uptake and reuptake of noradrenaline; **usage**: antihypertensive, centrally acting sedative

reserve something held back for later use

alkali reserve carbon dioxide binding capacity of the arterial blood; previously used as a parameter for assessing the acid-base balance, but now replaced by the standard bicarbonate

coronary reserve difference between the amount of oxygen supplied by the coronary blood flow and the requirements of the heart musculature

resistance *Syn: airway resistance*; resistance of the airways to the air stream that must be overcome during breathing; it is determined by whole body plethysmography; with steady mouth breathing, it is ap-

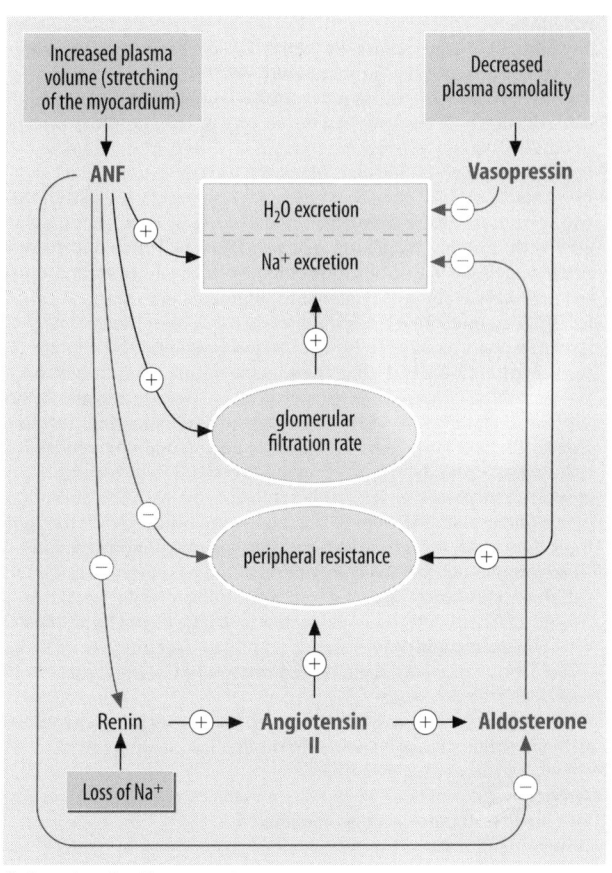

Renin-angiotensin-aldosterone system

proximately 2 cm of $H_2O/l/s$ [0.2 kPa/l/s]

antibiotic resistance natural or acquired resistance of microorganisms to antibiotics; **natural** or **primary antibiotic resistance** is due to genetically determined insensitivity, whereas **secondary** or **acquired antibiotic resistance** relates to selection pressure of the antibiotic; sensitive organisms die off, whereas those insensitive organisms found in any population grow unimpeded; the antibiotic can also induce changes in metabolism or structure and thereby trigger resistance; from these two considerations, it is clear that frequent use of antibiotics is associated with a higher likelihood that resistance will develop; the most important mode of resistance development is chromosomal mutation; in any bacterial colony, spontaneous mutations occur at a rate of 10^{-6} to 10^{-9}, i.e., mutations are always arising that alter metabolism, wall structure, etc.; most of these die off, but antibiotic use can act as a means of selection and offer the mutant optimal conditions; bacteria can inherit or pass on resistance genes in 3 ways: **transformation** [uptake of free DNA from the environment], **transduction** [transmission of the resistance gene by bacteriophages], and **conjugation** [direct transmission by means of sex pili from one cell to another]; the resistance mechanisms are divided into enzymatic inactivation [most common mechanism, e.g., β-lactamase], modification of the target molecule, modification of cell wall permeability, improved elimination from the cell, and overproduction of the target molecule

capillary resistance resistance of the capillary wall; measured by means of suction techniques or blood congestion [Rumpel-Leeds test]; reduced capillary resistance [**capillary fragility**] leads to petechial hemorrhage; occurs in inborn or acquired [allergic causes, vitamin C deficiency] forms

erythrocyte resistance *Syn: erythrocyte fragility, fragility of blood*; resistance of the erythrocytes, e.g., to mechanical loading

resistant not susceptible, immune

resonance sound produced when air is present

  amphoric resonance → *amphorophony*

  cavernous resonance → *amphorophony*

resorcinolphthalein → *fluorescein*

respirable suitable for inhalation, breathable

respiration 1. breathing **2.** → *cell respiration*

  amphoric respiration *Syn: amphoric breathing, amphorophony, cavernous respiration, cavernous breathing*; hollow-sounding breath

sound audible over large lung cavities
auxiliary respiration → *auxiliary breathing*
bronchial respiration → *bronchial breathing*
bronchovesicular respiration → *bronchovesicular breathing*
cavernous respiration → *amphoric respiration*
cell respiration *Syn: internal respiration, respiration, tissue respiration*; gas exchange between cells and their environment and the biologic oxidation of fuel to generate energy
Cheyne-Stokes respiration *Syn: Cheyne-Stokes breathing, Cheyne-Stokes sign, periodic breathing, tidal respiration, periodic respiration*; respiratory rhythm with an increasing and decreasing depth of breathing and possibly breathing pauses; it occurs, for example, in sleep, in chronic hypoxia, or opiate poisoning
diaphragmatic respiration *Syn: diaphragmatic breathing, diaphragmatic respiration*; a type of breathing in which inspiration occurs through contraction of the diaphragm and expiration is supported by contraction of abdominal wall muscles [abdominal press]
difficult respiration → *dyspnea*
diffusion respiration *Syn: apneic oxygenation*; oxygen exchange between pulmonary alveoli and blood by diffusion, e.g., in respiratory arrest
external respiration *Syn: respiration, pulmonary respiration*; the totality of convective gas transport in the lungs [inspiration], diffusion of respiratory gases through alveolar membranes into the blood, convective transport in the blood to tissues, diffusion from capillaries into cells, back diffusion from cells into capillaries, convective transport with the blood to the lungs, diffusion from the blood through alveolar membranes into the lungs, and convective removal of the gases [expiration]
harsh respiration → *bronchovesicular breathing*
internal respiration → *cell respiration*
Kussmaul-Kien respiration *Syn: Kussmaul breathing, Kussmaul-Kien breathing, Kussmaul's respiration, air hunger*; rhythmic respiration with deep breaths, e.g., in metabolic acidosis
labored respiration → *dyspnea*
periodic respiration → *Cheyne-Stokes respiration*
puerile respiration *Syn: puerile breathing*; harsh breath sounds in thin adolescents with a thin chest wall or deeper breathing in emotional excitement or physical exertion

pulmonary respiration →*external respiration*
rude respiration →*bronchovesicular breathing*
tidal respiration →*Cheyne-Stokes respiration*
tissue respiration →*cell respiration*
transitional respiration →*bronchovesicular breathing*
vesicular respiration →*vesicular breathing*

respiratory relating to or associated with breathing/respiration

restoration restitution, reconstitution
restoration to life →*resuscitation*

resuscitation *Syn: restoration to life*; totality of all measures for restoring sufficient circulatory and respiratory function after cardiovascular and/or respiratory arrest

cardiac resuscitation resuscitation after cardiac standstill

cardiopulmonary resuscitation *Syn: cardiorespiratory resuscitation, heart-lung resuscitation*; resuscitation during cardiovascular arrest; the procedure depends on the specific situation; basic measures [clearing of airways, rescue breathing, cardiac massage] are performed first; more extensive measures [defibrillation, intubation, drug therapy] can be instituted as soon as the situation improves or treatment by an emergency physician is available; however, it must be determined first whether the patient is conscious, and breathing and circulation must be checked; a cardiac massage is performed in circulatory arrest and rescue breathing [mouth-to-mouth, mouth-to-nose resuscitation] in respiratory arrest; during the ventilation, the circulation must be checked at 1-minute intervals; in the case of respiratory arrest and circulatory arrest, the emergency services must be notified immediately; combined rescue breathing and cardiac massage are then begun: **one-person method**: 15 chest compressions at a rate of 80/min, followed by 2 ventilations, **two-person method**: 5 chest compressions at a rate of 80/min alternating with 1 ventilation

cardiorespiratory resuscitation →*cardiopulmonary resuscitation*
heart-lung resuscitation →*cardiopulmonary resuscitation*

intrauterine resuscitation measures to improve the uteroplacental perfusion and thereby the oxygen delivery to the fetus; mostly needed in the setting of prolonged contractions [labor storm] or too frequent contractions; generally achieved by means of i.v. administration of β-sympathomimetics to break the labor storm or increase the duration of pauses between contractions; this usually achieves improved fetal oxygenation and normalization of the fetal heart

mouth-to-mouth resuscitation *s.u. transanimation*

mouth-to-nose resuscitation *s.u. transanimation*

pulmonary resuscitation *Syn: respiratory resuscitation*; resuscitation in respiratory arrest; *s.u. cardiopulmonary resuscitation*

respiratory resuscitation *Syn: pulmonary resuscitation*; resuscitation in respiratory arrest; *s.u. cardiopulmonary resuscitation*

rete net, network

arterial rete →*arterial network*

arterial rete mirabile →*arterial network*

rete arteriosum →*arterial network*

articular rete venous or arterial vessel plexus of a joint

rete lymphocapillare *Syn: lymphocapillary network*; network of lymphatic capillaries, lymphatic capillary plexus

lymphocapillary rete *Syn: lymphocapillary network*; network of lymphatic capillaries, lymphatic capillary plexus

rete mirabile vascular tuft consisting of the smallest arteries or capillaries

venous rete mirabile →*venous rete*

rete vasculosum articulare →*articular rete*

rete venosum →*venous rete*

venous rete *Syn: venous rete mirabile*; venous plexus, venous network

reteplase genetically produced deletion mutation of human tissue plasminogen activator

retinopathy *Syn: retinosis*; any disease of the retina

angiospastic retinopathy form of hypertensive retinopathy with spastic narrowing of vessels; mainly occurs in young patients with renal hypertension or pheochromocytoma

arteriosclerotic retinopathy form of hypertensive retinopathy with preponderance of vessel changes; typical features include hourglass constrictions of the veins at their crossing points with arteries [**Gunn crossing sign**] or arcuate deflection of the veins [**Salus sign**]; sometimes also lipid deposition in the retina

hypertensive retinopathy retinopathy due to persistent high blood pressure, which consists of two components: **1.** sclerosis of the retinal arteries [arteriosclerotic retinopathy] and **2.** spastic narrowing of vessels and changes to the retinal parenchyma [angiospastic retinopathy]; combined, they result in a typical ophthalmoscopic picture with narrowing of the arteries [**silver wiring**], **cotton-wool spots**, retinal hemorrhages, lipid exudates, **Gunn crossing sign** and **Salus signs**

retractometry hematologic method, which measures the contraction [retraction] of blood clots following primary clotting

retrocardiac behind the heart

revascularization 1. restoration of perfusion by capillary budding **2.** restoration of perfusion by operation, intraluminal angioplasty, or medical removal of an obstruction

reversal turning in an opposite direction or position

    adrenaline reversal *Syn: epinephrine reversal*; adrenaline activates both the α- and the β-receptors in the cardiovascular system; since the excitation of the α-receptors predominates, the blood pressure rises; if one blocks the α-receptors with phentolamine, then adrenaline injection leads to a reduction in blood pressure due to activation of the β-receptors

    epinephrine reversal → *adrenaline reversal*

    shunt reversal *Syn: reversed shunt*; reversal of the direction of flow within a shunt due to changes in the pressure relationships

rhesus-negative *s.u. Rhesus blood groups*

rhesus-positive *s.u. Rhesus blood groups*

rheumapyra → *rheumatic fever*

rheumatism rheumatic disease

    acute articular rheumatism → *rheumatic fever*

    articular rheumatism → *arthritis*

    inflammatory rheumatism → *rheumatic fever*

rheumatopyra → *rheumatic fever*

rhonchi → *rales*

    sibilant rhonchi *Syn: sibilant rales*; *s.u. dry rales*

    sibilant and sonorous rhonchi → *dry rales*

    sonorous rhonchi *Syn: sonorous rales*; *s.u. dry rales*

rhythm the regular recurrence of an action or function

    atrioventricular rhythm *Syn: A-V nodal rhythm, atrioventricular nodal rhythm, AV rhythm, nodal rhythm*; escape rhythm arising in the atrioventricular node with a fundamental frequency of 40–60 beats/min; the AV node takes over rhythm formation if the sinoatrial node fails or if conduction is blocked [SA block]

    atrioventricular nodal rhythm → *atrioventricular rhythm*

    AV rhythm → *atrioventricular rhythm*

    A-V nodal rhythm → *atrioventricular rhythm*

    bicircadian rhythm *s.u. circadian rhythm*

    biological rhythm → *biorhythm*

body rhythm →*biorhythm*
cantering rhythm →*gallop*
circadian rhythm endogenously controlled variation in the body's metabolism and preparedness for reaction, which roughly corresponds to a 24-hour cycle; in rare cases, there may also be a 48-hour cycle [**bicircadian rhythm**]
coupled rhythm *Syn: bigeminal pulse, bigeminus, coupled beat, paired beat, coupled pulse; s.u. bigeminy*
escape rhythm heart rhythm when the sinoatrial node malfunctions; e.g., AV rhythm
gallop rhythm →*gallop*
idioventricular rhythm automatism of heart excitation located in the automatic center of the ventricular myocardium; develops if the sinoatrial node fails or in third-degree AV-block as well as in ventricular tachycardia
nodal rhythm →*atrioventricular rhythm*
normal cardiac rhythm automatism of heart excitation and rhythm
parasystolic rhythm *Syn: parasystole, parasystolic beat*; simultaneous occurrence of two pacemaker centers in the heart
SA rhythm →*sinus rhythm*
sinus rhythm *Syn: SA rhythm*; normal heart rhythm arising in the sinoatrial node
trigeminal rhythm →*trigeminy*
rhythmless →*arrhythmic*
rhythmogenesis formation of a physiologic or biologic rhythm, e.g., of a circadian rhythm or an autonomous heart rhythm
ring →*circle*
fibrous ring of heart →*fibrous annulus*
Lower's ring →*fibrous annulus*
Ringer's lactate *Syn: Ringer's lactate solution*; modification of Ringer's solution with sodium, potassium, magnesium, and calcium chlorides and sodium lactate
rub →*friction sound*
friction rub →*friction sound*
pericardial rub →*pericardial friction sound*
rubefacient 1. an agent with rubefacient properties 2. provoking hyperemia, reddening the skin
rule principle; law
Wahl's rule one only hears a systolic murmur over an arterial aneu-

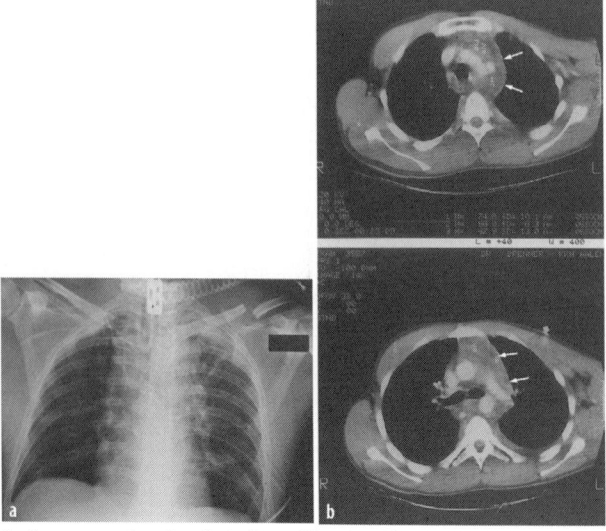

Aortic rupture. **a** enlarged mediastinal cavity [chest X-ray]; **b** mediastinal hematoma [CT]

rysm, whereas a continuous murmur with systolic loudening is heard over an arteriovenous fistula

rupture tearing or breaking of tissue

rupture of an artery → *arteriorrhexis*

aortic rupture acute life-threatening rupture of the usually already damaged aorta [aneurysm, arteriosclerosis] during accidents; in approx. 70% of cases, the rupture proves fatal; since there are usually additional traumas [head injury, open fractures, intra-abdominal bleeding], the aortic rupture is often overlooked; the surgical **therapy** consists either of implantation of a stent prosthesis or aortic oversewing, possibly with interposition of a prosthesis

cardiac rupture → *myocardial rupture*

chorda tendinae rupture rupture of the chordae tendinae of the mitral or tricuspid valve; leads to development of valve insufficiency

myocardial rupture *Syn:* cardiac rupture, cardiorrhexis; rupture of the heart wall due to trauma or extensive myocardial infarction; generally leads to immediate pericardial tamponade and death of the patient

rupture of the myocardial wall *Syn:* cardiorrhexis; rupture of the heart wall due to trauma or extensive myocardial infarction; generally leads to immediate pericardial tamponade and death of the patient

rupture of the papillary muscles *s.u. myocardial infarction*

plaque rupture *s.u. atherosclerosis*

septum rupture *s.u. myocardial infarction*

S

sac bag-like structure, pouch
    heart sac → *pericardial sac*
    pericardial sac *Syn: capsule of heart, heart sac, pericardium*; the pericardial sac consists of an outer **fibrous pericardium** and the inner **serous pericardium**; the **fibrous pericardium** contains both dense collagen fiber chains, which are orientated like folding grilles, as well as elastic fiber networks, which permit stretching by around 30%; the fibrous pericardium is connected to the adjacent parts of the pleura and sends the sternopericardial ligaments to the sternum and the **bronchopericardial membrane** to the tracheal bifurcation; the **serous pericardium** consists of two layers, the **visceral layer** and the **parietal layer**; the **visceral layer** lies directly on the myocardium [which is why it is also called the **epicardium**], i.e., it forms the outermost layer of the heart wall; the **parietal layer** is firmly attached to the fibrous pericardium; between it and the visceral layer is the pericardial cavity filled with serous fluid [**liquor pericardii**]

saluretic diuretic that promotes electrolyte excretion in the urine

sanative → *curative*

sanatory → *curative*

sangui- combining form denoting relation to blood

sanguifacient → *hemopoietic*

sanguification → *blood formation*

sanguinopoietic → *hemopoietic*

scan *Syn: scintiscan*; image or other visual display of data obtained by scintigraphy or sonography
    continous-wave Doppler scan *s.u. Doppler ultrasonography*

scanning the act of imaging by using a sensing device
    color scanning scintigraphy in which the impulse rates in the scintigram are converted to colors; since the human eye can only perceive 16–20 grey shades, but can differentiate substantially more colors, the scintigrams obtained can be subjectively better interpreted

myocardial scanning scintigraphy for the assessment of cardiac perfusion

scar *Syn: cicatrix*; a mark left by a healed wound, sore, or burn

    cardiac scar → *myocardial scar*

    myocardial scar *Syn: cardiac scar*; scar in the heart muscle following tissue destruction [e.g., myocardial infarct]

schistocyte → *helmet cell*

schistocytosis *Syn: schizocytosis*; appearance of schistocytes in the blood; mainly in mechanical injury [artificial heart valve], anemia, and hemolysis

schizocyte → *helmet cell*

schizocytosis → *schistocytosis*

scintigraphy imaging process using radionuclides or radionuclide-labeled pharmaceuticals; the distribution of activity of the radionuclide in the body or tissues permits assessment of, e.g., the function of particular organs or parts of organs or demonstrates changes in their storage properties [e.g., hot or cold nodules]; the activity is measured with, e.g., a gamma camera and displayed using a mechanical [strip scintigram, color scintigram] or optical [photoscintigram] system; the impulses can also be processed digitally [computer scintigraphy]

scleratogenous → *sclerogenous*

sclero- combining form denoting relation to hard

sclerogenic → *sclerogenous*

sclerogenous *Syn: scleratogenous, sclerogenic*; causing sclerosis

scleroid → *sclerotic*

sclerosal → *sclerotic*

sclerosed → *sclerotic*

sclerosis induration, hardening

    arteriolar sclerosis → *arteriolosclerosis*

    coronary sclerosis → *coronary arteriosclerosis*

    coronary artery sclerosis → *coronary arteriosclerosis*

    endocardial sclerosis → *endomyocardial fibrosis*

    Mönckeberg's sclerosis *Syn: Mönckeberg's arteriosclerosis, Mönckeberg's calcification, Mönckeberg's degeneration, Mönckeberg's medial calcification, Mönckeberg's mesarteritis*; clasp-like calcification of the tunica media of arteries in the extremities, which predominantly affects men and patients with diabetes mellitus and leads to the formation of so-called **gooseneck lamp arteries**

    nodular sclerosis → *atherosclerosis*

primary pulmonary sclerosis → *Ayerza's syndrome*

sclerosis of the pulmonary artery arteriosclerosis of the pulmonary artery and its branches

valvular sclerosis fibrotic thickening of a heart valve leading to heart valve insufficiency; the mitral valve is most commonly affected

sclerotic *Syn: scleroid, sclerosal, sclerous, sclerosed*; relating to or affected with sclerosis

coronary sclerotic relating to, marked by or caused by coronary artery sclerosis

sclerous → *sclerotic*

screening → *screening test*

section incision, cut

four-chamber section concept from 2D-echocardiography; describes an imaging plane in which both the ventricles and atria are displayed; the patient lies in a left lateral position and the probe is placed on the cardiac apex

segment *Syn: segmentum*; part, section

ST-segment *s.u. electrocardiogram*

selectins adhesion molecule that sits in the membrane of leukocytes [**L-selectins**], platelets [**P-selectins**], and in the endothelium of the vessels [**E-selectins**]; transmembrane glycoproteins, which are responsible for e.g., the binding of lymphocytes or granulocytes to the endothelium in the setting of inflammatory reactions

semi- combining form denoting relation to one half

senselessness → *unconsciousness*

separation act or instance of separating or the state of being separated

separation of circulation *s.u. tricuspid atresia*

plasma separation method of separating plasma from the blood cells; mostly by centrifugation or membrane filtration

sepsis *Syn: septicemia, septemia, septic intoxication, blood poisoning, hematosepsis*; generalization of a disease caused by the entry of pathogens into the bloodstream [septicemia]; the most frequent form is **bacterial sepsis**; viruses, parasites, and fungi are also possible causative agents of the basic infection; **clinical picture**: hyperthermia or hypothermia, intermittent fever, chills, tachycardia, hypotension, tachypnea, sweating, nausea, vomiting, reduced general health, slight enlargement of the liver and spleen, and signs of toxic organ damage; **diagnostic procedures**: (independent) history, clinical picture, drawing of several blood cultures [aerobic, anaerobic], primarily with a rise in temperature or chills; additional cultures [stool, urine, sputum, abscess puncture fluid, and wound smears]; rapid tests for bacterial antigens; **therapy**: nonspecific initial therapy with broad-spectrum antibiotics or more selective antibiotic administration based on the suspected form of sepsis and probable causative agent; selective antibiotic therapy after culturing results are available; treatment of septic foci

candida sepsis *Syn: disseminated candidiasis*; hematogenous dissemination of candida species [candidemia] to different organs and formation of multiple microabscesses in the kidneys, brain, myocardium, liver, and spleen; it usually originates from catheters or is the result of burns, antibiotic therapy, or chemotherapy; **therapy**: amphotericin B and flucytosine i.v.

sepsis lenta creeping sepsis generally following subacute bacterial endocarditis

pneumococcal sepsis → *pneumococcemia*

septal *Syn: septile*; relating to a septum

septemia → *septicemia*

septic *Syn: septicemic*; relating to or caused by sepsis

septicemia *Syn: blood poisoning, hematosepsis, septemia, septic fever, septic intoxication*; generalized disease with the appearance of pathogens [bacteria, viruses, fungi] or their toxins in the blood; usually equated with sepsis

septicemic → *septic*

septile → *septal*

septostomy surgical creation of an opening in a septum

balloon septostomy procedure introduced by Rashkind and Miller as a palliative measure in transposition of the great vessels; a balloon catheter is advanced through the inferior vena cava into the right atrium then through the foramen ovale into the left atrium; the balloon is inflated and jerked back and this forces open the foramen ovale

septum dividing structure, partitioning

atrioventricular septum muscle-free part of the ventricular septum [interventricular septum] between the right atrium and left ventricle

septum atrioventriculare → *atrioventricular septum*

interatrial septum *Syn: interauricular septum*; diaphragm between the right and left cardiac atria

septum interatriale → *interatrial septum*

interauricular septum → *interatrial septum*

interpulmonary septum → *mediastinum*

interventricular septum *Syn: ventricular septum*; separating wall between the right and left ventricles; the lower portion is muscular [**pars muscularis**], the upper membranous [**pars membranacea**]

ventricular septum *Syn: interventricular septum*; diaphragm between the right and left ventricles; the lower portion is muscular [**pars muscularis**], the upper membranous [**pars membranacea**]

serodiagnosis *Syn: diagnostic serology, immunodiagnosis, serum diagnosis*; diagnosis of diseases by analysis of the blood serum, e.g., using immunoassays [ELISA, RIA, RAST]

serology the branch of medical science that deals with the properties and reactions of serums, especially blood serum

    diagnostic serology → *serodiagnosis*

serosanguineous both serous and bloody

serozyme → *prothrombin*

serum 1. *Syn: blood serum*; fibrin-free blood plasma, which is therefore unable to clot **2.** serum containing antibodies, which is used for passive immunization and in serodiagnostic tests

    blood serum → *serum 1.*

serum glutamic oxaloacetic transaminase → *aspartate aminotransferase*

serumuria → *proteinuria*

shadow shade or comparative darkness, as in an area

    erythrocyte shadows effete, i.e., depleted of their hemoglobin, erythrocytes in the blood smear or urine sediment

sheath case, covering

    carotid sheath connective tissue sheath around the neck vessels [common carotid artery, internal jugular vein] and nerves [vagus nerve]

shift a change or transfer from one place, position, direction, etc., to another

    leftward shift → *deviation to the left*

shock acute circulatory failure due to a disparity between actual and necessary perfusion; it is characterized by a drop in blood pressure, tachycardia, and microcirculation disturbances; there are **three potential causes: 1.** reduced blood volume [hypovolemic shock] **2.** reduced cardiac output [cardiogenic shock] **3.** impaired vasomotor function in septicemia [septic shock] or anaphylaxis [anaphylactic shock]; all of these causes lead to a drop in arterial blood pressure, which in turn leads to disturbance of the microcirculation and hypoperfusion of tissues with a subsequent lack of oxygen and nutrients; the decrease in blood pressure stimulates sympathetic nervous system and adrenal medulla; a constriction of arteries and veins develops which causes a further decrease in perfusion and venous drainage; this congestion combined with the damage to the capillary walls [**capillary leak**] leads to a fluid loss into the interstitial space; the slow circulation promotes erythrocyte and platelet aggregation, which, together with the contents of dying cells and endotoxins, facilitate the development of disseminated intravascular coagulation; activation of the sympathetic nervous system causes centralization of the circulation as this secures perfusion of vital organs, such as heart, lung, and brain; as long as these mechanisms succeed, a state of **compensated shock** exists; the tissue hypoxia or anoxia leads to anaerobic glycolysis and metabolic acidosis, which counteracts the effect of the sympathetic nervous system; the blood vessels dilate and **decompensated shock** develops; regardless of the type of shock, the **clinical picture** always consists of cold, pale and moist skin, dyspnea, hyperventilation, restlessness and impaired consciousness; physical examination finds tachycardia, low blood pressure, and a marked temperature difference between core and periphery; **diagnosis** includes hemodynamic parameters [pulse, blood pressure, central venous pressure], chest X-ray, ultrasonographic examination of the abdomen, urine output, and blood analysis [cell count, electrolytes, creatinine, urea, lactate, coagulation tests]; the first goal of **therapy** is to re-establish oxygen supply to the organs and to increase cardiac output; oxygen is usually given via a nasal tube [4–6 l/min] or via a tube after intubation; in hypovolemic shock cardiac output can be increased by volume substitution; in cardiogenic shock reduction of preload and afterload as well as administration of catecholamines [dopamine] and digitalis glycosides will increase cardiac output; in septic and anaphylactic shock volume substitution, catecholamines, and steroids will achieve good results; once these steps have been successful further treatment focuses on improving symptoms and removal or treatment of the underlying cause

allergic shock →*anaphylactic shock*

anaphylactic shock *Syn: allergic shock, anaphylaxis, generalized anaphylaxis, systemic anaphylaxis*; shock state during an anaphylactic reaction; histamine release causes dilatation of vessels and increased membrane permeability; this leads to pooling of fluid in the low-pressure system [**relative intravascular volume deficiency**], loss of water into the tissues and perivascular edema [**absolute volume deficiency**]; the mainstays of therapy are therefore normalization of the vessel reg-

ulation and volume replacement
cardiac shock → *cardiogenic shock*
cardiogenic shock *Syn: cardiac shock, cardiovascular shock*; state of shock in myocardial damage [acute myocardial infarction, myocarditis, and toxic cardiomyopathy], disturbances in stimulus formation and conduction [tachycardia, bradycardia, and block], or impairment of ventricular filling or emptying [pulmonary embolism, pericardial effusion, pericardial tamponade, and tension pneumothorax]
cardiovascular shock → *cardiogenic shock*
compensated shock *s.u. shock*
decompensated shock *s.u. shock*
hematogenic shock → *hypovolemic shock*
hemorrhagic shock form of hypovolemic shock caused by massive blood loss; mostly due to injury or gastrointestinal bleeding; the reduction in intravascular volume leads to a reduction in the cardiac minute volume and to the secretion of catecholamines; these lead to vasoconstriction, increased heart rate, and centralization of the circulation; if the blood loss exceeds 20–25%, these mechanisms are insufficient and a shock state develops
hypovolemic shock *Syn: hematogenic shock, oligemic shock, oliguric shock*; shock as a result of blood loss to the outside or internally [hemorrhagic shock], plasma loss [predominantly in burns, widespread intra-abdominal wounds] or water and electrolyte losses [e.g., ileus, vomiting, ascites, enteritis with diarrhea, diabetes mellitus, or insipidus]
oligemic shock → *hypovolemic shock*
oliguric shock → *hypovolemic shock*
osmotic shock cell rupture by swelling in a hypotonic medium
septic shock sepsis with hypotension [systolic value < 90 mmHg], disturbances of microperfusion, lactic acidosis, oliguria, and impaired consciousness
traumatic shock shock developing following an injury; usually involves hypovolemic shock, but the cause may also be neuroendocrine dysregulation, disturbances of the microcirculation, consumptive coagulopathy, or sepsis
shortage → *deficit*
shortened → *contracted*
shortfall → *deficit*
shortness a deficiency or the amount of a deficiency

shortness of breath → *dyspnea*

shunt 1. functional or anatomic short circuit between vessels or hollow organs; e.g., arteriovenous shunt **2.** operative connection between vessels or hollow organs

arteriovenous shunt operative connection of an artery and a vein

left-to-right shunt shunt in which blood flows from the arterial side of the circulation to the venous side; e.g., in ventricular septal defect

right-to-left shunt *Syn: reversed shunt*; passage of blood from the venous system into the arterial system, e.g., in ostium secundum defects

Spitz-Holter VA shunt form of ventriculo-auriculostomy using a special valve [Holter valve]

transjugular intrahepatic portosystemic shunt *s.u. portal hypertension*

ventriculoatrial shunt → *ventriculoatriostomy*

Waterston shunt operative connection of the aorta and the pulmonary artery in congenital cyanotic heart defects

siderophages *Syn: heart failure cells, siderophores*; alveolar macrophages laden with hemosiderin and occurring in the sputum in heart-related pulmonary congestion

siderophores → *siderophages*

siderosis a disease caused by deposition of iron in tissue or cells

myocardial siderosis disease caused by deposition of iron in the setting of hemosiderosis; leads to cardiomyopathy and cardiac insufficiency

sign → *symptom*

Aschner's sign → *Aschner's reflex*

bandage sign *Syn: Hecht phenomenon, Leede-Rumpel phenomenon, Rumpel-Leede phenomenon, Rumpel-Leede sign*; *s.u. Rumpel-Leede test*

Cheyne-Stokes sign → *Cheyne-Stokes respiration*

de Musset's sign *Syn: Musset's sign*; pulse-synchronous nodding in severe aortic valve insufficiency; first observed by Depeuch in the French poet Alfred de Musset

Duroziez's sign → *Duroziez's murmur*

Ewart's sign *Syn: Pins' sign*; bronchial breathing or increased breath sound and dullness at the left inferior angle of the scapula in massive pericardial effusion

Gunn crossing sign *s.u. arteriosclerotic retinopathy*

Hill's sign elevation of the blood pressure in the femoral artery by 60–100 mmHg above the value in the upper arm in aortic valve insufficiency and patent ductus arteriosus

Homans' sign pains in the calf and hollow of the knee on passive dorsiflexion of the foot as a sign of thrombosis in the deep veins of the calf

Jaccoud's sign *Syn: Jaccoud's syndrome*; indrawing of the intercostal spaces during systole due to adhesions with the pericardium

Mahler's sign ladder pulse [i.e., stepwise increase in the pulse] at constant body temperature as an early sign of thrombosis or embolism

signs of maturity bodily developmental characteristics of the newborn, which allow determination of the gestational age; among other features, body length, weight, lanugo hair, fingernails, nose, and ear cartilage are assessed

McGinn-White sign temporary ECG changes in acute cor pulmonale, primarily in pulmonary embolism; P-pulmonale, SI/QIII type, and ST segment depression are seen

Musset's sign → *de Musset's sign*

Nicoladoni's sign slowing of the heart rate [bradycardia] and increase in the blood pressure [hypertension] in response to compression of a cirsoid aneurysm or an arteriovenous fistula of an extremity

Oliver's sign *Syn: Porter's sign, tracheal tugging*; palpable downward tugging of the windpipe or the gently elevated thyroid cartilage in aortic arch aneurysm or mediastinal processes

Osler's sign → *Osler's nodes*

Payr's sign pressure sensitivity of the inside of the foot as an early sign of thrombosis or thrombophlebitis of the leg veins

Pins' sign → *Ewart's sign*

Porter's sign → *Oliver's sign*

Quincke's sign → *Quincke's pulse*

Rumpel-Leede sign *Syn: bandage sign, Hecht phenomenon, Leede-Rumpel phenomenon, Rumpel-Leede phenomenon*; s.u. Rumpel-Leede test

Salus sign *Syn: Salus' arch*; s.u. arteriosclerotic retinopathy

Traube's sign → *Traube's double tone*

single pill combination the combination of two or more therapeutic agents in one pill

sinoatrial → *sinuatrial*

sinoauricular → *sinuatrial*

sinoventricular → *sinuventricular*
sinuatrial *Syn: sinoatrial, sinoauricular, sinuauricular*; realting to the sinus node and the cardiac atrium
sinuauricular → *sinuatrial*
sinus cavity, hollow space, recess, or pocket

aortic sinus *Syn: Petit's sinus, sinus of Morgagni, sinus of Valsalva, Valsalva's sinus*; pocket-like outpouchings between the semilunar valves and the aortic wall; point of origin of the right coronary artery [in the right aortic sinus] and the left coronary artery [in the left aortic sinus]

carotid sinus *Syn: carotid bulbus*; dilatation of the common carotid artery at the carotid bifurcation

sinus coronarius → *coronary sinus*

coronary sinus generic term for coronary veins on the posterior surface of the heart, which drain blood into the right atrium

sinus of Morgagni → *aortic sinus*

oblique sinus of pericardium outpouching of the pericardial cavity between the right and left pulmonary veins

sinus obliquus pericardii → *oblique sinus of pericardium*

Petit's sinus → *aortic sinus*

phrenicomediastinal sinus → *phrenicomediastinal recess*

pleural sinus → *pleural recesses*

transverse sinus of pericardium *Syn: Theile's canal*; outpouching of the pericardial cavity between the aorta and pulmonary veins

sinus transversus pericardii → *transverse sinus of pericardium*

sinus of Valsalva → *aortic sinus*

Valsalva's sinus → *aortic sinus*

sinus of venae cavae smooth area of the wall of the right atrium between the openings of the two great veins [ostia of the superior and inferior venae cavae], in which the blood from the two veins mixes

sinus venarum cavarum → *sinus of venae cavae*

sinus venosus venous sinus

sinuventricular *Syn: sinoventricular*; relating to sinus node and ventricle of the heart

skeocytosis → *deviation to the left*

slowness lack of speed

slowness of the pulse → *bradysphygmia*

sludging reversible aggregation of erythrocytes due to changes in the flow characteristics of the blood; mainly in hyperviscosity syndrome and in shock

sodium *Syn: natrium, natrum*; soft, extremely reactive alkali metal; sodium is the main ion in the extracellular compartment and very important in osmoregulation and the bioelectric potentials of the cell membrane; approx. 98% of the total body content of sodium is found in the extracellular compartment, of which approx. 40% is in the bones; sodium is at particularly high concentration in the interstitial fluid [144 mmol/l], the plasma [142 mmol/l], the pancreatic juice [140 mmol/l], the bile [130–165 mmol/l], and the small bowel secretions [82–148 mmol/l]; the daily intake is in the range 70–350 mmol and is almost exclusively in the form of NaCl [5–29 g] in drinks and food

  sodium apolate heparin-like substance; **usage**: hematomas, sprains, thrombophlebitis

  sodium nitroferricyanide → *nitroprusside sodium*

  sodium nitroprusside → *nitroprusside sodium*

sodium-potassium adenosinetriphosphatase → Na^+-K^+-*ATPase*

sodium-potassium-ATPase → Na^+-K^+-*ATPase*

solution a liquid, usually water, in which a medication is dissolved

  hypertonic solution solution with higher osmotic pressure than blood plasma

  hypotonic solution solution with lower osmotic pressure than blood plasma

  Ringer's solution → *Ringer's mixture*

  Ringer's lactate solution → *Ringer's lactate*

  Rous' solution aqueous solution of sodium citrate and glucose for conservation of erythrocytes

sonography ultrasound examination; non-invasive technique in which electrical energy is converted into sound waves with a frequency of 2–10 MHz; absorption, reflection and refraction of the sound waves in the tissues generate specific images that are displayed on a screen; the different techniques include **1. impulse echo technique**, in which the probe serves as both transmitter and receiver; the transmitted sound waves are reflected from structures in the insonated area and registered as echo signals; in the simplest case, the echo signals are represented as Amplitudes on a time base; the **A-mode image** obtained in this way relates the size of the amplitude to the intensity of the echo [the bigger, the more intense], whereas the distance to the amplitude indicates the distance from the probe and thereby the position in the body; because of the great advantages of the two-dimensional representation [B-mode image], the A-mode is hardly used now; in the **B-mode image**, the amplitude is converted into a spatially encoded, point Brightness, from which a two-dimensional gray-scale image is constructed on the screen; modern machines store the echo signals in digital form and thereby permit variations in the image preparation and quantitative analysis; in **M-mode** [Motion], the probe is held still, which results in moving interfaces appearing on the monitor as moving lines; M-mode is predominantly used in cardiology to investigate the heart and heart valves; all three processes are described as **real-time** since events can be observed directly on the monitor; 2. **Doppler sonography** registers the frequency changes of sound waves reflecting from moving objects [Doppler effect]; can operate with either continuous sound waves [**continuous-wave Doppler sonography**] or with sound impulses [**impulse Doppler sonography**]; the main area of use is in the investigation of the heart and vessels; in combination with B-mode imaging one can obtain sectional images that only show vessels containing flowing blood [**Doppler angiography**]

impulse Doppler sonography s.u. *Doppler ultrasonography*

sotalol non-selective β-blocker; class-III antiarrhythmic; **usage**: ventricular extrasystoles, ventricular tachycardia, WPW syndrome, paroxysmal supraventricular tachycardia

sound *Syn: murmur*; a noise heard on auscultation, e.g., heart murmur or breath sound

    additional heart sounds sounds arising in addition to the normal heart sounds, e.g., 3. heart sound, 4. heart sound, systolic click

    adventitious sounds → *rales*

    atrial sound → *fourth heart sound*

    bottle sound → *amphorophony*

    breath sound *Syn: respiratory sound*; sound over the lung, bronchi, and trachea produced by air flowing in and out

    bronchial breath sound → *bronchial breathing*

    bronchovesicular breath sound → *bronchovesicular breathing*

    dry adventitious sounds → *dry rales*

    ejection sounds → *ejection murmurs*

    first heart sound dull sound, which marks the start of systole; arises fundamentally from the vibrations of the ventricular wall and the closure of the mitral and tricuspid valves; weakened in mitral insufficiency, decompensated cardiac insufficiency, myocardial infarction, and in worsening of the conduction of sound [adiposity, pericardial effusion, lung emphysema, pneumothorax]; a louder 1. heart sound is found in mitral stenosis, hyperthyroidism, bradycardia, and states of increased sympathetic tone

fourth sound → *fourth heart sound*

fourth cardiac sound → *fourth heart sound*

fourth heart sound *Syn: atrial sound, fourth cardiac sound, fourth sound*; additional tone generated by increased stretching and contraction of the atrium in, e.g., left heart hypertrophy and in the acute phase of myocardial infarction; frequently occurs together with a 3. heart sound as a **summation gallop**

friction sound *Syn: friction murmur, friction rub, rub*; noise produced by rubbing together of two serous surfaces, e.g., pleural rub

heart sounds physiologic sounds occurring due to the movements of the muscle and valves; the 1. and 2. heart sounds are physiologic, additional sounds or splitting of the 1. or 2. heart sounds are described as extra sounds

Korotkoff sounds *s.u. Riva-Rocci method*

moist adventitious sounds → *moist rales*

pericardial friction sound *Syn: pericardial fremitus, pericardial murmur, pericardial rub*; fibrin exudation due to rubbing or inflammation of the pericardium, which leads to a characteristic rubbing sound on auscultation; the character of the sound is rough and proximate, and is partly perceived as a vibration; the rubbing sound is audible both during systole and diastole; as soon as an effusion forms [moist pericarditis], the rub disappears

pistol-shot sound → *Traube's double tone*

respiratory sound → *breath sound*

second heart sound marks the start of diastole and originates from the snapping shut of the aortic and pulmonary valves; due to the pressure difference between the two circulations, the aortic sound is earlier and louder than the pulmonary sound; the aortic sound is increased in arterial hypertension, high levels of sympathetic tone, sclerosis of the aorta or aortic valve, and following an extrasystole; it is reduced in arterial hypotension, aortic valve stenosis, aortic insufficiency, and left heart insufficiency; the pulmonary sound is increased in pulmonary hypertension and left-to-right shunting [e.g., atrial septal defect] and weakened in pulmonary stenosis; **splitting of the 2. heart sound** is physiologic during inspiration; abnormally wide splitting can be caused by right bundle branch block, atrial septal defect, and left ventricular extrasystoles; **paradoxical splitting of the 2. heart sound** [the pulmonary sound comes before the aortic sound] can be due to left bundle branch block, transvenous pacemakers, high-grade aortic valve stenosis, aortic isthmus stenosis, and volume overload of the left ventricle due to aortic insufficiency

third heart sound physiologic in juveniles, especially after heavy physical activity; in adults, a sign of increased ventricular filling [e.g., in mitral insufficiency] or impaired ventricular compliance [e.g., in cardiac insufficiency]

tracheal breath sound *Syn: tracheal breathing sound, tracheal breathing*; normal breath sound over the trachea

tracheal breathing sound → *tracheal breath sound*

vesicular breath sounds → *vesicular breathing*

space a demarcated area

complemental spaces → *pleural recesses*

H space → *Holzknecht's space*

Holzknecht's space *Syn: H space, prevertebral space, retrocardiac space*; space between the heart and spinal column

mediastinal space → *mediastinum*

perivascular space the space around the blood vessels

prevertebral space → *Holzknecht's space*

reserve spaces → *pleural recesses*

retrocardiac space → *Holzknecht's space*

retrosternal space space between the sternum and the pericardial sac in an X-ray image

transcellular space includes all extracellular spaces, which are separated from the interstitium by a membrane, i.e., pleural, pericardial, and peritoneal cavities, amniotic cavity, eye chambers, as well as the lumens of glands, stomach, intestinal, and urogenital tracts; normally constitutes about 2% of the extracellular space, but can in pathologic circumstances [e.g., ileus] increase several fold and lead to hypovolemia and hypotension

spasm sudden, involuntary contraction of muscles; cramp

clonic spasm → *clonus*

coronary spasm spasm of the heart arteries; causes an attack of angina pectoris

SPC → *single pill combination*

sphacelation → *necrosis*

sphygmo- combining form denoting relation to the pulse
sphygmogram → *pulse curve*
sphygmography registration of the pulse curve
sphygmomanometer an instrument for measuring blood pressure

  Riva-Rocci sphygmomanometer apparatus for non-invasive measurement of the blood pressure; the measurement is normally performed on the upper arm of the seated patient; the site of measurement should be at roughly heart height; the arm is slightly bent, the stethoscope applied loosely over the brachial artery and the cuff [12 cm wide, 30 cm long] is rapidly inflated until the pressure is about 30 mmHg higher than the systolic pressure; the pressure in the cuff is then slowly released until pulse-synchronous sounds can be heard over the artery [**Korotkoff sounds**]; the pressure on the manometer corresponds to the systolic blood pressure; with further release of air, the sounds become very quiet or disappear altogether; this pressure corresponds to the diastolic blood pressure; in obese patients or patients with extremely strong upper arms, high values are often measured; after physical or emotional stress, or in hyperthyroidism, anemia, and aortic insufficiency, the sounds are often audible right down to a cuff pressure of zero and determination of the diastolic value is difficult; measurement of the blood pressure in the thigh requires a special large cuff [18 cm wide, 60–80 cm long]; the measurement is performed in a lateral or prone position; the values are 10–30 mm higher than in the arms

sphygmomanometry the blood pressure can be measured directly or indirectly; in **direct** or **invasive blood pressure measurement**, a catheter is inserted into an artery and connected to measuring equipment; although it makes continuous measurement possible, the method is only used on intensive care units or during major operations; **indirect** or **bloodless blood pressure measurement** mostly relies upon the method of Riva-Rocci, even though more and more semi-automatic or electronic measurement devices are being used

sphygmoscope apparatus for demonstrating the pulse waveform
sphygmoscopy recording and assessment of the pulse waveform
spiramycin *Syn: foromacidin*; macrolide antibiotic derived from **Streptomyces ambofaciens**; has similar action to erythromycin
spironolactone the most important aldosterone antagonist; potassium-sparing diuretic; competitively displaces aldosterone from its receptor at the end-organ [the distal convoluted tubule]; has no effect upon the normal secretion of adrenal steroids; increases the Na^+ and lowers

the K⁺ excretion; **usage**: primary and secondary hyperaldosteronism, ascites in liver cirrhosis, cardiogenic, nephrotic, and cirrhotic edema; **side effects**: hyperkalemia, hyperchloremic acidosis, gynecomastia, impotence, amenorrhea; **contraindication**: pregnancy, acute renal failure, advanced renal insufficiency, hyperkalemia, hyponatremia; **Interactions**: acetylsalicylic acid reduces the diuretic effect; simultaneous administration of NSAIDs can worsen the hyperkalemia; simultaneous administration of ACE-antagonists or other potassium sparing diuretics can cause life-threatening hyperkalemia; neomycin inhibits reabsorption of spironolactone

spot a small, circumscribed mark

cotton wool spots *Syn*: cotton wool exudates, cotton wool patches; small, bright exudates in the fundus of the eye in a variety of eye diseases [hypertensive retinopathy, diabetic retinopathy, venous branch occlusions, central vein occlusion]

squatting *Syn*: squatting position; typical position of children with tetralogy of Fallot; it increases resistance in the systemic circulation and thereby also pulmonary blood flow and blood oxygen saturation

stabilizer anticoagulant used in the conservation of blood, which does not change the natural properties of the blood, e.g., ACD stabilizer

stagnancy → *stagnation*

stagnation *Syn*: stagnancy; standstill; stasis, congestion

staltic → *styptic*

standstill complete cessation of activity or progress

    cardiac standstill → *cardiac arrest*

    sinus standstill → *sinus arrest*

staph → *Staphylococcus*

staphylococci → *Staphylococcus*

    coagulase-negative staphylococci s.u. *Staphylococcus*

    coagulase-positive staphylococci s.u. *Staphylococcus*

    novobiocin-resistant staphylococci → *Staphylococcus saprophyticus group*

    novobiocin-susceptible staphylococci → *Staphylococcus epidermidis group*

Staphylococcus *Syn*: staph, staphylococcus, staphylococci; genus of gram-positive, nonmotile cocci, which join to form racemose clusters and multiply under both aerobic and anaerobic conditions; the production of free coagulase is used to subdivide these bacteria into **coagulase-positive staphylococci** [three species, of which only Staphylococcus aureus is clinically important] and **coagulase-negative staphylococci**, which were called Staphylococcus albus until the end of the 1960s; today these include 33 species, about a third of which can be pathogenic; they are divided based on their susceptibility or resistance to novobiocin into a **Staphylococcus saprophyticus group** [novobiocin-resistant staphylococci] and **Staphylococcus epidermidis group** [novobiocin-susceptible staphylococci]

Staphylococcus. Species and infections

Species	Infection(s)
coagulase-positive staphylococci	
S. aureus	purulent skin diseases [staphyloderma], wound infections, food poisoning, staphylogenic Lyell's syndrome, sepsis, endocarditis
coagulase-negative staphylococci	
S. epidermidis group	
– S. epidermidis	wound infections, endocarditis, sepsis, peritonitis
– S. hominis	
– S. haemolyticus	
– S. warneri	
– S. capitis	
S. saprophyticus group	
– S. saprophyticus	urinary tract infections
– S. xylosus	
– S. cohnii	

Staphylococcus albus → *Staphylococcus epidermidis*
Staphylococcus aureus Syn: staph, Staphylococcus pyogenes; causative agent of purulent skin diseases [staphyloderma], wound infections, food poisoning, and staphylogenic Lyell's syndrome, as well as other conditions; Staphylococcus aureus synthesizes a number of products with extracellular activity, which are responsible for the spread of the infection [e.g., coagulase, staphylokinase, DNase, hyaluronidase, staphylolysins, and leukocidin] or for specific clinical pictures [staph-

ylococcal enterotoxin, toxic shock syndrome toxin-1, and exfoliatin]; **diagnosis**: pathogen identification by culturing [blood agar]; pus, sputum, smears, blood, cerebrospinal fluid, etc., are suitable specimens for tests; **therapy**: it is susceptible to all β-lactam antibiotics [penicillin, cephalosporins], erythromycin, and aminoglycoside antibiotics; up to 80% of all strains produce penicillinases, which can be blocked by clavulanic acid, sulbactam, or tazobactam

Staphylococcus auricularis s.u. *Staphylococcus epidermidis group*

Staphylococcus capitis s.u. *Staphylococcus epidermidis group*

Staphylococcus cohnii s.u. *Staphylococcus saprophyticus group*

Staphylococcus delphini s.u. *Staphylococcus epidermidis group*

Staphylococcus epidermidis *Syn*: *Staphylococcus albus*; a staphylococcus species that inhabits the skin and mucous membranes; it cannot be differentiated clinically and with difficulty culturally from other members of the Staphylococcus epidermidis group; it is an important opportunistic causative agent of wound infections, endocarditis, septicemia, and biomaterial-associated infections; **diagnosis**: identification of the causative agent by culturing in pus, sputum, smears, blood, cerebrospinal fluid, or on plastic material [e.g., cathether tips]; **therapy**: it is generally susceptible to vancomycin, teicoplanin, rifampicin and fosfomycin; 80% of the hospital strains are penicillin- and oxacillin-resistant

Staphylococcus epidermidis group *Syn*: *novobiocin-susceptible staphylococci*; includes, in addition to Staphylococcus epidermidis, also Staphylococcus haemolyticus, S. hominis, S. warneri, S. capitis, S. lugdunensis, S. schleiferi, S. simulans, S. auricularis, S. intermedius, S. delphini, S. hyicus, and other species, which play a clinical role only in rare instances

Staphylococcus haemolyticus s.u. *Staphylococcus epidermidis group*

Staphylococcus hominis s.u. *Staphylococcus epidermidis group*

Staphylococcus hyicus s.u. *Staphylococcus epidermidis group*

Staphylococcus intermedius s.u. *Staphylococcus epidermidis group*

Staphylococcus lugdunensis s.u. *Staphylococcus epidermidis group*

Staphylococcus pyogenes → *Staphylococcus aureus*

Staphylococcus saprophyticus group *Syn*: *novobiocin-resistant staphylococci*; this group also includes Staphylococcus xylosus and Staphylococcus cohnii

Staphylococcus schleiferi s.u. *Staphylococcus epidermidis group*

Staphylococcus simulans s.u. *Staphylococcus epidermidis group*

Staphylococcus warneri *s.u. Staphylococcus epidermidis group*
Staphylococcus xylosus *s.u. Staphylococcus saprophyticus group*
staphylokinase enzyme that increases the formation of plasmin from plasminogen; in the earliest phase of infection, plasmin dissolves the fibrin capsule formed under the influence of coagulase and thereby permits the spread of infection in the tissues
stasis *Syn: stagnation, stoppage*; congestion, standstill, e.g., of the circulation
steady → *continuous*
steal → *steal phenomenon*
   subclavian steal → *subclavian steal syndrome*
stenocardia → *angina pectoris*
stenochoria → *stenosis*
stenosal → *stenotic*
stenosed affected by stenosis, narrowed
stenosing leading to stenosis, narrowing, constricting
stenosis *Syn: narrowing, stenochoria, stricture*; congenital or acquired narrowing of vessels, hollow organs, or origins/openings
   stenosis of the anterior interventricular branch stenosis of the anterior interventricular branch of the left coronary artery; frequent cause of anterior wall infarction or apical infarcts; **therapy**: angioplasty, aortocoronary bypass

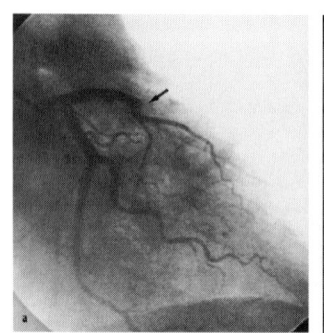

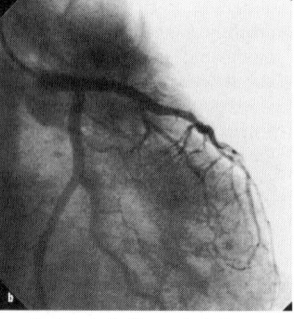

Stenosis of the anterior interventricular branch. **a** acute stenosis; **b** after angioplasty

aortic stenosis 1. *Syn: aortarctia, aortartia, aortostenosis*; inborn or acquired narrowing of the aorta or the aortic valve [aortic stenosis]; sub-valvular, valvular, and supravalvular aortic stenosis can be differentiated depending upon the level **2.** *Syn: aortarctia, aortartia*; congenital or acquired [rheumatic or bacterial endocarditis] narrowing of the aortic valve orifice; the pressure loading of the left ventricle leads to left heart hypertrophy and left heart insufficiency; the **clinical picture** is mainly determined by the degree of stenosis; at auscultation, the aortic component of the 2. heart sound is diminished and there is an ejection systolic murmur with the maximal point in the right 2. intercostal space; the ECG is mostly unremarkable, while the echocardiogram demonstrates the stenosis and allows assessment of the hemodynamics; **therapy**: dilatation with a balloon catheter [**balloon valvuloplasty**] or commissurotomy are the methods of choice; if there is restenosis or the development of insufficiency, then aortic valve replacement

aortic isthmus stenosis *Syn: isthmus stenosis, aortic coarctation, coarctation of aorta*; relatively frequent [5% of connatal angiocardiopathies] congenital narrowing of the aortic isthmus above [**preductal aortic isthmus stenosis**] or below [**postductal aortic isthmus stenosis**] the opening of the ductus arteriosus

arteriosclerotic renal artery stenosis *Syn: atherosclerotic renal artery stenosis; s.u. renal artery stenosis*

atherosclerotic renal artery stenosis *Syn: arteriosclerotic renal artery stenosis; s.u. renal artery stenosis*

buttonhole mitral stenosis → *fishmouth stenosis*

carotid stenosis *Syn: carotid occlusive disease*; stenosis of the common carotid artery or internal carotid artery; initially asymptomatic, subsequently may lead to disturbances of cerebral perfusion to the point of complete ischemic hemicranial infarct; in rare cases, an **external carotid artery stenosis** may display the same symptoms; **therapy**: angioplasty

central pulmonary stenosis *s.u. supravalvular pulmonary stenosis*

congenital mitral stenosis congenital stenosis combined with anemia, enteroptosis, and hemorrhoids

congenital stenosis of mitral valve → *Duroziez's disease*

coronary stenosis narrowing of the coronary vessels mostly caused by sclerotic processes; coronary stenoses are divided into three types based upon the angiographic features; this subdivision reflects the degree of stenosis and its position and provides an estimate of the success rate for interventional therapies

external carotid artery stenosis stenosis of the external carotid artery; the clinical picture depends upon the degree of stenosis; **therapy**: angioplasty

fishmouth stenosis *Syn: buttonhole deformity, buttonhole mitral stenosis, fishmouth mitral stenosis, mitral buttonhole*; generally acquired, mostly post-endocarditic, high-grade narrowing of a heart valve; most frequently affects the aortic and mitral valves

fishmouth mitral stenosis → *fishmouth stenosis*

infundibular stenosis → *subvalvular pulmonary stenosis*

infundibular pulmonary stenosis → *subvalvular pulmonary stenosis*

internal carotid artery stenosis stenosis of the external carotid artery; the clinical picture [among others, disturbances to vision or balance, contralateral hemiparesis] depends upon the extent of the stenosis; **therapy**: angioplasty

isthmus stenosis → *aortic isthmus stenosis*

mitral stenosis congenital or acquired narrowing of the mitral valve orifice; the most common cause [> 50%] is still rheumatic fever; only in approx. 50% of cases does pure mitral stenosis occur; in approx. 40% of cases, there is also significant mitral insufficiency; the prevention of diastolic filling of the left ventricle leads to enlargement of the left atrium, right ventricle, and pulmonary trunk with impairment of performance; **clinical**: the patients complain of reduced exercise capacity and exertional dyspnea; the typical **mitral facies** is striking, with reddish, livid discoloration of the cheeks and sometimes cyanosis; **auscultation** reveals a loud 1. heart sound, systole is clear, the **mitral opening sound** occurs approx. 0.08–0.11 s after the 2. heart sound; in severe stenosis, pulmonary hypertension develops leading to accentuation of the pulmonary segment of the 2. heart sound; **diagnosis**: echocardiography, cardiac catheterization; **therapy**: mild forms and inoperable patients are managed conservatively [diuretics, digitalis, β-blockers, verapamil]; of the operative procedures, **percutaneous balloon valvuloplasty** is the method of choice, although some still prefer open **commissurotomy**; **mitral valve replacement** is only rarely indicated

muscular subaortic stenosis congenital form of subvalvular aortic stenosis

peripheral pulmonary stenosis *s.u. supravalvular pulmonary stenosis*

pulmonary stenosis *Syn: pulmonary artery stenosis, pulmonary valve stenosis*; usually congenital stenosis of the pulmonary valve, frequently associated with other anomalies [tetralogy of Fallot]; depending on the location of the stenosis, pulmonary stenosis is divided into **subvalvular**, **valvular**, and **supravalvular**; **clinical picture** and **diagnosis**: most stenoses [apart from severe congenital stenoses] remain asymptomatic for a long time; in the long term, however, right-ventricular outflow obstruction leads to right ventricular loading and right ventricular hypertrophy; cyanosis develops only after decompensation; **auscultation**: typical systolic ejection murmur with the point of maximum impulse in the second-third intercostal space parasternal on the left side; the early diastolic pulmonary ejection sound is a so-called "ejection click", which is audible primarily in moderate stenosis; the pulmonary component of the second heart sound is weakened; **ECG**: signs of right ventricular hypertrophy and frequently a P dextrocardiale; **echocardiography** and **angiocardiography** further define the extent of the stenosis, flow impairment, and hypertrophy of the right ventricle; **therapy**: balloon valvuloplasty is the method of choice today; open commissurotomy or valve replacement is reserved for special cases

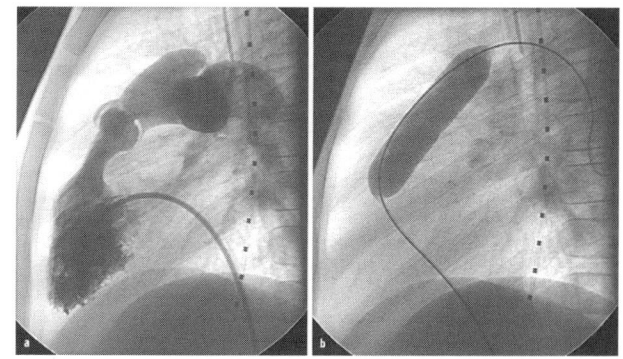

Pulmonary stenosis. Angiography and balloon valvuloplasty of a valvular stenosis

pulmonary artery stenosis → *pulmonary stenosis*
pulmonary valve stenosis → *pulmonary stenosis*

renal artery stenosis complete or incomplete narrowing of one or both renal arteries; mostly a partial symptom of more generalized arteriosclerosis [**atherosclerotic renal artery stenosis**]; leads to the development of renal hypertension and renal insufficiency

subaortic stenosis →*subvalvular aortic stenosis*

subvalvular stenosis →*subvalvular aortic stenosis*

subvalvular aortic stenosis *Syn: aortostenosis, subaortic stenosis, subvalvular stenosis*; narrowing of the outflow tract of the left ventricle lying below the aortic valve; the congenital form is referred to as **idiopathic hypertrophic subaortic stenosis**; clinical and therapeutic features are essentially the same as for aortic valve stenosis

subvalvular pulmonary stenosis *Syn: infundibular stenosis, infundibular pulmonary stenosis*; congenital narrowing of the outflow tract of the right ventricle by hypertrophied muscle bundles, which constrict the outflow tract [primarily during systole]; it occurs frequently together with tetralogy of Fallot; **therapy**: resection of the hypertrophied muscle bundles; possibly dilatation of the outflow tract

supravalvular aortic stenosis inborn [**Williams-Beuren syndrome**] or acquired true aortic stenosis; the clinical course mirrors that of aortic valvular stenosis

supravalvular pulmonary stenosis *Syn: pulmonary artery stenosis*; stenosis above the pulmonary valve; it occurs extremely rarely isolated but usually combined with tetralogy of Fallot or atrial septal defect; stenoses located directly above the valve are called **central pulmonary stenoses**, and those on the other side of the bifurcation, **peripheral pulmonary stenoses**

tricuspid stenosis congenital or acquired [inflammatory] narrowing of the tricuspid valve with back-damming in the superior and inferior vena cava; **isolated tricuspid valve stenoses** are very rare, and mostly there is also mitral and aortic valve stenosis; **secondary** or **relative tricuspid valve stenoses** are generally a result of increased blood volume in the pulmonary circulation; **functional tricuspid valve stenosis** is a narrowing of the tricuspid orifice [e.g., due to thrombi or tumors] or of the atrium from the outside [e.g., in pericardial effusion]; **clinical**: tricuspid valve stenosis is usually clinically silent, since the symptoms of the other heart defects predominate; **auscultation**: presystolic crescendo-decrescendo murmur in the 4.–5. intercostal space over the sternum and left parasternal area; **echocardiography**: permits assessment of the degree of stenosis and the flow dynamics; it has replaced

right cardiac catheterization as the method of choice; **therapy**: conservative management of the right heart insufficiency; the question of operative therapy [balloon dilatation, valve replacement] depends upon the accompanying deficits

valvular stenosis *Syn: stenotic valvular disease*; disease of a heart valve that leads to narrowing of its aperture; may be inborn or acquired [heart valve inflammation]; **relative** or **functional cardiac valve stenosis** there is a mismatch between the diameter of a healthy valve and the volume flowing through it; *s.a. aortic stenosis, pulmonary stenosis, mitral stenosis, tricuspid valve stenosis*

valvular pulmonary stenosis stenosis in the area of the semilunar valves; it is the most frequent form of pulmonary stenosis

stenotic *Syn: stenosal*; relating to or affected with stenosis, narrowed

coronary stenotic relating to, marked by or caused by coronary stenosis

stent spiral wire prosthesis to keep open vessels or hollow organs; predominantly **intracoronary stents**, which are widely used nowadays to keep coronary arteries open; there are two types: **self-expanding stents**, which open up to a predefined diameter following removal of the protective sheath and then maintain this size, and **balloon-expandable stents**, which are dilated using a balloon catheter

sterile 1. pathogen free; aseptic **2.** barren, infertile

sternalgia → *angina pectoris*

sternodynia → *angina pectoris*

sternopericardial relating to or associated with the sternum and pericardium

steroids natural or synthetic compounds, which have a core structure made up of three hexameric rings and one pentameric ring [perhydrocyclopentanophenanthrene]; important natural steroids include, e.g., cholesterol, steroid hormones, bile acids, vitamin D, and cardiac glycosides

stethoscope instrument for listening to [auscultation of] the functional sounds of organs, body cavities, vessels, and the like

stethoscopic relating to a stethoscope, by means of a stethoscope

stimulation the effect of a stimulus (on nerves or organs etc.)

AAI-stimulation *s.u. pacemaker*

DDD-stimulation *s.u. pacemaker*

DDI-stimulation *s.u. pacemaker*

VVI-stimulation *s.u. pacemaker*

stone concretion, calculus
  vein stone → *phlebolith*
stoppage → *stasis*
Streptococcus *Syn: streptococcus*; gram-positive, non-motile cocci occurring in pairs or chains; they are divided into α-, β-, and γ-hemolytic streptococci based on the hemolysis behavior in blood-containing culture media; this division is clinically important, because the α-hemolytic or **viridans streptococci**, with the exception of Streptococcus pneumoniae, are normal mucosal flora and are merely opportunistic pathogens, whereas β-hemolytic streptococci are obligate pathogens; γ-hemolytic or **non-hemolytic streptococci** play only a minor role in human medicine; equally important is the further subdivision of the β-hemolytic streptococci according to the C polysaccharide into **Lancefield groups**, of which groups A, B, C, D, F, G, and N are important for humans
Streptococcus agalactiae *Syn: Streptococcus mastitidis, group B streptococci*; β-hemolytic streptococci in Lancefield group B, which usually infect animals and less often humans; they can cause wound infections, meningitis [newborn], and inflammations of the nasopharynx; **diagnosis**: culturing [blood-containing Columbia agar] and serotyping; **therapy**: highly susceptible to penicillin G and cephalosporins
Streptococcus erysipelatis → *Streptococcus pyogenes*
Streptococcus hemolyticus → *Streptococcus pyogenes*
Streptococcus mastitidis → *Streptococcus agalactiae*
Streptococcus pneumoniae *Syn: pneumococcus, pneumonococcus, Diplococcus pneumoniae, Diplococcus lanceolatus*; lanceolate diplococci classified as α-hemolytic streptococci; surrounded by a polysaccharide capsule; it is the classic causative agent of pneumonia, meningitis, sepsis, and infections of the eyes and in the ear-nose-throat area; the presence and thickness of the capsule are important for the virulence of the pneumococci; encapsulated strains form smooth, glossy colonies and, for this reason, are also called the **S form** [smooth]; colonies of nonencapsulated, avirulent strains have a dull and rough appearance; for this reason, they are called the **R form** [rough]; **diagnosis**: identification of the pathogen in the specimen; identification of the capsular antigen; **therapy**: usually susceptible to penicillins, cephalosporins, macrolide antibiotics, and clindamycin
Streptococcus pyogenes *Syn: Streptococcus erysipelatis, Streptococcus hemolyticus, Streptococcus scarlatinae, group A streptococci*; β-hemolytic

streptococci from Lancefield group A are the causative agents of local infections, respiratory tract infections, scarlet fever, and erysipelas, among other conditions; the secondary diseases arising after the acute illnesses, for example rheumatic fever or glomerulonephritis, are also important; group A streptococci produce a number of products with extracellular activity [streptolysins, hyaluronidases, streptodornases, streptokinases, and erythrogenic toxin], which are important in the pathogenesis of various diseases and are therapeutically beneficial in some cases; **diagnosis**: culturing from specimens [blood agar] and serotyping; **therapy**: highly susceptible to penicillin G and cephalosporins

Streptococcus scarlatinae → *Streptococcus pyogenes*
Streptococcus viridans → *α-hemolytic streptococci*
streptococcus → *Streptococcus*
group A streptococci → *Streptococcus pyogenes*
group B streptococci → *Streptococcus agalactiae*
α-hemolytic streptococci *Syn: viridans streptococci, Streptococcus viridans*; streptococcus group producing a green zone on blood agar [α-hemolysis]; they are part of physiological mucosal flora; they are facultatively pathogenic causative agents of dental diseases [caries] and endocarditis [primarily endocarditis lenta]; the most important species are Streptococcus bovis, S. mutans, S. sanguis, and S. anginosus; **diagnosis**: culturing on blood agar and biochemical differentiation [test kits]; **therapy**: they are usually susceptible to penicillin G, aminopenicillins, and cephalosporins

α-hemolytic streptococci. Species and infections

Species	Infection(s)
S. bovis group	sepsis, endocarditis
S. mutans group	endocarditis, tooth decay
S. sanguis group	sepsis, endocarditis
S. anginosus group	abscess, sinusitis, meningitis

viridans streptococci → *α-hemolytic streptococci*
streptokinase *Syn: streptococcal fibrinolysin*; globulin produced by β-hemolyzing streptococci, which, together with plasminogen in the body, forms an activator complex for fibrinolysis; **usage**: as a fibrin-

olytic in acute peripheral arterial embolism and thrombosis, pulmonary embolism, venous thrombosis, myocardial infarction, retinal vessel occlusion, priapism; **side effects:** bleeding, microhematuria, anaphylactic reaction, shivering, and fever with late thrombolysis as a result of the release of pyrogens or toxins; **contraindications:** manifest or recent bleeding, local bleeding tendency [e.g., ulcerative disorders], hypertension, postoperatively, sepsis, subacute endocarditis, severe diabetes with retinopathy, apoplectic insult

stricture → *stenosis*

stroke a sudden attack of illness
  apoplectic stroke → *cerebrovascular accident*
  heart stroke → *angina pectoris*
  ischemic stroke s.u. *cerebrovascular accident*

strophanthin cardiac glycoside obtained from Strophanthus species
  k-strophanthin-α → *cymarin*

stypsis *Syn: hemostasia, hemostasis*; cessation of bleeding, hemostasis

styptic *Syn: hematostatic, hemostatic, hemostyptic, antihemorrhagic, anthemorrhagic*; **1.** an agent with styptic properties **2.** arresting hemorrhage

sub- combining form denoting relation to inferior to, below, or beneath

subacute moderately acute, not running an acute course

subareolar situated below the areola

subendocardial situated beneath the endocardium

subepicardial situated below the epicardium

subfebrile mildly feverish; (*temperature*) slightly elevated

sublymphemia → *lymphopenia*

subpericardial situated beneath the pericardium

subpulmonary *Syn: infrapulmonary*; (situated) beneath the lung(s)

substitute alternative, replacement, equivalent
  blood substitute aqueous solution of salts or organic substances for volume replacement in hypovolemia

subvalvular situated below a valve

suffusion larger, areal bleeding

suggillation areal bleeding into the skin

sulbactam β-lactamase inhibitor; used in combination with ampicillin

sulcus furrow, groove
  anterior interventricular sulcus *Syn: anterior interventricular groove, anterior longitudinal sulcus of heart*; groove on the anterior surface of the heart that defines the border between the right and left ventricles;

in it, the anterior interventricular branch of the left coronary artery runs to the apex of the heart

anterior longitudinal sulcus of heart → *anterior interventricular sulcus*

atrioventricular sulcus → *coronary sulcus of heart*

coronary sulcus of heart *Syn: atrioventricular groove, auriculoventricular groove, atrioventricular sulcus*; groove at the atrioventricular border in which the coronary vessels run [right and left coronary arteries]

inferior interventricular sulcus → *posterior interventricular sulcus*

sulcus interventricularis anterior → *anterior interventricular sulcus*

sulcus interventricularis posterior → *posterior interventricular sulcus*

posterior interventricular sulcus *Syn: inferior interventricular groove, inferior interventricular sulcus, posterior longitudinal sulcus of heart*; groove on the back of the heart that defines the border between the right and left ventricles; in it runs the posterior interventricular branch of the right coronary artery running to the cardiac apex

posterior longitudinal sulcus of heart → *posterior interventricular sulcus*

sulcus terminalis cordis → *terminal sulcus of right atrium*

terminal sulcus of right atrium groove on the outside of the right atrium between the superior and inferior vena cava

sulfinpyrazone pyrazole derivative; inhibitor of cyclooxygenase; **usage**: inhibitor of thrombocyte aggregation; uricosuric

sulfonamides aromatic amide of sulfonic acid, which can be used as a bacteriostatic antibiotic, oral antidiabetic, diuretic, and carbonic anhydrase inhibitor; the **sulfonamide antibiotics** are divided into **short-acting sulfonamides** with a half-life of 2–8 h [e.g., sulfadimidine, sulfafurazole], **intermediate-acting sulfonamides**, with a half life of 9–12 h [e.g., sulfamethoxazole, sulfamoxole], **long-acting sulfonamides**, with a half life of up to 60 h [e.g., sulfadoxine, sulfamerazine] and **non-reabsorbable sulfonamides** [e.g., sulfaguanol, sulfaguanidine]

super- combining form denoting relation to above, beyond, more than normal, or excessive

superacute → *hyperacute*

supercarbonate → *bicarbonate*

supra- combining form denoting relation to above or over

supracardiac *Syn: supracardial*; situated above the heart

supracardial → *supracardiac*

suprarenal → *adrenal*

suprarene → *adrenal gland*
supraseptal situated above a septum
supravalval → *supravalvular*
supravalvular *Syn: supravalval*; situated above a valve
supravascular situated above a vessel
supraventricular situated above the ventricle(s)
surface external aspect
   diaphragmatic surface of heart the lower surface of the heart
   pulmonary surface of heart the side of the heart turned toward the right [**facies pulmonalis cordis dextra**] or left [**facies pulmonalis cordis sinistra**] lung
   sternocostal surface of heart the anterior surface of the heart that faces the breastbone [sternum]
surgery treatment, as an operation, performed by a surgeon
   coronary surgery operative intervention to improve the perfusion of the heart muscle, e.g., by aortocoronary bypass or coronary angioplasty
suture 1. the process of joining two surfaces or edges of a wound or the like by stitching **2.** a particular method of doing this **3.** the line or stitch so formed **4.** the fine thread or other material used
   suture of an artery → *arteriorrhaphy*
swelling the act of swelling or the condition of being swollen
   pre-edematous swelling increased water storage, which has not yet presented as edema
switch transfer, shift, change
   arterial switch *Syn: arterial switch operation; s.u. transposition of the great vessels*
swoon 1. → *faint* **2.** → *syncope*
swooning → *syncope*
sympathectomy *Syn: sympathetectomy, sympathicectomy*; partial or complete removal of the ganglia of the sympathetic chain
   lumbar sympathectomy removal of lumbar sympathetic ganglia in disturbances of perfusion in the lower extremity
   periarterial sympathectomy → *Leriche's operation*
   thoracic sympathectomy removal of thoracic sympathetic ganglia in disturbances of perfusion in the upper extremity
sympathetectomy → *sympathectomy*
sympathetic 1. relating to the sympathetic nervous system **2.** encroaching upon a non-diseased organ

sympatheticomimetic → *sympathomimetic*

sympatheticotonia → *sympathicotonia*

sympathicectomy → *sympathectomy*

sympathico- combining form denoting relation to the sympathetic nervous system

sympathicolytic → *sympatholytic*

sympathicomimetic → *sympathomimetic*

sympathicotonia *Syn: sympatheticotonia*; increased excitability of the sympathetic nervous system; leads for example to increased sweating [hyperhidrosis], reduced gastric and intestinal peristalsis, tachycardia, mydriasis

sympatho- combining form denoting relation to the sympathetic nervous system

sympatholytic *Syn: sympathicolytic, sympathoparalytic, adrenolytic, antiadrenergic, antisympathetic*; **1.** an agent with antiadrenergic properties **2.** exciting the sympathetic system, having a stimulatory action on the sympathetic system increasing the action of adrenaline; inhibiting the sympathetic system

β-**sympatholytic** → *beta-blocker*

sympathomimetic *Syn: sympatheticomimetic, sympathicomimetic, adrenergic, adrenomimetic*; **1.** an agent that stimulates the sympathetic system; **direct sympathomimetics** act like adrenaline or noradrenaline; **indirect sympathomimetics** promote the release of noradrenaline from the presynaptic vesicles of adrenergic neurons **2.** exciting the sympathetic system, having a stimulatory action on the sympathetic system

alpha **sympathomimetic** → *alphamimetic*

sympathoparalytic → *sympatholytic*

symptom sign, manifestation of disease

Duroziez's symptom → *Duroziez's murmur*

symptoms of backward failure *s.u. chronic heart failure*

symptoms of forward failure *s.u. chronic heart failure*

partially reversible ischemic neurologic symptoms *s.u. cerebrovascular accident*

reversible ischemic neurologic symptoms *s.u. cerebrovascular accident*

symptomatology totality of disease symptoms

syn- combining form denoting relation to union or association

synapse contact site for transfer of information between nerve cells and other cells; depending upon the location, subdivided into, among others, **interneuronal synapses**, **neuromuscular synapses** [muscle end-plate], and **neuroglandular synapses**; synapses are subdivided depending upon the mechanism of transmission into **chemical** and **electrical synapses**, whereby chemical synapses are substantially more frequent; synapses are also classified as **excitatory** or **excitatory synapses** and **inhibitory** or **inhibitory synapses** depending upon their function

bioelectrical synapse →*electrical synapse*

chemical synapse most common form of synapse, in which the electric signal is transferred from the axon to the target organ via a second messenger [transmitter]; the axon ending forms a terminal bulb, which contains synaptic vesicles containing the neurotransmitter; if an action potential reaches the terminal bulb, the contents of the vesicles are discharged through the so-called **presynaptic membrane** of the axon into the **synaptic cleft** between the axon and the target organ; the transmitter binds to receptors on the **subsynaptic membrane** and leads to a change in the permeability of the membrane to sodium and potassium ions; this converts the chemical signal into an electric one; the transmitter is broken down enzymatically or taken back up into the axon

electrical synapse *Syn: bioelectrical synapse, ephapse*; at electric synapses, the current flows directly from one cell to the next across so-called **gap junctions**; electric synapses are found both in the central nervous system and also in functional syncytia, such as smooth muscle and heart muscle for example

synchronous *Syn: homochronous*; simultaneous, concurrent

syncopal *Syn: syncopic*; relating to syncope

syncope *Syn: deliquium, faint, fainting, ictus, swooning, swoon*; sudden, transient, and spontaneously reversible loss of consciousness with loss of tone due to a reduction in the cerebral perfusion and the lack of oxygen that this causes; the pathogenic cause is either insufficient vasoconstriction [e.g., vasovagal syncope, hypotonia with syncope] or inadequate pumping performance of the heart [e.g., cardiogenic syncope]; the **diagnosis** is based upon history, functional tests, and diagnostic tests for arrhythmias

cardiac syncope an inadequacy of the pumping performance can be due to a mechanical impairment of outflow [**mechanical cardiogenic syncope**] or else a disturbance of rhythm [**rhythmogenic syncope**]

carotid sinus syncope 1. *s.u. vasovagal syncope* **2.** → *carotid sinus syndrome*

emotional syncope *s.u. vasovagal syncope*

micturition syncope *s.u. vasovagal syncope*

pain syncope *s.u. vasovagal syncope*

situational syncope *s.u. vasovagal syncope*

Stokes-Adams syncope → *Adams-Stokes syndrome*

vasovagal syncope generic term for all forms of syncope that are caused by action of the vagus nerve; this includes, among others, **carotid sinus syncopes** in carotid sinus syndrome, **visceral reflex syncopes** [e.g., sneeze/micturition/pain syncopes], **centrally induced syncopes** [situational syncope, emotional syncope], and **neurocardiogenic syncopes**; in all forms, the main goal of treatment is to avoid the trigger factor

visceral reflex syncope *s.u. vasovagal syncope*

syncopic → *syncopal*

syndrome symptom complex; earlier designation for a group of symptoms characteristic for a specific disease; today the term is used more and more often for diseases with several or complex symptoms

abdominal muscle deficiency syndrome *Syn:* prune-belly syndrome; syndrome with congenital absence or underdevelopment of the abdominal wall musculature; often combined with other malformations [gastrointestinal malrotation, dilated uropathy, lung hypoplasia, heart abnormalities]

Abercrombie's syndrome → *amyloidosis*

Adams-Stokes syndrome *Syn:* Adams' disease, Adams-Stokes disease, Morgagni's disease, Morgagni's syndrome, Spens' syndrome, Morgagni-Adams-Stokes syndrome, Stokes' syndrome, Stokes-Adams disease, Stokes-Adams syncope, Stokes-Adams syndrome; acute, life-threatening loss of consciousness due to bradycardic or extremely tachycardic disturbances of heart rhythm with underperfusion of the brain; mainly found in high-grade valvular aortic stenosis, subclavian steal syndrome, carotid sinus syndrome, hypovolemia, and in laugh, cough, or micturition syncope

air-block syndrome *Syn:* air block; combination of dyspnea and cyanosis during compression of the inferior and superior vena cava by collection of air in the mediastinum and lung tissue

Alagille's syndrome malformation syndrome with hypoplasia of the bile ducts, pulmonary stenosis, facial malformations, and vertebral body anomalies; the prognosis is usually good, since liver cirrhosis only develops rarely

aortic arch syndrome umbrella term for diseases characterized by stenosis or occlusion of vessels arising from the aortic arch; it is often equated with Takayasu syndrome

aortic steal syndrome as a result of increased diastolic blood drainage out of the aorta, there is underperfusion of the brain [dizziness] and myocardium [angina]; the cause can be congenital [persistent ductus arteriosus] or acquired [Blalock-Taussig anastomosis]

asplenia syndrome *Syn: Ivemark's syndrome, Polhemus-Schafer-Ivemark syndrome*; congenital absence of the spleen in combination with other malformations [situs inversus, angiopathies, lung and heart malformations]

autoerythrocyte sensitization syndrome →*erythrocyte autosensitization syndrome*

Ayerza's syndrome *Syn: primary pulmonary sclerosis, Ayerza's disease, plexogenic pulmonary arteriopathy*; arteriosclerosis of pulmonary vessels of unknown etiology; it proceeds with dyspnea, cyanosis, right ventricular hypertrophy, and hepatosplenomegaly

Barlow syndrome →*mitral valve prolapse syndrome*

Beals' syndrome →*congenital contractural arachnodactyly*

Beau's syndrome →*cardiac arrest*

Bernard-Soulier syndrome *Syn: Bernard-Soulier disease, giant platelet disease, giant platelet syndrome*; autosomal recessive disturbance of thrombocyte formation with giant thrombocytes and purpura; the thrombocyte count is normal or mildly reduced, the bleeding time markedly prolonged

Bland-White-Garland syndrome *Syn: BWG syndrome*; malformation syndrome with the left coronary artery arising from the pulmonary artery; **clinical**: presents in infancy with restlessness, heavy nocturnal sweating, over-excitability, dyspnea, and ashen-sallow skin discoloration; **therapy**: implantation of the artery into the ascending aorta or anastomosis of the artery with the subclavian or internal thoracic artery; the operative risk is high and the long-term prognosis uncertain

Bouillaud's syndrome rheumatic endocarditis and pericarditis

Bouveret's syndrome *Syn: Bouveret's disease, paroxysmal tachycardia*; transient tachycardia without extrasystoles

brachial syndrome →*thoracic outlet syndrome*

Budd's syndrome →*Budd-Chiari syndrome*

Budd-Chiari syndrome *Syn: Budd's syndrome, Budd-Chiari disease, Chiari's disease, Chiari's syndrome, Chiari-Budd syndrome*; inflammation of unknown etiology which leads to occlusion of the hepatic veins

Bürger-Grütz syndrome *Syn: Bürger-Grütz disease, familial apolipoprotein C-II deficiency, familial fat-induced hyperlipemia, familial hyperchylomicronemia, familial lipoprotein lipase deficiency, familial hypertriglyceridemia, familial LPL deficiency, idiopathic hyperlipemia, type I familial hyperlipoproteinemia*; very rare, autosomal recessive lipid storage disease with a tendency to form eruptive xanthomata on the back, breast, arms, and gluteal region, hepatosplenomegaly and central nervous system damage; the arteriosclerosis risk is minimal; with dietary management, the prognosis is very good

BWG syndrome →*Bland-White-Garland syndrome*

cardiophobia syndrome clinical symptom complex [dizziness, strong palpitations, nausea, feeling of trepidation, fear of death] expressed in cardiac neurosis

cardiopulmonary syndrome of obesity →*pickwickian syndrome*

carotid sinus syndrome *Syn: carotid sinus reflex, carotid sinus syncope, Charcot-Weiss-Baker syndrome, pressoreceptive mechanism, pressoreceptor reflex*; bradycardia provoked by a blow to or pressure over the carotid sinus; may also cause hypotension or loss of consciousness; if the bradycardia predominates, this is the **cardioinhibitory type**, if the fall in blood pressure dominates, this is the **vasodepressor type**; **clinical**: the reflex may be triggered by, e.g., abrupt turning of the head and excessive stretching of the neck, shaving, buttoning up a shirt collar, etc.; it causes feelings of unsteadiness and weakness, giddiness, and possibly brief syncope; **therapy**: the cardioinhibitory type with syncopes is an indication for implantation of a pacemaker; in the vasodepressor type, the main focus of treatment is in the avoidance of the trigger factor

cat's-eye syndrome rare, partial tetrasomy 22q with coloboma, hypertelorism, accessory auricles, kidney malformations, heart defects, and anal atresia; mental development is generally normal

cerebral salt-losing syndrome disturbance of the central regulation of sodium balance and osmoregulation leads to hypernatremia, hypertonic hyperhydration, and interstitial edema; found in, e.g., head injury, brain hemorrhage, brain tumors, encephalitis

cerebral salt-retention syndrome →*sodium retention syndrome*

Charcot's syndrome → *intermittent claudication*
Charcot-Weiss-Baker syndrome → *carotid sinus syndrome*
Chiari's syndrome → *Budd-Chiari syndrome*
Chiari-Budd syndrome → *Budd-Chiari syndrome*
Churg-Strauss syndrome *Syn: allergic granulomatous angiitis, allergic granulomatosis*; systemic, necrotizing vasculitis of unknown etiology; the changes correspond to those in polyarteritis nodosa, but all vessels are affected with granuloma formation; eosinophilia and bronchial asthma also occur; **therapy**: prednisone, possibly in combination with cyclophosphamide; dose tapering only after 6–12 months of stable remission; **prognosis**: if untreated, the outcome is fatal in 50% within a year

costobrachial syndrome → *costoclavicular syndrome*

costoclavicular syndrome *Syn: costobrachial syndrome*; thoracic outlet syndrome caused by a narrowing of the space between first rib dorsally and clavicle ventrally; it can be caused by a cervical rib or congenital or acquired thoracic deformities [e.g., scoliosis] or tumors in the area of the pleural cupula; depending on the extent of compression, sensory and motor deficits of the brachial plexus, and circulatory disorders with weak pulse, cyanosis, or paleness of the fingers in certain movements [especially abduction and retroversion of the arm, pulling down of the shoulder] occur

DaCosta's syndrome → *neurocirculatory asthenia*

defibrination syndrome increased tendency to bleed in fibrin deficiency [fibrinogenopenia] or excessive degradation of fibrin [hyperfibrinolysis]

Degos' syndrome *Syn: Degos' disease, Köhlmeier-Degos disease, malignant atrophic papulosis*; disease of uncertain etiology, characterized by thrombosis of small arteries and formation of papules, which carries a poor prognosis; there are sporadic and familial forms as well as mild and protracted courses; **clinical**: stepwise development of disseminated papules, which become necrotic and heal with scar formation; more grave is the involvement of the internal organs [heart, kidney, lungs, liver, pancreas] and of the eye and brain; leads to colics, hematemesis, fever, and death mostly due to intestinal infarction with perforation

Determann's syndrome *Syn: intermittent dyskinesia*; intermittent failure of muscle groups due to angiosclerotic disturbances of perfusion or functional vascular diseases [vasospasms]

DiGeorge syndrome *Syn: pharyngeal pouch syndrome, third and fourth pharyngeal pouch syndrome, thymic-parathyroid aplasia, thymic hypoplasia*; congenital absence of or gross underdevelopment of the thymus; mostly combined with other malformations [aortic arch anomalies, conotruncal heart defects, facial dysmorphism, microgenia, cleft palate]; in some of patients, the problem is a microdeletion syndrome [10p13-14]; leads to disturbances of cellular immunity; **therapy**: transplantation of fetal thymus tissue

disseminated intravascular coagulation syndrome → *disseminated intravascular coagulation*

Dressler's syndrome *Syn: postmyocardial infarction syndrome*; complex of chest pain, fever, pericarditis, and pleuritis arising days to weeks [or sometimes months] after a heart infarct; occurs in approx. 4% of all patients, mainly after large infarcts and anticoagulant therapy; it is important to differentiate it from re-infarction; **diagnosis**: echocardiography, ECG, laboratory tests; **therapy**: analgesics, nonsteroidal anti-inflammatories, usually resulting in spontaneous cure

effort syndrome → *neurocirculatory asthenia*

Eisenmenger's syndrome → *Eisenmenger's tetralogy*

elfin facies syndrome → *Williams' syndrome*

EMC syndrome *Syn: encephalomyocarditis*; inflammation of brain and muscle caused by the **EMC virus**; extremely rare disease, which leads to loss of consciousness, motor pareses, and cardiac insufficiency

erythrocyte autosensitization syndrome *Syn: autoerythrocyte sensitization syndrome, Gardner-Diamond syndrome, painful bruising syndrome*; syndrome that occurs almost exclusively in women, with recurrent, painful bleeding into the skin; in addition to an allergic cause [autoantibodies against erythrocytes], psychogenic triggers are also under discussion [conversion neurosis]

Fallot's syndrome → *Fallot's tetrad*

Fanconi's syndrome → *Fanconi's anemia*

floppy mitral valve syndrome → *mitral valve prolapse syndrome*

Friderichsen-Waterhouse syndrome *Syn: acute fulminating meningococcemia, Waterhouse-Friderichsen syndrome*; hyperacute sepsis in meningococcal infection with massive bleeding into the skin, mucous membranes, and internal organs, circulatory shock, acute adrenal insufficiency, consumptive coagulopathy, acute interstitial myocarditis, or pericarditis with pericardial tamponade; occurs in 15% of all patients with meningococcal septicemia and proves fatal in more than

85% of cases

Gaisböck's syndrome *Syn: benign polycythemia, Gaisböck's disease*; polycythemia combined with hypertension

Gardner-Diamond syndrome →*erythrocyte autosensitization syndrome*

gastrocardiac syndrome functional chest pains in meteorism of the stomach and intestines, high-lying diaphragm and upward displacement of the heart; it leads to chest pains, tightness in the chest, possibly angina pectoris-like pains, extrasystoles, paroxysmal dyspnea, bouts of sweating, stomach pains, nausea, drops in blood pressure

giant platelet syndrome →*Bernard-Soulier syndrome*

Hageman syndrome →*Hageman factor deficiency*

heart-hand syndrome →*atriodigital dysplasia*

hemangioma-thrombocytopenia syndrome *Syn: Kasabach-Merritt syndrome*; in giant hemangiomas, thrombosis in the angioma can give rise to thrombocytopenia and consumptive coagulopathy; the mortality is 20–30%; **therapy**: anticoagulation, replacement of thrombocytes and factors, irradiation of the giant angioma

Holt-Oram syndrome →*atriodigital dysplasia*

Horton's syndrome →*Horton's arteritis*

hyperviscosity syndrome symptoms caused by increased viscosity of the blood, including e.g., headaches, dizziness, deafness, angina pectoris; **therapy**: reduction of the plasma viscosity by plasmapheresis or hemodilution by blood-letting

hypomagnesemia syndrome hypomagnesemia leads to muscle weakness, agitation, neuromuscular excitability, atrial tachycardia or fibrillation, ventricular and supraventricular disturbances of rhythm, ventricular fibrillation, calf cramps, more rarely also cramp attacks or delirium; **therapy**: oral or parenteral magnesium replacement

hypoplastic left heart syndrome congenital heart defect with underdevelopment of the left ventricle and usually also the ascending aorta; the aortic and mitral valves are narrowed or occluded and the ductus arteriosus generally remains open after birth; while still in the uterus, the right ventricle takes over the supply of blood to the whole body; **clinical**: in the first hours following birth, central and peripheral cyanosis, tachypnea, dyspnea, sweating, and poor drinking develop; if the ductus arteriosus closes, acute life-threatening cyanosis develops; **diagnosis**: echocardiography; **therapy**: maintenance of an open ductus arteriosus by infusion of prostaglandin E_1 or stent implantation;

Norwood operation: production of a functional aorta from a pulmonary artery branch and hypoplastic aorta; closure of the pulmonary artery bifurcation and onlay of an aortopulmonary shunt; heart transplantation would be the method of choice, but there are unfortunately insufficient donor hearts for infants

syndrome of inappropriate secretion of antidiuretic hormone causes of increased ADH secretion or increased efficacy of antidiuretic hormone [ADH] include increased secretion in cerebral diseases [encephalitis, meningitis, head injury, brain hemorrhage], effects of various medications [tricyclic antidepressants, carbamazepine, vincristine, vinblastine, cyclophosphamide], or ectopic hormone production in malignant tumors [bronchus, thymus, pancreas] or lymphomas; additional causes include chronic lung diseases [tuberculosis, pneumonia], diseases with sodium retention and edema formation [nephrotic syndrome, cardiac insufficiency, liver cirrhosis, hypothyroidism] and diseases that lead to hypovolemia or hypotension [adrenal cortical insufficiency, excessive fluid and electrolyte losses]; in **laboratory tests**, one finds hyponatremia and a marked reduction in the serum osmolality; water excretion is reduced, creatinine, urea, uric acid, and albumin levels are normal or reduced; **therapy**: in acute water intoxication, furosemide i.v. until the serum osmolality normalizes; thereafter, water restriction [800 ml/24 h] and treatment of the cause

ischemic syndrome description of acute ischemia and the symptoms it causes

Ivemark's syndrome → *asplenia syndrome*

Jaccoud's syndrome → *Jaccoud's sign*

Jervell and Lange-Nielsen syndrome *Syn: surdocardiac syndrome*; autosomal recessive prolongation of the QT-interval in the ECG with simultaneous inner ear deafness; leads to syncopes during sudden physical or emotional stress in childhood; **therapy**: pacemaker implantation

Kasabach-Merritt syndrome → *hemangioma-thrombocytopenia syndrome*

Kearns' syndrome → *Kearns-Sayre syndrome*

Kearns-Sayre syndrome *Syn: Kearns' syndrome*; rare, inherited mitochondrial myopathy with chronic progressive external ophthalmoplegia, retinitis pigmentosa, and disturbances of conduction of excitation in the heart

leopard syndrome → *multiple lentigines syndrome*

Leriche's syndrome *Syn: aorticoiliac occlusive disease*; underperfusion of the legs caused by occlusion of the aortic bifurcation and the symptoms that this causes [leg pains, pallor, intermittent claudication]; it requires operative removal of the cause [embolus, thrombus] or bypass for atherosclerosis

Libman-Sacks syndrome → *non bacterial thrombotic endocarditis*

Löffler's syndrome → *Löffler's endocarditis*

Lown-Ganong-Levine syndrome pre-excitation syndrome with a normal ventricular complex in the ECG; the excitation is partially conducted to the ventricular muscle by the James bundle, bypassing the AV node; this leads to a short QT-interval with a normal QRS complex

low output syndrome typical combination of hypotension, oliguria, and pale, cool skin with increased preload and reduced cardiac index, stroke volume, and stroke work index seen in cardiogenic shock or decompensated cardiac insufficiency

low salt syndrome → *salt-depletion syndrome*

low sodium syndrome → *salt-depletion syndrome*

Lutembacher's syndrome → *Lutembacher's disease*

Maffucci's syndrome rare constitutional mesodermal dysplasia of unknown etiology, with multiple cavernous hemangiomas, chondromas, and asymmetric bone chondromatosis with skeletal malformations; in approx. 20% of patients, there is malignant transformation and formation of, among others, angiosarcomas or chondrosarcomas

Marfan's syndrome → *Marfan's disease*

Martorell's syndrome → *brachiocephalic arteritis*

Minot-von Willebrand syndrome → *von Willebrand's syndrome*

mitral valve prolapse syndrome *Syn: Barlow syndrome, floppy mitral valve syndrome*; balloon-like systolic bulging of one or both mitral valve cusps into the left atrium, which mainly affects women and whose etiology is uncertain; usually asymptomatic, but with a prevalence of 2–6%, it is one of the most common valve anomalies; **diagnosis**: echocardiography, angiography; **therapy**: asymptomatic cases do not need treatment; in symptomatic patients, thromboprophylaxis [coumarin derivatives] and β-blockers for treatment of arrhythmias; operative reconstruction is only rarely indicated

Morgagni's syndrome → *Adams-Stokes syndrome*

Morgagni-Adams-Stokes syndrome → *Adams-Stokes syndrome*

Moya-Moya syndrome rare, partially congenital disease with inflam-

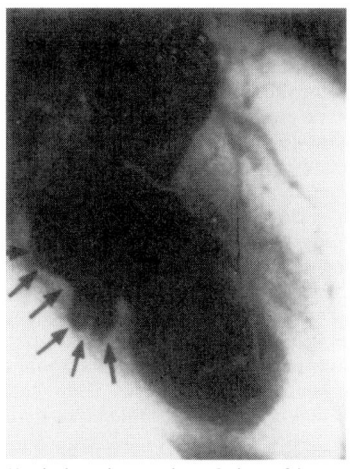

Mitral valve prolapse syndrome. Prolapse of the posterior mitral cusp [angiography]

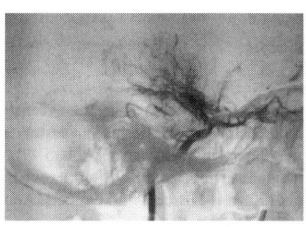

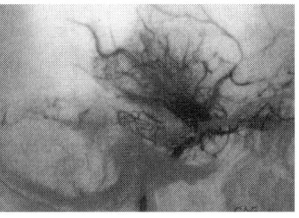

Moya-Moya syndrome. Stenosis of the left internal carotid

mation and severe stenosis of the internal carotid artery and of the proximal portion of the circle of Willis, as well as a network of abnormal collaterals; leads to relapsing ischemic syndromes, mostly in young patients; **therapy**: inhibitors of thrombocyte aggregation, cortisone, possibly bypass surgery

multiple lentigines syndrome *Syn: leopard syndrome*; rare, autosomal dominant syndrome with multiple Lentigines, Excitation conduction defects, Ocular hypertelorism, Pulmonary stenosis, Abnormal genitalia [hypogonadism], Retardation of growth, and Deafness

Naffziger's syndrome → *scalenus anticus syndrome*

Nygaard-Brown syndrome arterial occlusive disease with calf pain, intermittent claudication, and recurrent thromboses in the legs, later also in the abdominal and pelvic vessels with tendency to collapse and hematuria

Ortner's syndrome left-sided recurrent laryngeal nerve palsy due to compression of the recurrent laryngeal nerve by a dilated left atrium [mitral valve defect] or enlargement of the left pulmonary artery

outlet syndrome → *thoracic outlet syndrome*

pacemaker-twiddler syndrome *Syn: twiddler's syndrome*; repeated rotation of a cardiac pacemaker leads to disconnection of the probe and ineffective impulse transmission

Paget-von Schroetter syndrome *Syn: effort-induced thrombosis*; thrombosis of the subclavian vein leads to more or less acute venous engorgement of the arm with swelling and livid discoloration, feeling of pressure in the armpit, and a feeling of tightness and heaviness; usually develops following unusual exertion [tennis, swimming], with the most common cause being narrowing of the veins in the vicinity of the first rib; **therapy**: conservative [thrombolysis, elevation, anticoagulation], more rarely operative [thrombectomy]

painful bruising syndrome → *erythrocyte autosensitization syndrome*

pancytopenia-dysmelia syndrome → *constitutional infantile panmyelopathy*

Penfield's syndrome paroxysmal hypertension in brain tumors, particularly in the area of the thalamus

pharyngeal pouch syndrome → *DiGeorge syndrome*

Pickwick syndrome → *pickwickian syndrome*

pickwickian syndrome *Syn: Pickwick syndrome, cardiopulmonary syndrome of obesity*; combination of obesity and hypersomnia episodes with muscle twitching and cardiovascular disorders; it improves with weight loss

Polhemus-Schafer-Ivemark syndrome → *asplenia syndrome*

postcardiotomy syndrome → *postpericardiotomy syndrome*

postcommissurotomy syndrome → *postpericardiotomy syndrome*

postmyocardial infarction syndrome → *Dressler's syndrome*

postpericardiotomy syndrome *Syn: postcardiotomy syndrome, postcommissurotomy syndrome*; syndrome of pericarditis, pericardial effusion, disturbances of heart rhythm, fever, and similar, which occurs after heart operations

postphlebitic syndrome → *post-thrombotic syndrome*

posttachycardia syndrome as a result of ventricular or [more rarely] supraventricular tachycardia that persists for days, occasionally reversible ECG changes can develop, which are caused by small subendocardial myocardial injuries; usually heals without consequences

post-thrombotic syndrome *Syn: postphlebitic syndrome*; skin manifestations mostly affecting the lower leg and foot following burnt out phlebothrombosis with the development of secondary varices, skin pigmentation, and stasis edema; caused by chronic venous insufficiency, which is caused by injuries to the vein wall and valves

preexcitation syndrome *Syn: ventricular preexcitation, Wolff-Parkinson-White syndrome*; premature excitation of parts of the ventricular muscle caused by an accessory bundle [bundle of Kent, bundle of Mahaim]; occurs in approx. 0.2–0.3% of the population and in the great majority remains asymptomatic or is a partial symptom of a disease syndrome [e.g., mitral valve prolapse, Ebstein anomaly]; in rare cases, paroxysmal orthodromic or antidromic tachycardias or atrial flutter or fibrillation may develop; if antegrade conduction only devel-

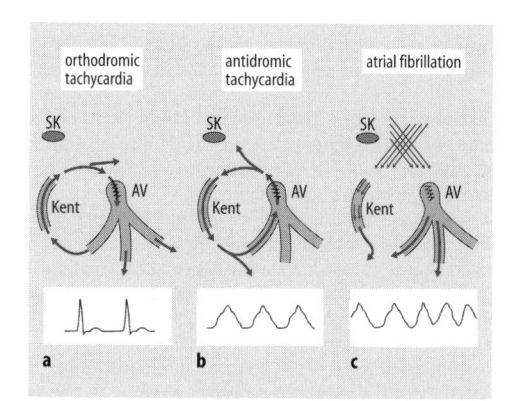

Preexcitation syndrome. **a** orthodromic tachycardia; **b** antidromic tachycardia; **c** atrial fibrillation

ops sporadically, then this is called **intermittent pre-excitation syndrome**; in **occult pre-excitation syndrome**, only retrograde impulses pass from the ventricle to the atrium

preinfarction syndrome the symptoms occurring before an infarct, particularly sudden chest pain with a characteristic feeling of constriction

prune-belly syndrome → *abdominal muscle deficiency syndrome*

Rendu-Osler-Weber syndrome → *Osler's disease*

Romano-Ward syndrome Syn: *Ward-Romano syndrome*; rare, autosomal dominant syndrome with marked prolongation of the QT-interval in the ECG; caused by changes in the genetic information for the potassium and sodium channels on 11p15.5

salt-depletion syndrome Syn: *low salt syndrome, low sodium syndrome, salt-depletion crisis*; disturbance of electrolyte balance caused by loss of sodium chloride with hyponatremia and hypochloremia; most commonly due to salt-wasting nephritis, but may also occur in chronic renal insufficiency, polyuria in acute renal failure, adrenal cortical insufficiency, osmotic diuresis, diabetes mellitus, diuretic abuse, burns, or gastrointestinal losses; **clinical**: headaches, dry skin, and mucous membranes, reduced skin turgor, weakness, lethargy, confusion; **therapy**: in mild cases, increased intake of salt in the diet [5–10 g/day]; in euvolemic hyponatremia, infusion of hypertonic NaCl solution [3%], in hypovolemic hyponatremia, isotonic NaCl-solution, and in hypertonic hyponatremia, restriction of water intake and loop diuretics

scalenus anticus syndrome Syn: *Naffziger's syndrome*; form of thoracic outlet syndrome caused by compression of the brachial plexus and subclavian artery at the posterior scalenus foramen between the anterior and medial scalenus muscles; depending upon the extent of compression, sensory and motor deficits of the brachial plexus and disturbances of perfusion with weakening of the pulse, cyanosis, or pallor of the fingers may develop with certain movements [mainly abduction and retroversion of the arm, traction of the shoulder]

scimitar syndrome combination of anomalous pulmonary venous drainage into the inferior vena cava [appears as scimitar-shaped shadow in the radiograph], pulmonary hypoplasia, bronchiectasis, and pulmonary sequestration; the prognosis is poor when patients develop pulmonary hypertension in childhood

Shy-Drager syndrome → *idiopathic orthostatic hypotension*

sick sinus syndrome symptom complex with various disturbances of rhythm [including persistent, inadequate sinus bradycardias, intermittent sinus arrest, or various forms of SA-block, as well as tachycardia-bradycardia episodes], which all reflect disturbances in sinoatrial node function; there is generally a structural abnormality of the region of the sinoatrial node, e.g., due to hypertensive and coronary heart disease, but primary degenerative processes in the impulse conduction system may be to blame; **clinical**: palpitations and racing heart as a result of tachycardic rhythms, weakness and tendency to collapse if bradycardia or asystole predominate; **therapy**: in symptomatic bradycardia, implantation of an AAIR pacemaker, in bradycardia-tachycardia syndrome pacemaker therapy with antiarrhythmic settings

Silverman's syndrome developmental anomaly of the sternum with premature synostosis; usually results in secondary pigeon breast [pectus carinatum]; mostly combined with congenital heart defects

sodium retention syndrome *Syn: cerebral salt-retention syndrome*; disturbance of the central regulation of sodium balance and osmoregulation leads to hypernatremia, hypertonic hyperhydration, and interstitial edema; found in, e.g., head injury, brain hemorrhage, brain tumors, encephalitis

Spens' syndrome → *Adams-Stokes syndrome*

Stokes' syndrome → *Adams-Stokes syndrome*

Stokes-Adams syndrome → *Adams-Stokes syndrome*

stroke syndrome → *cerebrovascular accident*

Stuart-Prower syndrome rare, autosomal recessive deficiency of factor X; leads to mild symptoms suggestive of hemophilia

subclavian steal syndrome *Syn: subclavian steal*; intermittent underperfusion of the brain with feelings of dizziness due to proximal occlusion of the subclavian artery; there is partial reversal of flow from the vertebral artery into the arm on the affected side; **clinical**: dizziness, syncope, visual disturbances, disturbances of hearing during exertion [predominantly of the affected side]; **diagnosis**: differences in blood pressure between the two sides, stenotic bruit over the subclavian artery, angiography, Doppler ultrasound; **therapy**: angioplasty, bypass

superior mesenteric artery syndrome *Syn: Wilkie's syndrome*; compression of the horizontal portion of the duodenum by the superior mesenteric artery; can lead to sporadic obstruction and even ileus

superior vena cava syndrome narrowing of the lumen of the superior vena cava from outside [bronchial, mediastinal tumors, lymph node enlargement, aortic arch aneurysm] or inside [thrombosis, rare] leading to flow congestion in the upper body with Stokes' collar, cyanosis, arm edema, dizziness, headache, chest pains, and air hunger; **diagnosis**: X-ray, CT, sonography; the **therapy** depends upon the cause

surdocardiac syndrome →*Jervell and Lange-Nielsen syndrome*

systemic inflammatory response syndrome systemic, inflammatory reaction to, among others, trauma, infection, ischemia, burns, shock, etc.; characterized by two or more of the following symptoms: hypo- or hyperthermia, tachycardia, tachypnea, leukocytosis

Takayasu's syndrome →*brachiocephalic arteritis*

TAR syndrome →*thrombocytopenia-absent radius syndrome*

Taussig-Bing syndrome *Syn: partial transposition of great vessels, Taussig-Bing disease*; congenital angiocardiopathy with incomplete transposition of the great vessels

third and fourth pharyngeal pouch syndrome →*DiGeorge syndrome*

thoracic outlet syndrome *Syn: brachial syndrome, outlet syndrome*; generic term for clinical symptoms due to compression of the neurovascular bundle at the thoracic outlet; the brachial plexus and subclavian artery can be narrowed from the outside by compression between the scalenus anterior and medius muscles, clavicle, first rib or a cervical rib, thoracic wall and pectoralis minor muscle, or by processes in the region of the dome of the pleura; depending upon the extent of compression, there may be sensory and motor deficits of the brachial plexus as well as disturbances of perfusion with a weak pulse, cyanosis or pallor of the fingers brought on by certain movements [particularly abduction and retroversion of the arm, traction on the shoulder]

thrombocytopenia-absent radius syndrome *Syn: TAR syndrome*; autosomal recessive combination of thrombocytopenia and bilateral total absence of the radii; often also combined with heart defects, hip dysplasia, foot deformities, or micrognathy; **therapy**: thrombocyte replacement prior to procedures or if there is a bleeding tendency; the thrombocytopenia usually improves over the course of the patient's life

thrombophlebitis syndromes generic term for diseases with recurrent inflammation of superficial veins; this includes thrombophlebitis migrans, Mondor phlebitis, and retinal phlebitis

Trousseau's syndrome *Syn: thrombophlebitis migrans*; s.u. *migrating phlebitis*

twiddler's syndrome →*pacemaker-twiddler syndrome*

von Willebrand's syndrome *Syn: angiohemophilia, constitutional thrombopathy, hereditary pseudohemophilia, Minot-von Willebrand syndrome, von Willebrand's disease, pseudohemophilia, Willebrand's syndrome*; autosomal dominant deficiency of von Willebrand factor with a bleeding tendency, which leads to hemorrhages particularly in the spring and fall; **clinical**: recurrent skin and mucous membrane bleeding, hyper- and polymenorrhea; more rarely, joint hemorrhages; injury or operations can cause difficult to control bleeding; **lab.**: prolonged bleeding time, factor VIII below 25%; reduction in the ristocetin cofactor; **DD**: idiopathic thrombocytopenic purpura, thrombocytopenia; **therapy**: fresh frozen plasma, cryoprecipitate; **prognosis**: good; usually the bleeding tendency declines after the age of 20

Ward-Romano syndrome → *Romano-Ward syndrome*

Waring-Blendor syndrome description of the shortened lifespan of erythrocytes and the increased formation of fragmentocytes as an expression of mechanical injury of the erythrocytes by artificial implants following operative correction of cardiac septal defects

Waterhouse-Friderichsen syndrome → *Friderichsen-Waterhouse syndrome*

Wegener's syndrome → *Wegener's granulomatosis*

Wilkie's syndrome → *superior mesenteric artery syndrome*

Willebrand's syndrome → *von Willebrand's syndrome*

Williams' syndrome *Syn: elfin facies syndrome*; microdeletion system with a frequency of 1:10,000 live births; leads to disturbances in calcium and vitamin D metabolism, elfin facies, hypertelorism, short nose, pouting lips, dental anomalies, short stature, heart defects [supravalvular aortic stenosis, pulmonary stenosis, ventricular septal defect], as well as mild mental retardation

Wolff-Parkinson-White syndrome → *preexcitation syndrome*

synephrine *Syn: oxedrine*; α-sympathomimetic, antihypotensive

syngeneic → *isologous*

syngenetic → *isologous*

synthetic → *artificial*

systaltic *Syn: pulsating*; contracting rhythmically, pulsating rhythmically

system a set of correlated and semi-independent parts that function together

absorbent system → *lymphatic system*

autonomic nervous system parts of the nervous system not controlled by will and consciousness; consists of the sympathetic nervous system [pars sympathica], parasympathetic nervous system [pars parasympathica], the abdominal segment of the vegetative nervous system [pars abdominalis plexus visceralis et ganglia visceralia], and intramural nerve fibers

cardiac conducting system *Syn: conduction system, conducting system*; autonomic system, which is responsible for the formation and spread of excitation in the heart muscle; consists of the **sinoatrial node**, **atrioventricular node**, and the **bundle of His**, which divides into the right and left **Tawara branches**; the Tawara branches run on both sides of the ventricular septum to the cardiac apex; their **subendocardial branches** penetrate the working muscle, where they form the final part of the excitation conduction system in the form of **Purkinje fibers**; individual Purkinje fibers can pass through the ventricular cavity as so-called **false tendons**

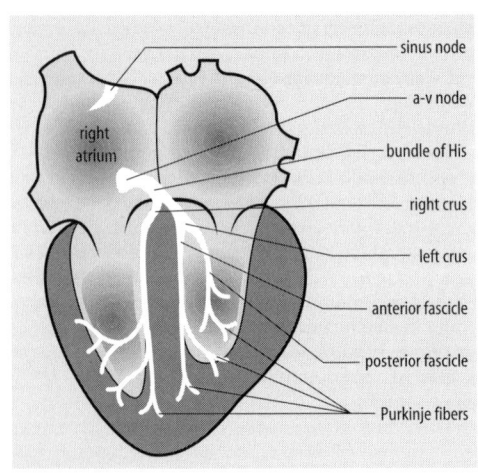

Cardiac conducting system

cardiovascular system includes heart [cor], arteries [arteriae], veins [venae], and the large lymphatic trunks [trunci et ductus lymphatici]
circulatory system → *circulation*
conducting system → *cardiac conducting system*

conduction system → *cardiac conducting system*
craniosacral system → *parasympathetic nervous system*
cytochrome system → *respiratory chain*
kallikrein system → *kallikrein-kinin system*
kallikrein-kinin system *Syn: kallikrein system, kinin system*; regulatory system responsible for the rapid release of kinins; kallikrein in the blood plasma [**plasma kallikrein**] releases bradykinin from the **tissue kallikrein** found in the granulocytes, salivary glands, tear glands, sweat glands, kidneys, pancreas, and intestines, in contrast to kallidin
Kidd blood group system → *Kidd blood groups*
kinin system → *kallikrein-kinin system*
low-pressure system part of the circulation with low pressure; it comprises all systemic veins, right atrium, right ventricle, pulmonary vessels, and left atrium, and during diastole the left ventricle as well; it contains about 85% of the total blood volume
lymphatic system *Syn: lymphatics, absorbent system, lymphoid system*; comprises primary [bone marrow, thymus] and secondary lymphatic organs [spleen, tonsillar ring], lymph follicles [noduli lymphoidei], and lymph nodes [nodi lymphoidei]; most of the cells of the immune system are formed or stored in them; they monitor the lymphatic vessels [lymph nodes], bloodstream [spleen], pharynx [Waldeyer's tonsillar ring], gastrointestinal tract [lymph follicles], and respiratory passages [lymph follicles] for foreign antigens and pathogenic microorganisms
lymphoid system → *lymphatic system*
MN blood group system → *MNSs blood group system*
MNSs blood group system *Syn: MN blood group system, MN blood groups, MNSs blood groups*; blood group system that only rarely causes transfusion reactions or hemolytic disease of the newborn
nervous system *Syn: systema nervosum*; totality of the nervous structures of the body; subdivided into the **central nervous system** and **peripheral nervous system**
parasympathetic nervous system *Syn: craniosacral system, parasympathetic part of autonomic nervous system*; parasympathetic portion of the autonomic nervous system; divided into a cranial portion [**pars cranialis**] and a pelvic portion [**pars pelvica**]; the transmitter substance in the parasympathetic system is acetylcholine; the fibers derived from the cranial portion run for the most part in the vagus nerve to the heart, lungs, esophagus, stomach, liver, pancreas, small intestine, and proximal colon; the rest supply the eye and the salivary

glands; the fibers derived from the pelvic portion run in the pelvic splanchnic nerves to the pelvic organs; in the neck, chest, abdominal, and pelvic areas, the sympathetic and parasympathetic nerves form a series of mixed plexuses, which surround the aorta and its branches

P blood group system → *P blood groups*

proteinate buffer system *Syn: protein buffer, protein buffer system, proteinate buffer*; part of the buffer system that maintains a constant blood pH; consists of the plasma proteins [buffering capacity: 5 mmol/l/pH] and hemoglobin [buffering capacity: 16 mmol/l/pH], which, due to its high concentration, contributes the major part of the buffering action

protein buffer system → *proteinate buffer system*

renin-angiotensin-aldosterone system major regulatory system keeping the blood volume, osmolality, and pressure constant; is closely connected with atrial natriuretic peptide and brain natriuretic peptide; hypovolemia, reduced pressure in the afferent glomerular arteriole and reduction in the sodium concentration in the serum lead to increased renin secretion, which leads to increased formation of angiotensin II and stimulation of aldosterone secretion and vasoconstriction

respiratory system → *respiratory tract*

Rh system → *Rhesus blood groups*

Rh blood group system → *Rhesus blood groups*

rhesus system → *Rhesus blood groups*

sympathetic nervous system *Syn: thoracicolumbar division of autonomic nervous system, thoracolumbar division of autonomic nervous system, thoracolumbar system*; sympathetic component of the vegetative nervous system; consists of the **sympathetic trunk**, paraganglia, prevertebral ganglia, and mixed sympathetic-parasympathetic nerve plexuses; the preganglionic neurons lie at C_8–$L_{2/3}$; their axons run in the ventral root and then in the **white ramus communicans** to the sympathetic chains; most fibers end here on postganglionic neurons, but a portion carry on to the prevertebral ganglia and mixed sympathetic-parasympathetic nerve plexuses; noradrenaline is the transmitter substance at the postganglionic sympathetic neurons

thoracolumbar system → *sympathetic nervous system*

systema system

systema nervosum → *nervous system*

systole *Syn: miocardia*; phase of the heart cycle in which the ventricular muscle contracts and the blood is pumped out of the heart into the systemic or pulmonary circulations; subdivided: **1. tension phase**: at the start of systole, tension in the myocardial fibers leads to deformation of the ventricle, an increase in pressure and immediate closure of the atrioventricular valve; since the volume in this phase doesn't change, it is described as isovolumetric contraction; one can further subdivide the **tension** phase into **deformation time** [start of the QRS-complex to the 1. heart sound] and the **pressure increase time** [start of the 1. sound to the start of ejection] **2. ejection phase**: as soon as the pressure in the ventricle exceeds the diastolic pressure in the aorta or pulmonary artery, the semilunar valves open and bloodstreams out of the ventricle into the vessels; the ventricular pressure initially continues to increase, then falls toward the end of systole; during this time, the volume falls from the **end-diastolic volume** of approx. 140 ml to the **residual volume** of approx. 50 ml, i.e., the **stroke volume** is approx. 90 ml and the **ejection fraction** is 0.64; the ejection phase ends with closure of the semilunar valves

extra systole → *extrasystole*
late systole → *prediastole*
premature systole → *extrasystole*
premature atrial systole → *atrial extrasystole*
premature ventricular systole → *ventricular extrasystole*
systolic relating to the systole

tachy- combining form denoting relation to swift or rapid

tachyarrhythmia *Syn: cardiac tachyarrhythmia*; tachycardia with arrhythmia

absolute tachyarrhythmia absolute arrhythmia with a frequency greater than 100/min; usually due to atrial fibrillation; can cause cardiac symptoms

cardiac tachyarrhythmia → *tachyarrhythmia*

tachycardia *Syn: heart hurry, polycardia, tachysystole*; elevation of the heart rate to more than 100/min at rest; the origin of the excitation can lie in the ventricular muscle [ventricular tachycardia], in the AV-node [AV-nodal tachycardia], the sinoatrial node [sinus tachycardia], and the atrium [atrial tachycardia]; depending upon the mechanism, tachycardias are divided into focal impulse formation and so-called circular excitations [re-entry tachycardia]; the **clinical picture** is mostly non-specific; the course is often asymptomatic or harmless [palpitations], but it can also provoke dizziness or syncopes; the goal of **therapy** is to remove the cause, normalize the ventricular rate [e.g., with β-blockers, calcium antagonists] and to minimize or prevent arrhythmias; operative therapy [catheter ablation] is only rarely necessary [mainly in WPW syndrome, therapy-resistant atrial flutter]

antidromic tachycardia *s.u. reentrant tachycardia*

atrial tachycardia *Syn: auricular tachycardia*; tachycardia arising in the atrium; can be idiopathic or occur in cardiac diseases [among others, acute myocardial infarction, cor pulmonale]; also frequently in digitalis overdose or intoxication when combined with hypokalemia; **therapy**: in digitalis overdose, cessation of the glycoside and potassium replacement; otherwise normalization of the ventricular rate [e.g., with β-blockers, calcium antagonists] and prevention or elimination of arrhythmias with antiarrhythmics

auricular tachycardia → *atrial tachycardia*

A-V nodal tachycardia tachycardia originating in the atrioventricular node; the majority arise as re-entry tachycardias [**AV-node re-entry tachycardia**]; in these cases, catheter ablation is the current treatment of choice

AV nodal reentrant tachycardia *s.u. reentrant tachycardia*

ectopic tachycardia tachycardia with a focus of excitation outside the sinoatrial node

normotopic tachycardia tachycardia with a focus of excitation in the sinoatrial node

orthodromic tachycardia *s.u. reentrant tachycardia*

paroxysmal tachycardia → *Bouveret's syndrome*

reentrant tachycardia in re-entry tachycardia, there is either a circulating excitation in the AV-node areal [AV-node re-entry tachycardia, AV-node re-entry] or the excitation is conducted from the atrium to the ventricles via an accessory conduction bundle [e.g., bundle of Kent] and thus begins to circle; if the conduction passes in the direction of normal conduction, it is known as **orthodromic tachycardia**, if it runs retrogradely as **antidromic tachycardia**

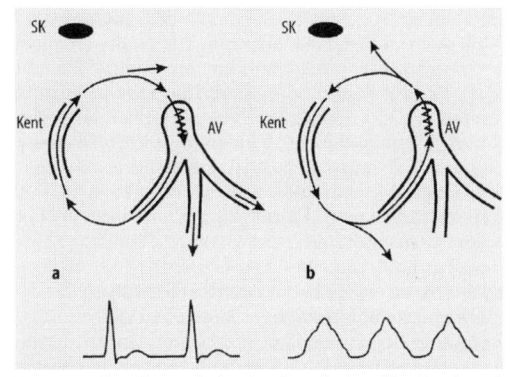

Reentrant tachycardia. **a** orthodromic tachycardia; **b** antidromic tachycardia

sinus tachycardia tachycardia arising in the sinoatrial node; occurs physiologically with physical or emotional stress, in small children and with elevated body temperature; often found as a symptom in inflammations of the heart [pericarditis, myocarditis], cardiac insufficiency, aortic insufficiency, anemia, cor pulmonale, hyperthyroidism, or ingestion of stimulants [alcohol, nicotine, caffeine] or medications [atropine, adrenaline]

supraventricular tachycardia generic term for sinus tachycardia, AV-nodal tachycardia, and atrial tachycardia; the large majority arise as re-entry tachycardias; in such cases, catheter ablation is the treatment of choice

ventricular tachycardia tachycardia with the origin of excitation in the Tawara branches; **acute therapy**: lidocaine or ajmaline are the agents of choice for acute medical management; if this is unsuccessful, anti-tachycardic stimulation or cardioversion

tachycardiac *Syn: tachycardic*; relating to tachycardia

tachycardic → *tachycardiac*

tachysystole → *tachycardia*

talinolol beta-blocker

tamponade *Syn: tamponage*; the use of a tampon, as to stop a hemorrhage

cardiac tamponade → *pericardial tamponade*

pericardial tamponade *Syn: cardiac tamponade*; filling of the pericardial sac with blood or exudate; the most common causes are uremic pericarditis, pericardial carcinosis, and acute myocardial infarction; leads to restriction of the motility of the musculature with elevation of the central venous pressure, reduction of the arterial blood pressure, tachycardia, tachypnea, dyspnea, and pulsus paradoxus; **diagnosis**: echocardiography, CT; **therapy**: pericardial puncture and drainage

T-cells → *thymus-dependent lymphocytes*

technique method, procedure

Dotter technique *s.u. angioplasty*

double-contrast barium technique → *double-contrast radiography*

impulse echo technique *Syn: pulse echography; s.u. sonography*

indicator-dilution technique → *indicator-dilution method*

Judkins technique Seldinger technique, in which the catheter is introduced via the femoral artery

MIDCAB technique *s.u. aortocoronary bypass*

Ouchterlony technique → *Ouchterlony test*

Oudin technique *Syn: Oudin test*; one-dimensional immunodiffusion in a tube containing agar gel

real-time technique *Syn: real-time sonographic examination*; imaging process [e.g., sonography], in which events can be observed directly on a monitor

Seldinger technique technique for retrograde catheterization of large blood vessels, e.g., for angiography or placement of a central venous catheter; **principle**: in the first step, puncture of a vein [e.g., internal jugular or subclavian vein] with a cannula; removal of the mandrel and introduction of a guidewire through the cannula; removal of the cannula; introduction of the catheter over the guidewire

Sones technique Seldinger technique, in which the catheter is introduced through the brachial artery

TECAB technique s.u. *aortocoronary bypass*

teicoplanin glycopeptide antibiotic derived from **Actinoplanes teichomyceticus**; active mainly against Gram-positive organisms; **side effects**: allergic reactions; raised transaminase levels

tela tissue layer; tissue

tela subserosa pericardii subserous layer of the serous pericardium

telangiectasia permanent dilatation and tortuosity of terminal vessels [capillaries, venules] that are visible through the epidermis

hereditary hemorrhagic telangiectasia → *Osler's disease*

telangiectatic relating to telangiectasia

tele- combining form denoting relation to the end or operating at a distance, or far away

telediastolic → *end-diastolic*

telelectrocardiography *Syn: radioelectrocardiography*; wireless electrocardiography with transmission of the measured values by radio transmitter

telesystolic → *end-systolic*

temocillin semisynthetic penicillin; it is effective especially against gram-negative causative agents

tendency an inclination, bent, or predisposition to something

thrombotic tendency *Syn: thrombophilia*; congenital or acquired tendency to thrombus formation due to disturbances in blood clotting or changes in the blood cells or vessel walls

tendon a fibrous cord of connective tissue by which muscles are connected to other structures

coronary tendon → *fibrous annulus*

tenebrimycin → *tobramycin*

tenecteplase 3. generation thrombolytic derived from human tissue plasminogen activator; binds preferentially to fibrin in thrombus and activates the plasminogen trapped in the thrombus to make plasmin

tenemycen → *tobramycin*

terazosin peripheral α$_1$-blocker; **usage**: arterial hypertension

terlipressin vasopressin analogue, hemostatic, vasoconstrictor; **usage**: bleeding esophageal varices

tertatolol beta-blocker

test examination, trial

ACTH test *Syn: ACTH stimulation test*; test of adrenal cortical function if adrenal cortical insufficiency is suspected; the cortisol level in the blood is measured before ACTH injection [250 µg i.v.] and 60 minutes after; the rise in level and the peak value are assessed; if the cortisol increases to > 550 nmol/l, then adrenal insufficiency is practically excluded; at values between 250 and 550 nmol/l, partial adrenal insufficiency is possible, at values < 250 nmol/l there is adrenal insufficiency

ACTH stimulation test → *ACTH test*

clot observation test global test for assessment of the clotting function of the blood; determination of the clotting time of 2–5 ml whole blood in an agitation tube [normal 6–12 min]; if it is prolonged then there is fibrin deficiency, if the clot dissolves within 10 min, a coagulopathy due to fibrin degradation products

cold pressure test *Syn: Hines and Brown test*; test of circulatory control during cold stress; a hand is immersed in ice-cold water for 1 minute; the blood pressure is recorded before and during the immersion; it is normal for it to increase by up to 10–25 mmHg during the cold stress and to return to normal within 2–3 minutes after ending the stress; the value is increased in pheochromocytoma and hypertension

Duke's test → *Duke's method*

fluorescent antibody test test using immunofluorescence to demonstrate antigens or antibodies; if the labeled antibodies bind directly to the antigen, it is called the **direct immunofluorescence test**; in the **indirect immunofluorescence test**, the antibodies bind to the antigen, which is then made visible with a second labeled antibody [sandwich technique]

forced expiration test *Syn: Tiffeneau's test, forced expiratory volume*; determination of the volume of air that can be exhaled in 1 second after a deep inhalation

hemagglutination-inhibition test → *hemagglutination-inhibition assay*

Hess' test → *Rumpel-Leede test*

Hines and Brown test → *cold pressure test*

latex agglutination test *Syn: latex agglutination assay, latex fixation assay, latex fixation test*; immunologic agglutination test with latex particles, which are coated in antigen or antibodies

latex fixation test → *latex agglutination test*

Master's test *Syn: Master's two-step exercise test, two-step exercise test*; old-fashioned test of the circulation in which the patient climbs up and down an approx. 25 cm high step for 90 seconds; pulse, blood pressure, and ECG are monitored following this exertion, and at 3 and 10 minutes; now replaced by ergometric testing

Master's two-step exercise test → *Master's test*

Ouchterlony test *Syn: double-diffusion in two dimensions, Ouchterlony technique*; two-dimensional immunodiffusion for investigation of antigen identities; antigen and antibody diffuse into each other; in the equivalence zone, immune complexes form, which appear as precipitates; if the two antigens are identical, they form a continuous line, if not then several lines may form

Oudin test → *Oudin technique*

passive hemagglutination-inhibition test → *indirect hemagglutination-inhibition assay*

prothrombin test → *Quick's value*

prothrombin-consumption test clotting test that measures the utilization of prothrombin during spontaneous clotting

Quick test → *Quick's value*

radioimmunosorbent test radioimmunoassay with antibodies applied to one surface, which absorb antigens [sandwich method]

Ratschow's test method of establishing the perfusion of extremities in arterial occlusive disease; **principle**: the patient performs foot movements for 2 minutes in the lying position with elevated legs; after sitting up, the legs are then allowed to hang down loosely; after 5–10 seconds, the skin will pink up due to reactive hyperemia if perfusion is normal, and after approx. 15 seconds, the veins on the dorsum of the foot will fill; in impaired perfusion, these signs are delayed and the hyperemia lasts longer

rheumatoid factor latex agglutination test → *RF latex*

Rose-Waaler test *Syn: Waaler-Rose test*; indirect test of inhibition of hemagglutination to demonstrate the presence of rheumatoid factors; sheep erythrocytes loaded with rabbit antibodies are agglutinated by rheumatoid factors

Rumpel-Leede test *Syn: Hess' test*; creation of blood congestion in the upper arm with a blood pressure cuff; if capillary resistance is impaired, this may lead to petechial hemorrhages in the skin [**Rumpel-Leede phenomenon**]

Schellong's test testing of the circulation by measurement of the pulse and blood pressure in lying and standing positions; three measurements of blood pressure and pulse in the supine patient within 5–10 minutes; then measurement at 1-minute intervals in the freestanding patient for 7–10 minutes; then repeated measurement lying down over 3 minutes; a drop in the systolic value of less than 10 mmHg with constant or slightly increased diastolic values is physiologic; a blood pressure drop of more than 20 mmHg systolic or 10 mmHg diastolic is clearly pathologic; the most important test when orthostatic hypotension is suspected

screening test *Syn: screening*; crude test that identifies asymptomatic carriers, or potential carriers/transmitters, of a disease

two-step exercise test → *Master's test*

Waaler-Rose test → *Rose-Waaler test*

tetracyclines group of semisynthetic, bacteriostatic, broad-spectrum antibiotics that inhibit protein biosynthesis in bacteria; they are derived from **tetracycline**, an antibiotic produced by Streptomyces aureofaciens; they are most effective against gram-negative pathogens [gonococci, Haemophilus influenzae, Escherichia coli, Salmonella, Shigella, and Klebsiella], and less effective against gram-positive streptococci, staphylococci, and pneumococci; **indications**: mixed infections of the gastrointestinal, upper respiratory, and urogenital tracts; **side effects**: liver damage, allergies, photosensitization, gastrointestinal symptoms, and damage to bone, nails, and teeth in fetuses and very young children; **contraindications**: pregnancy, nursing, children under 8 years of age, hepatic impairment, and renal failure

tetrad *Syn: tetralogy*; a complex of four symptoms

Fallot's tetrad *Syn: Fallot's disease, Fallot's syndrome, tetralogy of Fallot*; congenital heart defect [8% of all heart defects] with [subvalvular, valvular, supravalvular] pulmonary stenosis, high ventricular septal defect, overriding aorta, and hypertrophy of the right ventricle; the extent of the various anomalies is variable, but the pulmonary stenosis is the most important hemodynamic factor, since it determines the lung perfusion and indirectly the hypertrophy of the right ventricle and the size of the right-to-left shunt; associated malformations include atrial septal defect [Fallot's pentalogy], aplasia of the pulmonary valve and right aortic arch; **clinical**: cyanosis becomes apparent within the first weeks or months [blue baby]; there are frequent hypoxemic attacks when going from rest to activity; thus, sudden loss of consciousness with skin pallor and sometimes cramp attacks can follow a period of sleep; there is failure to thrive, poor drinking, developmental disturbances, clubbed fingers and hourglass nails; **diagnosis**: coarse systolic murmur over the 2. and 3. left parasternal intercostal spaces; signs of right ventricular hypertrophy in the ECG, echocardiography, cardiac catheterization, angiography, chest X-rays [clog-shaped heart]; **therapy**: β-blocker [propranolol, atenolol] to minimize the hypoxemic attacks; operative correction in the acyanotic form [pink Fallot] is undertaken at the end of the first year of life, in the cyanotic forms as soon as the weight reaches 4000–5000 g; the operation attempts to close the ventriculoseptal defect [using a pericardial patch from the right atrium] and to eliminate the pulmonary stenosis [sometimes just by commissurotomy of the narrowed valve, but mostly needing enlargement of the valve ring; the pulmonary insufficiency this causes is well tolerated]; the mortality associated with this operation is around 2–5%; the life expectancy following successful correction is good; re-operation is relatively rarely necessary

tetralogy *Syn: tetrad*; a complex of four symptoms

Eisenmenger's tetralogy *Syn: Eisenmenger's complex, Eisenmenger's disease, Eisenmenger's syndrome*; congenital heart defect with ventricular septal defect, overriding of the aorta, pulmonary hypertension, and enlargement of the right heart; the ventricular septal defect leads to a right-to-left shunt with cyanosis, polycythemia, finger clubbing, and hourglass fingernails

tetralogy of Fallot → *Fallot's tetrad*

theodrenaline antihypotensive agent

therapeutic *Syn: therapeutical*; relating to therapy or therapeutics, curative

therapeutical → *curative*

therapy treatment of signs, symptoms or causes of a disease

combination therapy antibiotic treatment with two or more substances

embolic therapy → *embolization*

thermometer apparatus for measuring temperature; classical thermometers use the expansion of fluids [mercury, alcohol] on heating;

nowadays, thermometers that generate electrical impulses, which are converted into a display, are used more and more; various temperature scales are used depending upon the area of application or the country [Celsius scale, Fahrenheit scale, Kelvin scale]

thesaurismosis *Syn: thesaurosis*; accumulation disease, storage disease
  amyloid thesaurismosis → *amyloidosis*
  water thesaurismosis → *edema*

thevetine cardiac glycoside derived from the nuts of Thevetia neriifolia; generally used if digitalis and strophanthin cannot be tolerated

thiabutazide → *buthiazide*

thoracicoabdominal → *thoracoabdominal*

thoraco- combining form denoting a relationship to the chest/thorax

thoracoabdominal *Syn: thoracicoabdominal, abdominothoracic*; relating to or associated with the thorax and stomach/abdomen

thoracograph → *thoracopneumograph*

thoracopneumograph *Syn: thoracograph*; device for recording respiratory movements of the chest

thoracoscope rigid endoscope for use in thoracoscopy

thoracoscopy endoscopic examination of the chest cavity or the pleural cavity

thoracostomy creation of an external thoracic fistula, e.g., for drainage of fluid

thoracotomy *Syn: pleuracotomy, pleurotomy*; surgical incision of the thorax; it is performed most frequently as a sternotomy, **anterolateral thoracotomy** [in the fifth intercostal space, possibly with removal of the fifth and sixth ribs], or **posterolateral thoracotomy**
  exploratory thoracotomy incision of the thorax for the diagnosis of diseases

throbbing → *pulsatile*

thromb- combining form denoting relation to a clot or thrombus

thrombapheresis *Syn: plateletpheresis, thrombocytapheresis*; separation of thrombocytes from the blood

thrombase → *factor IIa*

thrombasthenia → *Glanzmann's disease*
  Glanzmann's thrombasthenia → *Glanzmann's disease*
  hereditary hemorrhagic thrombasthenia → *Glanzmann's disease*

thrombectomy *Syn: thromboembolectomy*; surgical removal of an embolus; it is performed primarily in peripheral arterial embolism or [less often] in embolism of the pulmonary arteries [**pulmonary thrombectomy**]

thrombelastogram *Syn: thromboelastogram*; graphical representation obtained by thromboelastography

thrombelastography simultaneous measurement and recording of reaction times to the start of clotting, formation of clot, and maximal thrombus elasticity

thrombembolia → *thromboembolism*

thrombembolism → *thromboembolism*

thrombin → *factor IIa*

thrombo- combining form denoting relation to a clot or thrombus

thromboagglutination *Syn: platelet agglutination*; agglutination of thrombocytes by anti-thrombocyte antibodies

thromboangiitis → *thromboangitis*

   thromboangiitis obliterans → *Winiwarter-Buerger disease*

thromboangitic relating to or marked by thromboangitis

thromboangitis inflammation of the wall of an artery [thromboarteritis] or vein [thrombophlebitis]

thromboarteritic relating to or marked by thromboarteritis

thromboarteritis thrombosis combined with inflammation of an artery

thromboasthenia → *Glanzmann's disease*

thromboclasis → *thrombolysis*

thromboclastic → *thrombolytic*

thrombocytapheresis → *thrombapheresis*

thrombocytes *Syn: blood platelets, platelets*; small, non-nucleated, disc-shaped blood cells with a diameter of 1–4 µm and a thickness of 0.5–0.75 µm; the blood of healthy subjects contains about 150,000–450,000 platelets/µl; their residence time in the blood is 5–11 days, after which they are broken down in the liver, lung, and spleen; platelets circulating in the blood are in an inactive state; they are activated after contact with the surface of damaged vessels or with various coagulation factors; platelets are very important for blood coagulation and hemostasis

thrombocythemia permanent elevation in the thrombocyte count in the blood

   essential thrombocythemia → *megakaryocytic leukemia*

   hemorrhagic thrombocythemia → *megakaryocytic leukemia*

   idiopathic thrombocythemia → *megakaryocytic leukemia*

   primary thrombocythemia → *megakaryocytic leukemia*

thrombocytic relating to platelets

thrombocytolysis platelet disruption, thrombocyte disruption

thrombocytopathia → *thrombopathy*

thrombocytopathy → *thrombopathy*

thrombocytopenia *Syn: thrombopenia, thrombopeny*; reduced thrombocyte count [< 100,000/µl]; occurs as a result of reduced formation, increased utilization, disturbances of distribution or dilution of the blood [hemodilution]; leads to prolongation of the bleeding time and hemorrhagic diathesis [petechiae, nosebleeds, gastrointestinal or urogenital bleeding, prolonged and heavier menses]

essential thrombocytopenia → *idiopathic thrombocytopenic purpura*

immune thrombocytopenia thrombocytopenia caused by autoantibodies against thrombocytes

thrombocytopenic *Syn: thrombopenic*; relating to thrombocytopenia

thrombocytopoiesis → *thrombopoiesis*

thrombocytopoietic affecting or stimulating thrombopoiesis

thrombocytosis temporary elevation of the thrombocyte count in the blood

thromboelastogram → *thrombelastogram*

thromboembolectomy → *thrombectomy*

thromboembolia → *thromboembolism*

thromboembolism *Syn: thrombembolia, thromboembolia, thrombembolism*; embolism caused by a thrombus carried by the bloodstream; a pulmonary embolism is the most common

arterial thromboembolism the heart [80–90%; heart wall aneurysms, heart valve prostheses, mitral and aortic valve defects, bacterial endocarditis, atrial fibrillation] and proximal vessels [10–15%; aneurysms, atheromatous plaques] are the most common sources of emboli; most commonly affects the pelvic and leg arteries [80%] and generally presents as an acute ischemic syndrome often with threat to life

venous thromboembolism the thrombi generally stem from deep leg and pelvic veins or the right atrium and cause a pulmonary embolism

thromboendarterectomy → *endarterectomy*

thromboendocarditic relating to or marked by thromboendocarditis

thromboendocarditis rarely used description of endocarditis with thrombus formation

thrombogen → *prothrombin*

thrombogene → *accelerator globulin*

thrombogenesis → *thrombosis*

thrombogenic promoting thrombus formation

β-thromboglobulin factor with weak affinity for heparin contained in the α-granules of the thrombocytes; plasma levels increase in thrombosis and embolism

thromboid resembling a thrombus

thrombolymphangitic relating to or marked by thrombolymphangitis

thrombolymphangitis inflammation of lymphatic vessels with formation of a lymph clot

thrombolysis *Syn: thromboclasis*; dissolution of a thrombus

thrombolytic *Syn: thromboclastic*; **1.** an agent with thrombolytic properties **2.** affecting or promoting thrombolysis

thrombomodulin vascular endothelial receptor, which binds and inactivates thrombin

thrombopathia →*thrombopathy*

thrombopathic relating to thrombopathia

thrombopathy *Syn: thrombocytopathia, thrombocytopathy, thrombopathia*; disturbance of thrombocyte function

   constitutional thrombopathy 1. →*Glanzmann's disease* **2.** →*von Willebrand's syndrome*

thrombopenia →*thrombocytopenia*

thrombopenic →*thrombocytopenic*

thrombopeny →*thrombocytopenia*

thrombophilia →*thrombotic tendency*

thrombophilic relating to or caused by thrombophilia

thrombophlebitic relating to thrombophlebitis

thrombophlebitis inflammation of a vein wall (superficial veins) with occlusion of its lumen; can affect varicose [**varicothrombosis**] or normal veins; damage to a vein [mainly iatrogenic due to needles or catheters] is a frequent cause; it is important to note that in 20–40% of cases there is also simultaneous thrombosis of the deeper portions of the vein; **therapy:** compression bandages, possibly stab incision and expression of the pus for acute relief of pain; thromboprophylaxis

   thrombophlebitis migrans *Syn: Trousseau's syndrome; s.u. migrating phlebitis*

thromboplastic initiating or favoring the formation of a thrombus

thromboplastin *Syn: thrombokinase, platelet tissue factor, thrombozyme, prothrombin activator, prothrombinase*; protease that converts prothrombin to thrombin in the early stages of blood clotting

   tissue thromboplastin →*factor III*

thromboplastinogen →*factor VIII*

thrombopoiesis *Syn: thrombocytopoiesis*; thrombocytes are made in the bone marrow by megakaryocytes

thrombopoietin hemopoietic growth factor made by the hepatic and renal cells, which stimulates the formation of thrombocytes in the bone marrow

thrombosed affected by thrombosis

thrombosin → *factor IIa*

thrombosinusitic relating to or marked by thrombosinusitis

thrombosis *Syn: thrombus formation, thrombogenesis*; intravital thrombus formation in the arteries or veins; the clinical term also covers the resulting symptoms; thrombus formation is promoted especially by slow blood flow, changes in blood composition [especially hyperviscosity] and clotting behavior [hypercoagulability], and damage to vessel walls [trauma, surgery, ischemia, inflammation, neoplasms, and arteriosclerosis]; the deep leg and pelvic veins are affected most often; thromboses in the upper extremities are also seen after iatrogenic damage [i.v. injections, infusions], in vessel stenosis, or in neoplasms; because of the absence of symptoms, thrombosis is often not diagnosed and noted only with the occurrence of complications [pulmonary embolism]; **diagnosis**: medical history, examination, phlebography, and duplex sonography; **therapy**: fresh thrombi, i.e., those less than a week old, can be dissolved by local or systemic thrombolytic agents, such as streptokinase or urokinase; older thrombi are already organized and the goal of treatment is to prevent a postthrombotic syndrome; a thrombectomy is indicated only in very rare cases [phlegmasia coerulea dolens with arterial ischemia]

basilar artery thrombosis thrombosis of the basilar artery mostly caused by arteriosclerosis, which leads to extensive, often bilateral disturbances with loss of function in the lower cranial nerves [glossopharyngeal, vagus, accessory, hypoglossal], sensory pathways, severe ataxia, and hemi- or tetra-paresis]; mostly leads to respiratory paralysis and coma

cardiac thrombosis thrombus formation in the heart; most thrombi form in the cardiac auricle in atrial fibrillation, as parietal thrombi in the ventricular wall in myocardial infarcts or on the heart valves in endocarditis; the thrombi can break off and cause pulmonary emboli or cerebral or peripheral arterial emboli

coronary thrombosis thrombosis in the coronary vessels; leads to coronary stenosis and possibly to acute myocardial infarction

deep leg vein thrombosis *Syn: deep venous thrombosis of the leg;* common illness, which most often affects the deep veins in the legs and pelvis [**deep pelvic vein/leg vein thrombosis**]; because of the absence of symptoms, it is often not diagnosed and noted only with the occurrence of complications [pulmonary embolism]; in most cases, it is a symptomatic thrombosis with a known cause and less often an idiopathic disease; the most important predisposing factors are: age, cancer, obesity, and congenital or acquired blood coagulation disorders with thrombophilia; surgery, prolonged bed rest, immobilization, trauma, birth, prolonged sitting [**travel thrombosis**], and overexertion [**effort thrombosis**] are considered to be primary precipitating factors; **diagnosis**: medical history, examination, phlebography, duplex sonography; **therapy**: fresh thrombi, i.e., those less than a week old, can be dissolved by local or systemic thrombolytic agents, for example streptokinase or urokinase; older thrombi are already organized and the goal of treatment is to prevent a postthrombotic syndrome; treatment to prevent recurrence is then initiated depending on the cause; coumarin derivatives or platelet aggregation inhibitors, for example acetylsalicylic acid, are administered most often; a thrombectomy is indicated only in very rare cases [phlegmasia coerulea dolens with arterial ischemia]; if emboli recur, a vena cava filter can be used

deep vein thrombosis *Syn: deep venous thrombosis;* thrombosis usually affecting the large leg and pelvic veins; because of the absence of symptoms, thrombosis is often not diagnosed and noted only with the occurrence of complications [pulmonary embolism]; in most cases, it is a symptomatic thrombosis with a known cause and less often an idiopathic disease

deep venous thrombosis → *deep vein thrombosis*
deep venous thrombosis of the leg → *deep leg vein thrombosis*
effort thrombosis *s.u. deep leg vein thrombosis*
effort-induced thrombosis → *Paget-von Schroetter syndrome*
leg vein thrombosis *Syn: phlebothrombosis of the leg;* thrombosis most often affecting the deep leg veins; thrombosis of superficial leg veins [thrombophlebitis] occurs less often

pelvic venous thrombosis more frequent postoperative or postpartum thromboses of the great pelvic veins [external iliac vein, internal iliac vein]; often relates to **deep pelvic** or **leg vein thrombosis**

thrombosis prophylaxis coumarin derivatives or inhibitors of thrombocyte aggregation, such as acetylsalicylic acid, are mainly used as prophylaxis against recurrence; **postoperative** or **post-traumatic thromboprophylaxis** consists of medical prophylaxis [low-dose heparin 2–3 × 5,000 IU subcutaneously/day, low-molecular-weight heparin once daily] as well as general measures [mechanical prophylaxis], such as graduated compression stockings, physiotherapy, early or immediate mobilization, volume filling, elevation of the end of the bed, elevation of the legs, etc.

splenic vein thrombosis thromboses of the lienorenal veins are generally the result of local or transmitted inflammations, but can also be idiopathic or occur in the setting of generalized infection; the impaired drainage of blood leads to swelling of the spleen [splenomegaly], fever, mucosal bleeding [predominantly in the stomach and gastrointestinal tract], and later to liver swelling and portal hypertension

stagnant thrombosis thrombosis due to stagnation of blood flow

travel thrombosis *s.u. deep leg vein thrombosis*

ulnar artery thrombosis thrombosis of the ulnar artery

venous thrombosis *Syn: phlebemphraxis, phlebothrombosis*; non-inflammatory thrombosis, affecting the deep veins, with occlusion of the lumen; thrombosis of superficial veins is called thrombophlebitis

thrombospondin nectin formed by thrombocytes; comparable to fibronectin in its action

thrombotic relating to, affected with, or characterized or caused by thrombosis

coronary thrombotic relating to, marked by or caused by coronary thrombosis

thrombotic-thrombocytopenic characterized by both thrombosis and thrombocytopenia

thromboxanes substances belonging to the prostaglandin superfamily, which promote thrombocyte aggregation; they are mainly formed from prostaglandin H in the blood platelets

thromboxane A_2 causing bronchoconstriction, vasoconstriction, and thrombocyte aggregation; receptors for thromboxane A_2 have been found in thrombocytes, thymus, lungs, kidneys, and myocardium

thrombus *Syn: blood clot, clot*; blood clot developing in a blood vessel; in the first step of blood clotting, a white thrombus forms; this is replaced by a red thrombus that contracts and solidifies during thrombus maturation

atrial thrombus blood clot in the left atrium; mostly caused by atrial fibrillation or mitral stenosis; can lead to cerebral infarction or arterial embolism

ball thrombus free-floating thrombus, usually lying in the left atrium

blood platelet thrombus *Syn: plate thrombus, platelet thrombus*; pale thrombus consisting of thrombocytes

calcified thrombus → *phlebolith*

chicken fat thrombus → *bacon-rind clot*

coagulation thrombus → *red thrombus*

conglutination-agglutination thrombus → *washed clot*

laminated thrombus → *washed clot*

mixed thrombus → *washed clot*

pale thrombus → *washed clot*

plain thrombus → *washed clot*

plate thrombus → *blood platelet thrombus*

platelet thrombus → *blood platelet thrombus*

red thrombus *Syn: coagulation thrombus*; thrombus forming due to rapid blood clotting, which is colored red by erythrocytes

white thrombus → *washed clot*

thyrocardiac relating to thyroid and heart

ticarcillin oral penicillin with a rather broad spectrum; it is effective particularly against Pseudomonas aeruginosa, Proteus species, and Escherichia coli

ticlopidine inhibitor of thrombocyte aggregation; **usage**: if acetylsalicylic acid cannot be tolerated

time a particular period

bleeding time time between the placement of a stab incision and the cessation of bleeding; serves as a global test of primary hemostasis; the most convenient methods to estimate it are the **underwater bleeding time after Marx** [pricking of the finger pulp, immersion of the bleeding finger in lukewarm water, measurement of the time until the forming blood filament tears off] and the **bleeding time after Duke** [pricking of the finger pulp or ear lobe, gentle wiping of the blood with filter paper until the bleeding stops]; normal value is 2–5 minutes

clotting time *Syn: coagulation time*; time between sampling of blood and the clotting of the sample by the formation of solid fibrin

coagulation time → *clotting time*

heparin recalcification time global test of clotting, which tests both the endogenous clotting system and thrombocyte function

prothrombin time → *Quick's value*

Quick's time → *Quick's value*

recalcification time test of clotting in which the time to clotting is measured following addition of calcium ions

reptilase clotting time clotting test that measures the time from addition of reptilase to citrated blood to the start of clotting; normal range: 17–21 seconds; prolonged in fibrinogen deficiency, dysfibrinogenemia, hyperfibrinolysis, and consumptive coagulopathy

thrombin time *Syn: thrombin clotting time*; clotting test to assess the second phase of blood clotting

thrombin clotting time → *thrombin time*

thromboplastin time → *Quick's value*

timolol β-blocker; **usage**: eye drops for the treatment of glaucoma

tinzaparin sodium low-molecular weight heparin; **usage**: pre- and postoperative thromboprophylaxis

tirofiban high-affinity, selective antagonist of the GPIIb/IIIa receptor of the thrombocytes; inhibitor of thrombocyte aggregation; **usage**: unstable angina pectoris, myocardial infarction without ST-segment elevation; **side effects**: bleeding complications, thrombocytopenia, hypotension, bradycardia

tissue aggregation of specialized cells

muscle tissue *Syn: muscle, muscular tissue*; muscle tissue consists of cells that shorten and develop tension and are able to convert chemical energy directly into mechanical energy; all muscle cells contain the contractile proteins actin and myosin, which together make up the myofibrils; myoglobin is one of the proteins related to hemoglobin, which is responsible for the typical red coloration of muscles; subdivided into **smooth muscle tissue** and **striated muscle tissue**, which is itself further subdivided into **skeletal muscle** and **cardiac muscle** tissues; the division is based upon both morphologic [the striated muscles show cross banding under the light microscope, which is absent in smooth muscles] and functional aspects [smooth muscle is only innervated by the vegetative nervous system, striated predominantly by the somatic system; smooth muscle contracts slowly, striated quickly, etc.]

muscular tissue → *muscle tissue*

T-lymphocytes lymphocytes primarily formed in the thymus [and therefore called **thymus-dependent lymphocytes** or **thymus lymphocytes**], which are responsible for the cell-mediated immune response; following the first contact with an antigen, they differentiate into either **T-effector cells** or **T-memory cells**; the T-memory cells often circulate for years in the blood and when exposed to the antigen for a second time unleash a rapid and vigorous cellular immune response; the T-effector cells can be subdivided into two populations: **T_4-lymphocytes** and **T_8-lymphocytes**, the differentiation being based upon certain surface receptors; their role is to release cytokines and destroy the antigens; **T_4-lymphocytes** differentiate into T_H0-cells [H for T-helper cells] following contact with antigen presenting cells from which T_H1- and T_H2-cells then develop; T_H1-cells release cytokines that stimulate the cellular immune response, whereas T_H2-cells stimulate the B-lymphocytes and thereby the humoral immune response; the **T_8-lymphocytes** are destined to develop into **T-killer cells**; if they come upon an infected cell whose antigens match their own antigen receptor [T_3/T-receptor], they kill the cell

TM-mode *Syn: time-motion, M-mode; s.u. sonography*

tobramycin *Syn: tenebrimycin, tenemycen;* aminoglycoside antibiotic, produced by **Streptomyces tenebrarius**, with a broad action spectrum against gram-positive and gram-negative microorganisms [such as Bacillus, Listeria, staphylococci, Bordetella, Enterobacter, Escherichia coli, Mycoplasma, and Pseudomonas]

tocainide antiarrhythmic of lidocaine type

tolazoline direct α-sympatholytic, vasodilator; usage: peripheral disturbances of perfusion, disturbances of perfusion in the eye

tolerance 1. the act or capacity of enduring 2. acceptance of a tissue graft or transplant without immunological rejection

  ischemic tolerance capacity of an organ or tissue to tolerate transient, acute ischemia without lasting damage; varies widely from tissue to tissue or organ to organ

  tissue tolerance →*histocompatibility*

tomography techniques for making detailed X-rays of a predetermined plane section of a solid object

  cardial computer-tomography computer tomography of the heart, which is either triggered by the patient's ECG or is performed untriggered; it permits assessment of the internal spaces of the heart, septae, and the muscle tissue; partially replaced by MRI nowadays

  computer-tomography a method of examining body organs by scanning them with X rays and using a computer to construct a series of cross-sectional scans

  positron-emission tomography computer tomography-like procedure in which the photons emitted from positron emitters are registered; used in the diagnosis of disturbances of perfusion and metabolism in the brain or heart

tone quality or character of sound

Traube's double tone *Syn: pistol-shot sound, Traube's sign*; systolic double sound heard over the great vessels in aortic insufficiency

torsade a twisted cord

ventricular torsade special electrocardiographic form of polymorphic ventricular tachycardias on the background of congenital and acquired QT prolongation

toxanemia → *hemotoxic anemia*

toxemia → *toxicemia*

toxic *Syn: toxicant*; acting as a poison, containing poison(s), poisonous

toxicant → *toxic*

toxicemia *Syn: toxemia, toxicohemia, toxinemia*; damage of blood cells by toxins

toxicohemia → *toxinemia*

toxinemia *Syn: toxemia, toxicemia, toxicohemia*; overflow of bacterial toxins into the blood

trabecula a structural part resembling a small beam or crossbar

fleshy trabeculae of heart → *muscular trabeculae of heart*

muscular trabeculae of heart *Syn: fleshy columns of heart, fleshy trabeculae of heart*; net-like bands of muscle on the inner surface of the right and left ventricles [**trabeculae carneae**]

septomarginal trabecula *Syn: moderator band, septomarginal band*; ridge of muscle on the floor of the right ventricle stretching from the interventricular septum to the anterior papillary muscle

trabecula septomarginalis → *septomarginal trabecula*

trachea *Syn: windpipe*; a flexible tube, 10–12 cm long, which begins at the bottom of the cricoid cartilage [cartilago cricoidea] and branches into the right and left primary bronchus [bronchus principalis dexter and sinister] at the level of the fourth thoracic vertebra; it has a **cervical part** [pars cervicalis/colli], which continues at the superior thoracic aperture as the **thoracic part** [pars thoracica]; the wall of the trachea consists anteriorly of horseshoe-shaped cartilage rings [**cartilagines tracheales**], which are augmented posteriorly by a membranous posterior wall [**paries membranaceus tracheae**] and smooth muscles [**musculus trachealis**] into a tube; the individual cartilage rings are connected by ligaments [**ligamenta anularia trachealia**]; a cartilage spur [**carina tracheae**] projects into the lumen at the **tracheal**

bifurcation [bifurcatio tracheae]; the mucosa [**tunica mucosa**] has a ciliated epithelium, which is coated by goblet cells and mucus from the tracheal glands; the exterior of the trachea is covered by a tunica adventitia, which enables movement of the trachea during swallowing or coughing

tract a number of organs that are arranged in series and work together
respiratory tract *Syn: respiratory organs, respiratory system, respiratory apparatus, respiratory passages*; the totality of organs and structures that conduct air taken as a whole [mouth, nose, pharynx, larynx, trachea, and lungs]

tranexamic acid plasminogen activator inhibitor; **usage**: hemostatic in hemorrhage due to increased fibrinolysis or fibrinogenolysis

trans- combining form denoting relation to through, across, or beyond

transanimation *Syn: kiss of life*; direct artificial ventilation, i.e., mouth-to-mouth and mouth-to-nose ventilation; in **mouth-to-nose ventilation** the head of the patient to be ventilated is tilted back with one hand on the forehead/hair border [opening of the airway]; the other hand lifts the jaw and closes the mouth with the thumb; the air donor takes a deep breath in and then places their opened mouth firmly over the patient's nose; during inflation, a check is made to see that the chest wall rises; after the insufflation, the mouth is then removed from the nose and the escape of air from the lungs is observed [the thorax sinks]; at the beginning, 2–3 insufflations are performed quickly one after the other, in order to correct the O_2 deficit; thereafter, an interval of 5–6

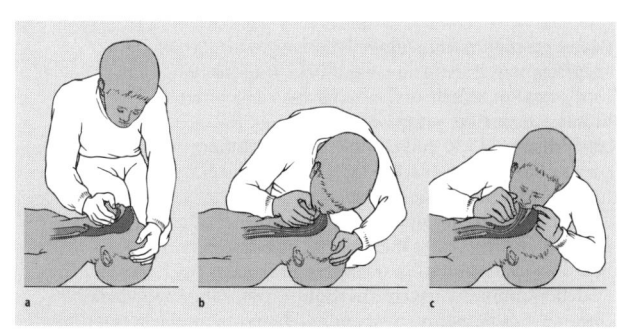

Transanimation. **a,b** mouth-to-nose ventilation; **c** mouth-to-mouth ventilation

seconds is maintained between breaths; **mouth-to-mouth ventilation** follows the same principles; the hands lie in the same initial position; the air donor seals their mouth tightly around that of the patient; the nasal opening can be closed with the cheek or by pinching together the nostrils with the upper hand

transaortic through the aorta

transatrial through the atrium

transformation change in form, appearance, nature, or character

    fast Fourier transformation *s.u. electrocardiogram*

transfusion *Syn: metachysis, blood transfusion*; transfer of blood or blood components from a donor to a recipient; in order to avoid incompatibility reactions, only AB0- and Rh-D type matched blood may be transfused; to exclude mistakes, incorrect typing or rare incompatibility to other blood group systems, a **crossmatch** must be carried out before each transfusion; in this test, the **major test** assesses the compatibility of donor erythrocytes and recipient serum, and the **minor test** the tolerance of recipient erythrocytes to donor serum

    blood transfusion →*transfusion*

    exchange transfusion *Syn: exsanguination transfusion, exsanguinotransfusion, replacement transfusion, substitution transfusion, total transfusion*; blood transfusion with simultaneous removal of recipient blood with the goal of replacing the recipient blood with donor blood so far as possible; performed using either a **single vessel method** [alternating blood removal and infusion using the same vessel] or a **two vessel method** [continuous removal and infusion using two different vessels]

    exsanguination transfusion →*exchange transfusion*

    replacement transfusion →*exchange transfusion*

    substitution transfusion →*exchange transfusion*

    total transfusion →*exchange transfusion*

transplant *Syn: graft*; transplanted organ or tissue

    combination transplant →*composite graft*

    composite transplant →*composite graft*

    multi-organ transplant →*composite graft*

transplantation the act of implanting a transplant

    cardiac transplantation →*heart transplantation*

    cardiopulmonary transplantation →*heart-lung transplantation*

    heart transplantation *Syn: cardiac transplantation*; replacement of a diseased heart with the heart of a deceased donor; divided into orthotopic heart transplantation [implantation at the same site] and **heterotopic heart transplantation** [implantation at another site]; usually performed for dilated or ischemic cardiomyopathy with end stage cardiac insufficiency and an estimated life expectancy of under 1 year; the **1-year survival rate** is more than 80%, the **5-year survival rate** is 60–70%, and the **10-year survival rate** in the region of 40–50%

heart-lung transplantation *Syn: cardiopulmonary transplantation*; transplantation performed in irreversible damage to heart and lungs; the most frequent surgical complication is failure of bronchial anastomoses in the early phase; the 1-year survival rate is about 80% and the 5-year rate 50–60%

heterologous transplantation →*heteroplasty*
heteroplastic transplantation →*heteroplasty*
xenogeneic transplantation →*xenotransplantation*

transport the act of transporting or conveying
reverse cholesterol transport *s.u. lecithin-cholesterol acyltransferase*

transposition displacement of an organ

transposition of the great vessels congenital angiocardiopathy, occurring in various forms, with the aorta arising from the right ventricle and the pulmonary artery from the left ventricle; as a result, the pulmonary and systemic circulation are connected parallel, i.e., venous blood flows through the right ventricle directly into the aorta and back to the systemic circulation, whereas the oxygenated blood of the pulmonary circulation is always pumped back to the lung; severe cyanosis results which is fatal if untreated; however, there are often shunts at the atrial level [atrial septal defect], ventricular level [ventricular septal defect], or between the great vessels [persistent ductus arteriosus], which cause the mixing of arterial and venous blood; **therapy**: today, an anatomic correction is performed in the first 2 weeks of life by switching the great arteries [**arterial-switch operation**] and the coronary arteries; the mortality associated with the surgery is 5%; the results are excellent and the children have an almost normal physical functional capacity; but there may be problems or complications later in adulthood

partial transposition of great vessels → *Taussig-Bing syndrome*

transseptal through a septum
transventricular through the ventricle(s)
trapping *s.u. intracranial aneurysm*
triacylglycerol *Syn: triglyceride*; glycerin ester, in which all three OH-

groups are esterified with saturated or unsaturated fatty acids

triad a group of three entities

acute compression triad →*Beck's triad*

Beck's triad *Syn: acute compression triad*; arterial hypotension, venous hypertension, and diminished heart wall pulsation in pericardial tamponade

Virchow's triad factors responsible for promoting thrombus formation, namely sluggish blood flow, injury to the vessel wall, and changes in the coagulability [hypercoagulability]

triamterene potassium-sparing diuretic; **usage**: hyperaldosteronism in liver cirrhosis, ascites, cardiac, hepatic and nephrotic edema

triangle a three-cornered structure

carotid triangle *Syn: carotid trigone, Gerdy's hyoid fossa, Malgaigne's fossa, Malgaigne's triangle*; triangle in the neck bounded by muscles [*cranially*: posterior digastric muscle; *dorsolateral*: sternocleidomastoid muscle; *ventromedial*: omohyoid muscle]; point of division of the common carotid artery into external and internal branches; the superior root of the ansa cervicalis passes between the external and internal carotid arteries through the carotid triangle; part of the anterior triangle of the neck

Einthoven's triangle *Syn: Einthoven's method; s.u. Einthoven's leads*

Malgaigne's triangle →*carotid triangle*

trichlormethiazide oral saluretic with a half-life of 2–3 hours

trichocardia →*hairy heart*

tricuspid *Syn: tricuspidal, tricuspidate*; having three ponts or cusps; relating to the tricuspid valve

tricuspidal →*tricuspid*

tricuspidate →*tricuspid*

trigeminy *Syn: trigeminal pulse, trigeminal rhythm*; disturbance of heart rhythm with two extrasystoles following each normal systole

triglyceride →*triacylglycerol*

trigone triangle

carotid trigone →*carotid triangle*

left fibrous trigone of heart triangular region of the heart between the left atrium and left ventricle made of fibro-cartilage

right fibrous trigone of heart triangular region of the heart between the right atrium and right ventricle made of fibro-cartilage

trigonum triangle

trigonum fibrosum dextrum →*right fibrous trigone of heart*

trigonum fibrosum sinistrum → *left fibrous trigone of heart*
trilogy a complex of three symptoms
   trilogy of Fallot congenital cardiac defect with high ventricular septal defect, pulmonary stenosis and hypertrophy of the right ventricle; **clinical** and **therapy** *s.a. Fallot's tetrad*
trinitrin → *nitroglycerin*
trinitroglycerin → *nitroglycerin*
trinitroglycerol → *nitroglycerin*
triterpenes terpene made up of 6 isoprene groups; mostly in the form of tetra- or pentacyclic aromatic compounds; these include, e.g., the steroid hormones, digitalis glycoside, and vitamin D
tropine tropate → *atropine*
troponin muscle protein in the thin filaments of the muscle fiber; binds to free calcium ions during muscle excitation and exposes the myosin binding site as a result of the conformational change that this produces, allowing contraction to proceed; consists of three subcomponents [**troponin I, C, T**], of which the troponin I and T have a role in the diagnosis of acute myocardial infarction; their serum concentration increases within 3–12 hours after the start of ischemia; troponin T reaches its peak after 12 to 48 h and troponin I after 24 h; normalization of the troponins follows after about one to two weeks; elevations in troponin independent of infarction can also occur in renal insufficiency, myocarditis, pulmonary embolization, hypertensive crisis, decompensated cardiac insufficiency, transplant rejection, and cardiac contusion
truncal relating to the trunk
truncus trunk; vascular trunk or nerve trunk
   truncus arteriosus common arterial trunk of the embryonal heart, which later divides into the aorta and pulmonary artery; in rare cases the division does not occur; the two ventricles have a shared vessel [**common arterial trunk**] with four valves; this congenital heart defect [< 1% of all disorders] is combined with a high-lying ventricular septal defect; **clinically** notable are cyanosis, dyspnea, and a loud pansystolic murmur on the left side over the 3.-4. intercostal space; **therapy** consists of operative correction of the defect
   truncus brachiocephalicus → *brachiocephalic trunk*
   truncus costocervicalis → *costocervical trunk*
   truncus fasciculi atrioventricularis → *trunk of atrioventricular bundle*
   truncus pulmonalis *Syn:* pulmonary trunk, pulmonary artery, arterial

vein; trunk of the pulmonary artery arising from the right ventricle; it divides into the right and left pulmonary arteries

truncus thyrocervicalis → *thyrocervical trunk*

trunk stem, body

atrioventricular trunk → *atrioventricular bundle*

trunk of atrioventricular bundle stem of the bundle of His [atrioventricular bundle]

basilar trunk → *basilar artery*

brachiocephalic trunk *Syn: brachiocephalic artery, innominate artery*; approx. 3 cm long arterial branch arising from the aortic arch; divides into right and left subclavian arteries and common carotid artery

costocervical trunk *Syn: costocervical arterial axis, costocervical axis*; conjoined trunk of the deep cervical and supreme intercostal arteries arising from the subclavian artery; arises from the back of the artery behind the scalenus anterior muscle

pulmonary trunk → *truncus pulmonalis*

thyrocervical trunk *Syn: thyroid axis*; arterial stem arising from the subclavian artery; gives off the inferior thyroid artery, ascending cervical artery, suprascapular artery, superficial cervical artery, and dorsal scapular artery

tube elongated hollow organ or instrument

Westergren tube *s.u. erythrocyte sedimentation rate*

tubercle *Syn: tuberculum*; nodular granuloma with epitheloid cells and Langhans' giant cells in tuberculosis; central necrosis [caseation] is possible

intervenous tubercle small swelling on the wall of the right atrium between the openings of the two great veins [ostia of the superior and inferior venae cavae]

tuberculum 1. protuberance, node, or nodule **2.** → *tubercle*

tuberculum intervenosum → *intervenous tubercle*

tugging a pulling (sensation)

tracheal tugging → *Oliver's sign*

tumid → *edematous*

tumor *Syn: neoplasm*; any new and uncontrolled growth; swelling

aneurysmal giant cell tumor *Syn: aneurysmal bone cyst, hemangiomatous bone cyst, hemorrhagic bone cyst*; multi-chambered, blood-filled cysts that occur in the metaphyses of the long bones; cause local pain and bone swelling; **therapy**: because of the risk of recurrence, en-bloc resection with reconstruction of the defect with spongy bone is the method of choice

glomus tumor → *angiomyoneuroma*

granulation tumor → *granuloma*

Lindau's tumor → *hemangioblastoma*

vascular tumor → *angioma*

tunic coat, covering

Bichat's tunic → *intima*

tunica tunic, coat, skin, or membrane

tunica externa *Syn: external coat, adventitial coat, adventitia;* outer layer of the vessel; in arteries it is called the tunica adventitia

tunica media → *media*

tunica serosa pericardii the serosa of the serous pericardium coated in serous fluid [**liquor pericardii**] filling the **pericardial cavity**

twinning → *bigeminy*

type variety

acral type of arterial occlusive disease *s.u. chronic arterial occlusive disease*

blood type → *blood group*

cardioinhibitory type *s.u. carotid sinus syndrome*

digital type of arterial occlusive disease *s.u. chronic arterial occlusive disease*

heart muscle type *s.u. creatine kinase*

horizontal type *s.u. electrocardiogram*

intermediate type *s.u. electrocardiogram*

left type *Syn: left axis deviation; s.u. electrocardiogram*

lidocaine type *s.u. antiarrhythmic*

lower arm type of arterial occlusive disease *s.u. chronic arterial occlusive disease*

lower leg type of arterial occlusive disease *s.u. chronic arterial occlusive disease*

Mobitz type type 2 2. degree AV-block

pelvic type of arterial occlusive disease *s.u. chronic arterial occlusive disease*

quinidine type *s.u. antiarrhythmic*

right type *Syn: right axis deviation; s.u. electrocardiogram*

sagittal type *s.u. electrocardiogram*

semihorizontal type *s.u. electrocardiogram*

shoulder girdle type of arterial occlusive disease *s.u. chronic arterial occlusive disease*

steep type *s.u. electrocardiogram*
thigh type of arterial occlusive disease *s.u. chronic arterial occlusive disease*
upper arm type of arterial occlusive disease *s.u. chronic arterial occlusive disease*
vasodepressor type *s.u. carotid sinus syndrome*

UACR → *urine albumin-to-creatinine ratio*
UAER → *urinary albumin excretion rate*

ulcer *Syn: ulceration, ulcus, fester*; a lesion of the skin or a mucous membrane

  leg ulcer ulcer of the skin on the lower leg or foot; mostly occurs as a consequence of chronic venous insufficiency [**ulcus cruris venosum**] or arterial occlusive disease [**ulcus cruris arteriosum**]; the typical venous ulcer on the lower leg sits in the region of the inside of the ankle joint and is surrounded by altered skin [indurated to calloused, usually eczematous]; it is solitary, round and only mildly tender; generally a so-called **mother varix** or **nutrient vein** leads away from the ulcer; the ulcers tend to spread and recur, with recurrent ulcers being more extensive, deeper, and more therapy-resistant; **therapy** is difficult and mostly prolonged; it is important to remove the engorgement with compression and ambulatory exercises in the daytime and elevation at night; in addition, the wound is treated with synthetic wound dressings; surgical coverage with mesh grafts is only appropriate and successful in individual cases; some authors recommend fasciectomy and/or wide excision of the ulcer

ultrasonography *Syn: echography, sonography*; non-invasive imaging procedure in which ultrasound is used as an impulse [**sonography**] or continuous tone [**Doppler method**]

  color duplex ultrasonography procedure of Doppler sonography, which permits assessment of vessel geometry and flow conditions

  Doppler ultrasonography ultrasound technique, which records the frequency changes when sound waves reflect from moving objects [Doppler effect]; can use either continuous sound waves [**wave-wave Doppler sonography**] or with sound impulses [**impulse Doppler sonography**]; the main area of use is in the investigation of the heart and vessels; in combination with B-mode imaging, sectional images, which only show vessels containing flowing blood [**Doppler angiog-**

raphy] can be obtained

duplex ultrasonography ultrasound technique in which a **Duplex probe** is used, which contains both a probe for B-mode and a probe for Doppler signals; this permits simultaneous B-mode imaging and Doppler sonography

unconsciousness *Syn: exanimation, insensibility, senselessness*; loss of consciousness; often equated with fainting or syncope [brief loss of consciousness]; a more prolonged loss of consciousness is described as coma

uninterrupted → *continuous*

unit any group of things regarded as an entity

colony-forming unit *s.u. blood formation*

uptake absorption and incorporation of a substance

oxygen uptake 1. the amount of oxygen taken up by the body from 1 l of air [about 30–45 ml at rest] **2.** → *oxygen utilization*

urapidil α_1-blocker, antihypertensive; **usage**: blood pressure crisis, hypertensive emergency

ureidopenicillins *Syn: acylaminopenicillins*; group of parenteral penicillins with a broad action spectrum against gram-positive and gram-negative pathogens; it includes apalcillin, azlocillin, mezlocillin, and piperacillin

urinary albumin/creatinine ratio → *urine albumin-to-creatinine ratio*

urinary albumin excretion rate *Syn: urine albumin excretion rate*; the amount of albumin excreted in urine in a pre-specified time interval, usually 24 hours; studies have shown that albuminuria is predictive of increased renal and cardiovascular morbidity and mortality

urine albumin excretion rate → *urinary albumin excretion rate*

urine albumin-to-creatinine ratio *Syn: urinary albumin/creatinine ratio*; estimates 24-hour urine albumin excretion; as a ratio between two measured substances it is unaffected by variation in urine concentration; reducing urine albumin to the normal or near-normal range can improve the prognosis of renal and cardiovascular diseases

urinative → *diuretic*

utilization the act of using

oxygen utilization *Syn: oxygen uptake, oxygen extraction*; the oxygen consumption by specific organs or tissues; it is the result of perfusion and the arteriovenous difference in oxygen partial pressure

V

vagal relating to the vagus nerve

vagotonia *Syn: vagotony, sympathic imbalance, sympathetic imbalance, parasympathicotonia, parasympathotonia*; increased excitability or predominance of the parasympathetic nervous system, e.g., in constitutional, autonomic lability; it leads to, e.g., hypotension, bradycardia, bronchospasms, miosis, and acceleration of gastrointestinal motor functions

vagotony → *vagotonia*

valsartan angiotensin-II blocker, antihypertensive

value estimated or assigned worth; valuation

    blood glucose value → *blood glucose level*

    fasting value blood levels of a substance after a 12-hour fast

    globular value → *blood quotient*

    glucose value → *blood glucose level*

    Quick's value *Syn: prothrombin test, prothrombin time, Quick test, Quick's method, thromboplastin time, Quick's time*; clotting test to diagnose disturbances in factors II, V, VII, and X; measures the formation of thrombus following activation with tissue thromboplastin; the normal range is 70–100%

valva valve, valve-like structure

    valvae cordis → *cardiac valves*

valve a structure that controls the flow of a fluid

    anterior semilunar valve anterior semilunar cusp of the pulmonary valve

    valve of aorta → *aortic valve*

    aortic valve *Syn: valve of aorta*; valve in the aortic orifice of the left ventricle made up of three strong valve cusps [semilunar valve]; it opens during systole and closes at the start of diastole; the closure causes the 2nd heart sound heard on auscultation

    artificial heart valve *Syn: prosthetic heart valve, prosthetic valve*; heart valve made from alloplastic or biologic material; the **mechani-**

cal heart valve prostheses are subdivided into **tilting disc prostheses** and **bileaflet prostheses**; the modern mechanical heart valve prostheses are extremely biocompatible and cause only minimal mechanical hemolysis; however, since they are thrombogenic, lifelong treatment with anticoagulants [coumarin derivatives] is required; **biologic heart valve prostheses** are either **xenogeneic heart valve prostheses** [mostly porcine heart valves] or **allogeneic heart valve prostheses** [cadaveric transplant]; biologic replacement valves have the advantage that no anticoagulation is required; on the other hand, they have a limited shelf life and allogeneic transplants can provoke a rejection reaction

atrioventricular valve *Syn: auriculoventricular valve*; heart valve between the right atrium and the right ventricle [right atrioventricular valve] or left atrium and left ventricle [left atrioventricular valve]

auriculoventricular valve → *atrioventricular valve*

bicuspid valve → *mitral valve*

bileaflet valve *s.u. artificial heart valve*

Björk-Schiley valve artificial heart valve with moveable flaps [tilting disc prosthesis]

cardiac valves *Syn: heart valves*; generic term for the valves between the right atrium and the right ventricle [tricuspid valve] or the left atrium and left ventricle [mitral valve] as well as the valve between the right ventricle and the pulmonary trunk [pulmonary valve] and the left ventricle and the aorta [aortic valve]

caval valve → *eustachian valve*

coronary valve *Syn: thebesian valve*; fold at the opening of the coronary sinus coronarius into the right atrium

eustachian valve *Syn: caval valve, valve of inferior vena cava, valve of Sylvius*; fold at the opening of the inferior vena cava into the right atrium

flap valve → *semilunar cusp*

valve of foramen ovale remnant of the embryonic septum primum in the atrial septum of the left atrium

heart valves → *cardiac valves*

valve of inferior vena cava → *eustachian valve*

left atrioventricular valve → *mitral valve*

left semilunar valve of aortic valve left semilunar cusp of the aortic valve

left semilunar valve of pulmonary valve → *valvula semilunaris sinistra valvae trunci pulmonalis*

mitral valve *Syn: bicuspid valve, left atrioventricular valve*; valve system between the left atrium and left ventricle consisting of two cusps [anterior and posterior cusps]; during systole, it prevents retrograde flow into the atrium and during diastole it lets blood out of the atrium into the ventricle

posterior semilunar valve posterior semilunar cusp of the aortic valve

prosthetic valve → *artificial heart valve*

prosthetic heart valve → *artificial heart valve*

pulmonary valve *Syn: pulmonary trunk valve*; cardiac valve consisting of three semilunar cusps [valvula semilunaris], at the entrance to the pulmonary trunk from the right ventricle; it opens during systole and closes at the start of the diastole; the closing causes the second heart sound audible on auscultation

pulmonary trunk valve → *pulmonary valve*

right atrioventricular valve → *tricuspid valve*

right semilunar valve of aortic valve right semilunar cusp of the aortic valve

right semilunar valve of pulmonary valve → *valvula semilunaris dextra valvae trunci pulmonalis*

semilunar valve → *semilunar cusp*

valve of Sylvius → *eustachian valve*

thebesian valve → *coronary valve*

tilting-disk valve artificial heart valve with disc-shaped moveable flap, e.g., Björk-Shiley prosthesis

tricuspid valve *Syn: right atrioventricular valve*; heart valve between the right atrium and right ventricle consisting of three cusps [anterior, posterior and septal cusps]; prevents backward flow of blood into the atrium and allows blood out of the atrium into the ventricle during diastole

valvoplasty *Syn: valvuloplasty*; plastic procedure on a heart valve to restore its function, e.g., in stenosis or insufficiency

valvotomy *Syn: cardiovalvotomy, cardiovalvulotomy, valvulotomy*; operative division of a stenotic heart valve

valvula a small valve or valvule

valvula foraminis ovalis → *valve of foramen ovale*

valvula semilunaris anterior → *anterior semilunar valve*

valvula semilunaris dextra valvae aortae → *right semilunar valve of aortic valve*

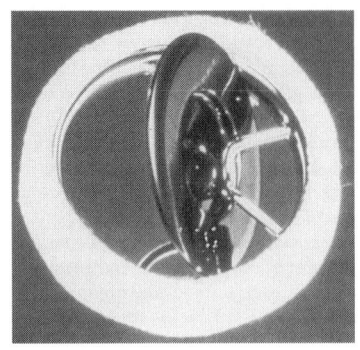

Tilting-disk valve

valvula semilunaris dextra valvae trunci pulmonalis *Syn: right semilunar valve of pulmonary valve*; right cusp of the pulmonary valve [valva trunci pulmonalis]

valvula semilunaris posterior valvae aortae →*posterior semilunar valve*

valvula semilunaris sinistra valvae aortae →*left semilunar valve of aortic valve*

valvula semilunaris sinistra valvae trunci pulmonalis *Syn: left semilunar valve of pulmonary valve*; left cusp of the pulmonary valve [valva trunci pulmonalis]

valvular relating to a valve or valves

valvulitic relating to or marked by valvulitis

valvulitis 1. inflammation of a valve **2.** inflammation of a cardiac valve, valvular endocarditis

rheumatic valvulitis →*Bouillaud's disease*

valvuloplasty →*valvoplasty*

balloon valvuloplasty disruption of a heart valve stenosis using a balloon catheter

valvulotomy →*valvotomy*

vancomycin bactericidal antibiotic produced by **Streptomyces orientalis**; it is effective primarily against gram-positive microorganisms [staphylococci, streptococci, Corynebacterium, enterococci, pneumococci, clostridia, and Listeria]; **indications**: alternative drug in resistant bacteria, pseudomembranous enterocolitis caused by Clostridium species

varicophlebitic relating to or marked by varicophlebitis

varicophlebitis inflammation of a (superficial) varicosity [varix]

vas → *vessel*

  vas afferens afferent vessel

  vas anastomoticum → *anastomotic vessel*

  vas efferens efferent vessel

  vasa sanguinea blood vessels; arteries and veins

  vasa sanguinea intrapulmonalia *Syn: intrapulmonary blood vessels*; branches of the pulmonary arteries and veins passing between lung segments

  vasa vasorum → *vessels of vessels*

vas- combining form denoting relation to a vessel

vasalgia *Syn: angiodynia*; pain in a vessel or along a vessel

vascular relating to (blood) vessels

vascularization *Syn: arterialization*; vessel supply, vessel formation

vasculitic relating to, affected with, or characterized by inflammation of a vessel/vasculitis

vasculitis inflammation of a vessel or the (entire) vessel wall

  allergic vasculitis *Syn: hypersensitivity vasculitis, localized visceral arteritis, leukocytoclastic vasculitis, leukocytoclastic angiitis*; a vascular inflammation belonging to the immune complex diseases, which can be triggered by medications, bacterial and viral infections, or may be idiopathic; affects mainly the post-capillary venules of the skin; the involvement of internal organs and the extent of systemic symptoms varies from case to case; **clinical**: acute or fluctuating course, often involves only the lower leg and ankle, in severe forms also the thigh and trunk; the petechiae coalesce to dark red, painful infiltrates, which regress within days or weeks, leaving behind a hyper-pigmented area [hemosiderin]; larger inflammatory lesions develop central necrotic blisters and ulcers; these need considerably longer to heal; organ involvement [joints, muscles, kidney, gastrointestinal tract, central nervous system] is generally mild and without major consequences; **therapy**: removal of the cause; in severe cases pulses of corticosteroids, on occasion cyclophosphamide

  hypersensitivity vasculitis → *allergic vasculitis*

  hypocomplementemic vasculitis rare form of immune complex vasculitis, which is characterized by a chronic fluctuating [years-decades], mild course; **therapy**: indomethacin, in exceptional cases cyclophosphamide

leukocytoclastic vasculitis → *allergic vasculitis*

necrotizing vasculitis → *necrotizing angiitis*

nodular vasculitis painful nodes found on the flexor surfaces of the lower leg in hypertensive patients

vasculo- combining form denoting relation to a vessel

vasculocardiac → *cardiovascular*

vasculogenesis development of a vascular system

vasculomotor → *vasomotor*

vasculopathy any disorder of blood vessels

vasculotoxic injuring blood vessels

vasifaction → *angiopoiesis*

vasifactive → *angiopoietic*

vaso- combining form denoting relation to a vessel

vasoactive influencing vascular tone

vasoconstriction constriction of blood vessels

vasoconstrictor *Syn: vasoconstrictive, vasohypertonic*; **1.** an agent with vasoconstrictor properties **2.** producing vasoconstriction, constricting vessels

vasodepression reduction in vascular resistance

vasodepressor 1. an agent with vasodepressor properties **2.** reducing the vascular resistance

vasodilatation → *vasodilation*

vasodilation *Syn: vasodilatation*; dilatation of vessels; described as **active vasodilatation** when the muscle in the vessel wall relaxes and as **passive vasodilatation** in overfilling

vasodilative *Syn: vasodilator, vasohypotonic*; affecting or provoking vasodilatation, dilating vessels

vasodilator *Syn: vasohypotonic*; **1.** a substance that widens vessels; used to improve the peripheral, central, and cerebral perfusion; the most important vasodilators are α-blockers, calcium antagonists, prostaglandins, ACE inhibitors, and organic nitrates **2.** causing dilatation of a blood vessel

coronary vasodilator → *coronary dilatator*

vasofactive → *angiopoietic*

vasoformation → *angiopoiesis*

vasoformative → *angiopoietic*

vasogenic arising from a vessel

vasohypotonic 1. → *vasodilator* **2.** → *vasodilative*

vasoligation obstruction of a vessel

vasomotor *Syn: angiokinetic, vasomotory, vasculomotor;* **1.** an agent with vasomotor properties **2.** affecting the caliber of (blood) vessels

vasomotoricity *Syn: angiokinesis, vasomotor function;* control of the dilation and constriction of vessels; vasomotor control is achieved predominantly by vasoconstrictor sympathetic neurones, which modify the basic tone of the vessels and thereby guide perfusion; the sympathetic nerve fibers run for the most part in the arterial vessels between the adventitia and media; the venous side of the terminal vascular bed only has a few sympathetic fibers; these postganglionic unmyelinated fibers contain multiple **varicosities**, in which are synaptic vesicles containing transmitters; there are specific receptors for these transmitters in the subsynaptic membrane of the smooth muscle cells of the vessel wall

vasomotory → *vasomotor*

vasoneuropathy disease of vessels due to loss of their nerve supply

vasoneurosis → *angioneurosis*

vasoneurotic relating to or marked by vasoneurosis

vasoparesis → *angioparesis*

vasopressin → *antidiuretic hormone*

vasopressor 1. an agent with vasopressor properties **2.** increasing the vessel tone or vessel pressure

vasorelaxation reduction in vessel tone

vasospasm → *angiospasm*

vasospastic *Syn: angiospastic;* affecting or producing vasospasm

vasotonia *Syn: angiotonia;* tone or tension of a vessel (wall)

vasotonic *Syn: angiotonic;* **1.** an agent with vasotonic properties **2.** increasing the vessel tone

vasotrophic *Syn: angiotrophic;* relating to vascular nutrition

vectorcardiogram graphical representation obtained by vectorcardiography

vectorcardiograph apparatus for vectorcardiography

vectorcardiography continuous representation of the integral vector of the heart's electrical activity in three dimensions

vein *Syn: vena;* vessel that conveys blood to the heart; all veins, other than the pulmonary veins, contain deoxygenated blood; the structure of the venous wall varies depending on the caliber and body region; however, it can generally be stated that veins have thinner walls and larger lumens than the corresponding arteries; the wall consists of three layers; the inner **intima** [tunica intima] consists of vascular endothelium and subendothelial connective tissue; only in large veins is it clearly separated from the **media** [tunica media] by the **internal elastic membrane** made of elastic fibers; this membrane consists of circular, spirally arranged, smooth muscle fibers, elastic networks, and collagen connective tissue; it is not clearly separated from the **adventitia** [tunica adventitia]

accessory hemiazygos vein upward continuation of the stem of the hemiazygos vein; runs to the right side and opens above the hemiazygos vein into the azygos

anterior cardiac veins heart vein running in the anterior wall of the right ventricle, which opens into the small cardiac vein

anterior interventricular vein vein in the anterior interventricular sulcus; opens into the great cardiac vein

anterior jugular vein collects blood from the chin and neck; opens into the external jugular vein or the subclavian vein

apical vein *s.u. superior right pulmonary vein*

apicoposterior vein *s.u. superior left pulmonary vein*

atrial veins venous branches of the right [**venae atriales dextrae**] and left atrial wall [**venae atriales sinistrae**]; drain into the small cardiac veins

atrioventricular veins veins at the atrioventricular border

axillary vein large vein arising from the upper arm veins [brachial, basilic veins]; becomes the subclavian vein at the lateral border of the first rib

azygos vein → *vena azygos*

basilic vein *Syn: ulnar cutaneous vein*; skin vein on the ulnar side of the forearm [**antebrachial basilic veins**] and upper arm; drains into the axillary vein

brachial veins veins accompanying the brachial artery, which together with the basilic vein form the axillary vein

brachiocephalic vein common venous stem of the internal jugular vein and subclavian vein; the angle between the internal jugular vein and subclavian is called the **venous angle** [angulus venosus]; on the left side, it is the point of entry of the thoracic duct; the right and left brachiocephalic veins join behind the right 1. costal cartilage to make the superior vena cava

cardiac veins the veins of the heart wall; open into the coronary sinus,

external jugular vein collects blood from the back of the head, neck and shoulder region; opens into the subclavian vein or the internal jugular vein

great cardiac vein vein running in the anterior interventricular sulcus, which joins with the oblique vein of the left atrium to form the coronary sinus

hemiazygos vein *Syn: hemiazygous vein, left azygos vein*; vein running parallel to the azygos vein, which runs upwards on the left side of the spinal column, before turning to the right side at the level of the eighth thoracic vertebra and running behind the aorta, thoracic duct, and esophagus to the azygos vein

hemiazygous vein → *hemiazygos vein*

inferior left pulmonary vein *Syn: vena pulmonalis sinistra inferior*; carries blood from the inferior lobe [lobus inferior] of the left lung; common final pathway of the superior vein of the inferior lobe, common basal vein, superior basal vein, anterior basal vein, and inferior basal vein

inferior right pulmonary vein *Syn: vena pulmonalis dextra inferior*; carries blood from the inferior lobe [lobus inferior] of the right lung; collecting vein for the superior vein of the inferior lobe, common basal vein, anterior basal vein, and inferior basal vein

inferior ventricular vein transmits blood from the temporal lobes to the basal vein [of Rosenthal]

internal jugular vein the vein collecting blood from brain, tongue, pharynx, and larynx; joining with the subclavian veins, it forms the brachiocephalic vein; it has two bulbs: the **superior jugular bulb** in the jugular fossa and the **inferior jugular bulb** before it joins with the subclavian vein

left azygos vein → *hemiazygos vein*

left marginal vein vein on the left heart border; opens into the great cardiac vein

left ventricular veins veins from the left ventricle; drain into the thebesian veins

lingular vein *s.u. superior left pulmonary vein*

vein of Marshall → *Marshall's oblique vein*

Marshall's oblique vein *Syn: oblique vein of left atrium, vein of Marshall*; small veins on the posterior wall of the left atrium

middle cardiac vein vein running in the anterior interventricular sul-

vein

cus, which opens into the coronary sinus

vein of middle lobe *s.u. superior right pulmonary vein*

nutrient vein *s.u. leg ulcer*

oblique vein of left atrium → *Marshall's oblique vein*

pericardiac veins take blood from the pericardium to the azygos or brachiocephalic veins

pericardicophrenic veins veins accompanying the pericardiophrenic artery; transmit blood from the pericardium and diaphragm to the brachiocephalic vein

posterior vein of left ventricle vein from the posterior wall of the left ventricle; drains into the coronary sinus

posterior vein of superior lobe *s.u. superior right pulmonary vein*

pulmonary veins *Syn: venae pulmonales*; the pulmonary veins carry oxygenated blood from the lung to the left atrium; each lung has a superior [vena pulmonalis dextra superior, vena pulmonalis sinistra superior] and an inferior pulmonary vein [vena pulmonalis dextra inferior, vena pulmonalis sinistra inferior]

radial veins veins accompanying the radial artery; drain into the brachial vein

right marginal vein vein on the right heart border; opens into the lesser cardiac vein

right ventricular veins veins from the right ventricle; drain into the thebesian veins

small cardiac vein collecting vein for the anterior cardiac veins and the right marginal vein; opens into the coronary sinus

smallest cardiac veins *Syn: thebesian veins, veins of Thebesius*; small heart veins that collect blood from the two atria and ventricles and deliver it to the coronary sinus

superior basal vein *s.u. inferior left pulmonary vein*

superior left pulmonary vein *Syn: vena pulmonalis sinistra superior*; carries blood from the superior lobe [lobus superior] of the left lung; collecting vein for the apicoposterior vein, anterior vein of the superior lobe, and lingular vein

superior right pulmonary vein *Syn: vena pulmonalis dextra superior*; carries blood from the superior [lobus superior] and middle lobe [lobus medius] of the right lung; common final pathway of the apical vein, anterior vein of the superior lobe, posterior vein of the superior lobe, and middle lobar vein

thebesian veins → *smallest cardiac veins*

veins of Thebesius → *smallest cardiac veins*
ulnar cutaneous vein → *basilic vein*
veinous → *venous*
ven- combining form denoting relation to a vein
vena → *vein*
vena axillaris → *axillary vein*
vena azygos *Syn:* azygos vein, azygos, azygous; large vein that extends on the right side of the vertebral bodies to the superior vena cava [vena cava superior]; it arises from the right ascending lumbar vein [vena lumbalis ascendens]; after passing through the diaphragm, it is directly adjacent to the vertebral column; it then bends forward and arches [arcus venae azygos] over the right primary bronchus [bronchus principalis dexter] to the vena cava; it drains the hemiazygos and accessory hemiazygos veins, as well as the esophageal, bronchial, pericardiac, and mediastinal veins, among others
vena basilica → *basilic vein*
venae brachiales → *brachial veins*
vena brachiocephalica → *brachiocephalic vein*
venae cardiacae minimae → *smallest cardiac veins*
vena cava filter *Syn:* vena caval umbrella filter; s.u. vena caval block
inferior vena cava *Syn:* postcava; great vein opening into the right atrium, which collects blood from the lower extremities and the abdominal and pelvic organs; arises through the union of the two common iliac veins at the level of the 4.-5. lumbar vertebra; it runs upwards on the right side of the abdominal aorta on the posterior abdominal wall, through the vena caval foramen in the diaphragm into the middle mediastinum, where it enters the right atrium from below
superior vena cava *Syn:* precava; short, unpaired collecting vein from the upper half of the body; arises at the junction of the right and left brachiocephalic veins behind the head of the right first rib; in its short [4–5 cm] course behind the right border of the sternum, it receives the azygos vein and discharges into the right atrium through the ostium of the superior vena cava
vena hemiazygos → *hemiazygos vein*
vena hemiazygos accessoria → *accessory hemiazygos vein*
vena interventricularis anterior → *anterior interventricular vein*
vena jugularis anterior → *anterior jugular vein*
vena jugularis externa → *external jugular vein*
vena jugularis interna → *internal jugular vein*

vena marginalis dextra → *right marginal vein*
vena marginalis sinistra → *left marginal vein*
venae pericardicophrenicae → *pericardicophrenic veins*
venae pulmonales → *pulmonary veins*
vena pulmonalis dextra inferior → *inferior right pulmonary vein*
vena pulmonalis dextra superior → *superior right pulmonary vein*
vena pulmonalis sinistra inferior → *inferior left pulmonary vein*
vena pulmonalis sinistra superior → *superior left pulmonary vein*
venae radiales → *radial veins*
venae ventriculares dextrae → *right ventricular veins*
venae ventriculares sinistrae → *left ventricular veins*
vena ventricularis inferior → *inferior ventricular vein*
vena ventriculi sinistri posterior → *posterior vein of left ventricle*

venectasia → *phlebectasia*

venectomy *Syn: phlebectomy*; operative removal of a vein

venesection 1. operative exposure and opening of a vein **2.** incision into a vein

venesuture → *phleborrhaphy*

veni- combining form denoting relation to a vein

venisuture → *phleborrhaphy*

veno- combining form denoting relation to a vein

venoatrial *Syn: venoauricular, venosinal*; relating to vena cava and right atrium

venoauricular → *venoatrial*

venogram → *phlebogram*

venography → *phlebography*

venoperitoneostomy operative connection of the great saphenous vein and peritoneal cavity for drainage of ascites

venosclerosis → *phlebosclerosis*

venosinal → *venoatrial*

venous *Syn: veinous, phleboid*; relating to a vein or veins

venovenostomy → *phlebophlebostomy*

venovenous connecting two veins

ventilation 1. *Syn: respiration*; pulmonary ventilation **2.** artificial ventilation of the lungs

    continuous mechanical ventilation → *long-term ventilation*

    CPAP ventilation *Syn: CPAP breathing, continuous positive airway pressure (breathing), continuous positive pressure breathing, positive pressure breathing/respiration*; form of positive pressure breathing used to support spontaneous breathing, in which the airway pressure is increased during both inspiration and expiration [continuous positive airway pressure, CPAP]; this opens collapsed sections of the lower respiratory passages, which increases the gas exchange surface area and reduces shunt blood flow; the work necessary for breathing is simultaneously reduced by the reduction in airway resistance

long-term ventilation *Syn: continuous mechanical ventilation*; artificial ventilation for more than 48 hours

positive pressure ventilation → *CPAP ventilation*

ventricle 1. chamber **2.** heart chamber, cardiac ventricle

aortic ventricle → *left ventricle*

left ventricle *Syn: aortic ventricle*; muscle-rich chamber that lies at the back of the heart and pumps oxygen-rich blood into the systemic circulation; on its inside there are prominent muscular ridges [**trabeculae carneae ventriculi sinistri**] and two **papillary muscles** [anterior and posterior papillary muscles], from which tendinous strands [chordae tendineae cordis] run to the two cusps of the aortic valve [valva aortae]; during diastole, blood flows into the left ventricle through the mitral valve and is then pumped through the aortic valve into the aorta during systole

right ventricle anteriorly placed heart chamber that pumps oxygen-poor blood from the body circulation through the pulmonary arteries into the pulmonary circulation; the right ventricular wall is significantly weaker than the left; on the inner surface, it contains a network of small muscle ridges [trabeculae carnae of the right ventricle] and 3 **papillary muscles** [anterior, posterior, and septal papillary muscles], from which tendinous threads [chordae tendinae] connect to the three cusps of the pulmonary valve [valve of the pulmonary trunk]; blood flows through the tricuspid valve during diastole into the right ventricle and is pumped during systole into the pulmonary arteries through the pulmonary valve [valve of the pulmonary trunk]; the **septomarginal trabecula** on the floor of the right ventricle separates the inflow and outflow channels

ventricular relating to a ventricle

ventriculitic relating to or marked by ventriculitis

ventriculitis inflammation of a ventricle

ventriculoatrial relating to ventricle and atrium

ventriculoatriostomy *Syn: ventriculoatrial shunt*; operative connection of the cerebral ventricle and the atrium of the heart for drainage of CSF in hydrocephalus

ventriculogram image obtained in ventriculography

ventriculography 1. X-ray demonstration of the heart chambers with contrast agent or radionuclides **2.** X-ray contrast demonstration of the cerebral ventricle; now hardly ever performed

radionuclide ventriculography scintigraphy of the ventricle of the heart with radionuclides

ventriculomyotomy incision through the ventricular muscle

ventriculonector → *atrioventricular bundle*

ventriculotomy incision into a cerebral ventricle or a cardiac ventricle

verapamil class IV antiarrhythmic; calcium antagonist, which reduces the oxygen requirements of the heart muscle; the excitability of the myocardium is reduced and the AV conduction slowed; **usage:** paroxysmal supraventricular tachycardia, extrasystoles, ventricular tachycardia due to ventricular fibrillation or flutter, atrial tachycardia, coronary heart disease, arterial hypertension

vertigo giddiness, dizziness

arteriosclerotic vertigo dizziness caused by arteriosclerotic changes in the brain vessels and the resultant hypoperfusion

vessel any channel or tube for carrying liquid

anastomotic vessel vessel that connects other vessels [arteries, veins, lymphatic vessels]

capillary vessel → *capillary*

collateral vessel vessel that runs in the same direction as another vessel and supplies a comparable area; in clinical practice, there is a division into naturally present collateral vessels [**primary** or **pre-existent collateral vessels**] and collateral vessels that are formed in response to a situation of need [load, chronic hypoxia] [**secondary collateral vessels**]

elastic vessel → *artery of elastic type*

intrapulmonary blood vessels → *vasa sanguinea intrapulmonalia*

silver-wire vessels → *silver-wire arterioles*

vessels of vessels *Syn: vasa vasorum*; smallest blood vessels, which supply the walls of bigger arteries and veins

vestibule *Syn: vestibulum*; atrium

aortic vestibule the area of the left ventricle below the aortic orifice

vestibulum → *vestibule*

vestibulum aortae → *aortic vestibule*

vibex striped bruise, striae, stria

virostatic → *virustatic*
virulent → *infectious*
virus minute infectious agent that replicates only in the cells of a living host; consist of a DNA or RNA core, a protein coat, and, sometimes, a surrounding envelope
  Coxsackie virus → *coxsackievirus*
virustatic *Syn: virostatic, virostatic agent*; antibiotic that inhibits the replication of viruses
viscerocardiac relating to viscera and heart
vitiligoidea → *xanthoma*
vitium 1. fault, defect **2.** → *heart defect*
volemia the current blood volume with respect to the body weight [normal approx. 75 ml/kg body weight or approx. 7.5% of the body weight]; held as constant as possible by the body [normovolemia]
voltage electromotive force or potential difference
  low voltage description of an abnormally small amplitude QRS complex in the ECG
volume amount of space occupied by an object or substance
  blood volume total blood volume of the body; in adults it is approx. 6–8% of the body weight or approx. 4–6 l; the majority of the blood volume [approx. 85%] is found in the venous system, which because of its high capacitance can accommodate volume changes; if, e.g., 500 ml blood are removed, only 5 ml of this derive from the arterial system, the remainder [495 ml] coming from the low-pressure system
  forced expiratory volume → *forced expiration test*
  mean corpuscular volume derived from the hematocrit divided by the erythrocyte count per liter; the normal range is 80–98 μm^3
  minute volume *Syn: cardiac output, minute output*; blood volume ejected per minute; at rest approx. 5 l and increases during exertion to 25 l or more; measurement mainly relies upon the Fick principle applied as an indicator dilution method or a thermodilution method
  red cell volume total volume of erythrocytes in the circulating blood; calculated from the hematocrit and the blood volume
  regurgitation volume the mass of blood that flows back into the atrium or ventricle during systole or diastole as a result of valvular insufficiency
  reserve volume the blood remaining in the heart at the end of systole
  stroke volume *Syn: systolic discharge*; the blood volume ejected per beat of the heart; generally approx. 70 ml

vortex whorl
   vortex of heart whorled arrangement of heart muscle fibers over the cardiac apex

W

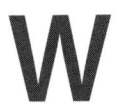

warfarin synthetic coumarin derivative that is used as an anticoagulant
wave a curved shape, outline, or pattern
    F waves *Syn: fibrillary waves*; flutter or fibrillation waves in the ECG
    fibrillary waves → *F waves*
    P wave excitation of the atrium in the ECG
    Q wave first negative wave/deflection in the ECG; start of ventricular excitation
    R wave positive wave in the QRS complex
    S wave *s.u. electrocardiogram*
    T wave last wave in the ECG
    U wave *s.u. electrocardiogram*
weakness → *asthenia*
windpipe → *trachea*
wrapping *s.u. intracranial aneurysm*

xanthelasma → *xanthoma*

xanthoma *Syn:* vitiligoidea, xanthelasma; benign skin tumor, which typically contains yellow lipid-rich cells [**xanthoma cells**]; xanthomas occur mainly in disorders of lipid metabolism (hyperlipoproteinemia, hypercholesterolemia) [**hyperlipidemic xanthomas**], but may also be found with normal lipid levels [**normolipidemic xanthomas**]; there is a degree of correlation between clinical manifestations [eruptive, tuberous, intertriginous xanthomas, tendinous xanthomas, hand line xanthomas], nevertheless, they cannot be described as specific for a particular lipoproteinemia

xanthomatosis *Syn:* xanthelasmatosis, lipoid granulomatosis, lipid granulomatosis; occurrence of widespread xanthomas, especially on elbows and knees; often associated with a disorder of lipid metabolism

familial hypercholesteremic xanthomatosis → *LDL-receptor disorder*

xenogeneic 1. *Syn:* xenogenous, xenogenic; caused by a foreign body, arising from outside; exogenous **2.** *Syn:* xenogenous, xenogenic, heterologous, heteroplastic, heterogeneic, heterogenic, heterogenous; (derived) from another species

xenograft → *heterotransplant*

xenotransplantation *Syn:* heterologous transplantation, heteroplastic transplantation, xenogeneic transplantation; plastic procedure with transfer of tissues from another species [e.g., porcine heart valves]

xipamide saluretic, antihypertensive

Z

zuckergussleber → *frosted liver*